TARGETED CANCER THERAPY

A HANDBOOK FOR NURSES

GAIL M. WILKES, MS, APRN-BC, AOCN
Oncology Clinical Instructor
Boston Medical Center
Boston, Massachusetts

JONES AND BARTLETT PUBLISHERS

Sudbury, Massachusetts

BOSTON   TORONTO   LONDON   SINGAPORE

World Headquarters
Jones and Bartlett Publishers
40 Tall Pine Drive
Sudbury, MA 01776
978-443-5000
info@jbpub.com
www.jbpub.com

Jones and Bartlett Publishers
Canada
6339 Ormindale Way
Mississauga, Ontario L5V 1J2
Canada

Jones and Bartlett Publishers
International
Barb House, Barb Mews
London W6 7PA
United Kingdom

Jones and Bartlett's books and products are available through most bookstores and online booksellers. To contact Jones and Bartlett Publishers directly, call 800-832-0034, fax 978-443-8000, or visit our website, www.jbpub.com.

Substantial discounts on bulk quantities of Jones and Bartlett's publications are available to corporations, professional associations, and other qualified organizations. For details and specific discount information, contact the special sales department at Jones and Bartlett via the above contact information or send an email to specialsales@jbpub.com.

The author, editor, and publisher have made every effort to provide accurate information. However, they are not responsible for errors, omissions, or for any outcomes related to the use of the contents of this book and take no responsibility for the use of the products and procedures described. Treatments and side effects described in this book may not be applicable to all people; likewise, some people may require a dose or experience a side effect that is not described herein. Drugs and medical devices are discussed that may have limited availability controlled by the Food and Drug Administration (FDA) for use only in a research study or clinical trial. Research, clinical practice, and government regulations often change the accepted standard in this field. When consideration is being given to use of any drug in the clinical setting, the health care provider or reader is responsible for determining FDA status of the drug, reading the package insert, and reviewing prescribing information for the most up-to-date recommendations on dose, precautions, and contraindications, and determining the appropriate usage for the product. This is especially important in the case of drugs that are new or seldom used.

Production Credits
Publisher: Kevin Sullivan
Acquisitions Editor: Emily Ekle
Acquisitions Editor: Amy Sibley
Associate Editor: Patricia Donnelly
Editorial Assistant: Rachel Shuster
Associate Production Editor: Katie Spiegel
Senior Marketing Manager: Barb Bartoszek
Marketing Manger: Rebecca Wasley
V.P., Manufacturing and Inventory Control: Therese Connell
Composition: Paw Print Media
Cover Design: Kristin E. Parker
Cover Image: © Les Cunliffe/Dreamstime.com
Printing and Binding: Malloy, Inc.
Cover Printing: Malloy, Inc.

Library of Congress Cataloging-in-Publication Data
Wilkes, Gail M.
  Targeted cancer therapy : a handbook for nurses / Gail M. Wilkes.
    p. ; cm.
  Includes bibliographical references and index.
  ISBN 978-0-7637-7211-6
  1. Cancer—Nursing. 2. Drug targeting. 3. Cancer—Cytopathology. 4. Cancer—Molecular aspects. I. Title.
  [DNLM: 1. Neoplasms—drug therapy—Nurses' Instruction. 2. Drug Delivery Systems—methods—Nurses' Instruction. 3. Neoplasms—nursing. 4. Neoplasms—physiopathology—Nurses' Instruction. 5. Signal Transduction—drug effects—Nurses' Instruction. QZ 267 W682t 2010]
  RC266.W55 2010
  616.99'4061—dc22

                          2009037358

6048

Printed in the United States of America
13 12 11 10 09   10 9 8 7 6 5 4 3 2 1

Contents

Introduction

Major strides are being made in understanding cancer and potential molecular flaws that can be targeted in its treatment. Cancer is a disease in which molecular flaws lead to abnormal cell proliferation, lack of controlled growth, and the ability of malignant cells to invade and metastasize.[1] Von Eschenbach, the former director of the National Cancer Institute, stated that understanding the abnormal signaling pathways in the cell and the process of metastasis is critical to reducing the many deaths from cancer and therein allowing patients to live with cancer as a "chronic disease."[2] With this focus in mind, cancer researchers continue to identify characteristics of the cancer process that may lead to therapeutic breakthroughs. For instance, we now know that solid tumors cannot grow beyond 1 to 2 mm, the diffusion distance of oxygen, without developing new blood vessels via the process of angiogenesis.[3] The concept of limiting tumor growth so that metastases does not occur is a new one, in which the tumor will remain small, and cancer then becomes a "chronic illness." This understanding has led to new anticancer agents, which target the different malignant flaws that cause tumors to grow, invade, and metastasize.

Nurses, who have provided the mainstay of care for patients receiving anticancer therapy, need to keep abreast of major developments in therapy, including targeted therapy. In many instances, nurses administer targeted therapies in the form of monoclonal antibodies such as trastuzumab (Herceptin), mTOR inhibitors (Torisel), or other targeted agents. In addition, they educate patients and families about what targeted therapy is, how it differs from chemotherapy, potential side effects, and self-care measures to help patients adhere and benefit from an often long course of oral therapy, as with erlotinib (Tarceva). Because the side effect profile of targeted therapy differs from that of chemotherapy, oncology nurses, defined as any nurse who cares for patients with cancer and their family, must understand the emerging pathophysiology of cancer, how these targeted agents work, their side effect profile, and measures to help patients minimize toxicity and maximize adherence to therapy.

Of these learning needs, understanding the emerging pathophysiology of cancer may be the most challenging. There has never been a more exciting time for oncology nurses. As our understanding of cancer rapidly evolves, we are offered new targets and opportunities to stop cancer for those patients who do not achieve cure and to make cancer a truly chronic disease for these patients. Nurses, however, have often forgotten much of basic cell biology, or they had a minimal exposure to it during their basic nursing education. This book is designed to help nurses understand the newly emerging science of cancer against a backdrop of normal cell biology, in a nonfrightening manner.

Because this complex material is best understood when combined with relevant nursing implications, the chapters are organized according to the corresponding tumor biology, which underpins the mechanisms of action of the drugs administered in cancer treatment. The categorization of these agents is based on the work of Ma and Adjei.[4] Chapter 1 provides a foundation for exploring cancer biology. It includes a discussion of inflammation and the microenvironment, together with the other six cardinal hallmarks of cancer.[5] Chapter 2 offers an overview of monoclonal antibodies; membrane-bound receptors and their signaling pathways; the agents that target these pathways, intracellular signaling kinases (including Hedgehog) and their pathways; heat shock proteins; and the ubiquitin–proteasome pathway and inhibitors. Chapter 3 addresses angiogenesis, angiogenesis inhibitors, hypoxia-inducible factor, m-TOR inhibitors, and epigenetic abnormalities. It also discusses agents that influence methylation and histone conformation. Chapter 4 addresses the microenvironment from the perspective of bone metastasis and describes ways of targeting flaws in the processes of apoptosis and mitosis. Chapter 5 discusses some of the challenges in supporting patients on oral anticancer therapies, including managing drug interactions in the P450 microenzyme system and adhering to oral regimens. Each chapter includes a discussion of the pathophysiology, key drugs that target malignant flaws, and nursing implications.

REFERENCES

1. Wilkes GM. Intravenous administration of antineoplastic drugs: review of basics and what's new in 2009. *J Inf Nurs.* 2009;32(5):1-10.

2. Von Eschenbach AC. NCI aims for cancer goal by 2015. *Science.* 2003;299(5611):1297-1298.

3. Folkman J. Tumor angiogenesis: therapeutic implications. *N Engl J Med.* 1971;285:1182-1186.

4. Ma WW, Adjei AA. Novel agents on the horizon for cancer therapy. *CA Cancer J Clin.* 2009;59(2):111-136.

5. Hanahan D, Weinberg RA. The hallmarks of cancer. *Cell.* 2000;100:57-90.

CHAPTER 1

Cancer Biology, Signaling Pathways, and Malignant Transformation

Cancer is a genetic disease, meaning that it involves genetic mutations, whether genetically inherited or acquired through the course of one's life. Normally cell birth equals cell death, and cells must stay in a prescribed area or undergo programmed cell death (apoptosis). With cancer, however, changes in the genome permit cells to override the intrinsic and deliberate safeguards that keep cell division in check.

A number of qualities, known as the "hallmarks of cancer," are required for a cell to become malignant and form a tumor. This process is multistep, and knowledge continues to grow in this area. Each of the steps involves a genetic mutation, and it is thought that there are at least four to seven major steps.[1] With each mutation, cells acquire a growth advantage that ultimately results in an aggressive malignant clone of cells with the ability to invade and metastasize. Understanding how cells become malignant will allow targets to be identified and therapies to be developed to destroy these targets. Thus, we may ultimately prevent cancer, or at the very least, prevent metastasis, as 90% of patients with cancer die from metastasis, not from the primary tumor.[2]

HALLMARKS OF CANCER

Hanahan and Weinberg describe six cardinal requirements for a cell to become malignant and for a malignant tumor to develop.[3] These common qualities are true of most, if not all, cancers and allow the cell to overcome anticancer protective mechanisms of the normal cells and tissues. They are as follows:

- Self-sufficiency in growth signals
- Insensitivity to antigrowth signals
- Ability to evade apoptosis (programmed cell death)
- Limitless replication potential
- Sustained angiogenesis
- Ability to invade and metastasize

In addition, Mantovani suggests that inflammation be added as a seventh hallmark of cancer.[4] This quality is inseparable from the microenvironment or stroma, so it will be added as a seventh hallmark of cancer.

APPLICATION OF THE HALLMARKS OF CANCER

Malignant Transformation

There are many differences between normal and malignant cells.

Normal cells look like the parent cell, with a distinct shape and appearance. The nucleus is small, and the nuclear to cytoplasmic ratio is small, as opposed to malignant cells where the ratio is high. The normal cell is differentiated with a clear function(s); for example, erythrocytes make hemoglobin. Normal cells bind closely together and stay put in their neighborhood. They stop dividing when they feel their neighbors (contact inhibition) and are not able to move from their neighborhood (anchorage dependency). Normal cells have a diploid number of chromosomes (23 pairs, or 46 individual chromosomes), which is called euploidy. In contrast, cancer cells may have fewer or more copies of the chromosome, called aneuploidy.

As stated previously, normal cells divide only when the body needs more cells. Once an individual is born, the body is very careful that cell birth equals death, so that cell division occurs only when needed. Proto-oncogenes are genes that drive cell division. One can think of them like the accelerator of a car, pushing the cell to divide when the body communicates the need. The safeguards of this are TSGs, which can be thought of as the brakes on cell division, so that when cell birth and death are equal, the TSGs stop the proto-oncogenes from pushing for cell division. Because millions of cells need to be replaced daily, many mistakes (mutations) can occur in the replication of the cells. DNA repair genes either excise or repair these mutations or mistakes in copies of the DNA when the cell is dividing; if unable to repair them, the cell is sent to programmed cell death (apoptosis). In cancer, there appear to be mutations in proto-oncogenes, forming oncogenes, TSGs, and the DNA repair genes. In this way, the accelerator on cell division becomes unopposed.

Let's get back to normal cell division. Mitosis is the division of the cell into two daughter cells. The normal cell cycle is tightly controlled, as has been briefly discussed. There are restriction points that allow the cell to check whether the cell has the right amount of DNA, whether it is correctly copied, and whether it divides properly. The cell cycle is controlled by proteins made by TSGs, and, unfortunately, many of them are mutated or silenced by cancer.

Not all cells are dividing. Some remain in the resting or G_0 phase of the cell cycle. When cells are in the G_0 phase, they are actually busy doing their daily jobs as differentiated cells. If the body says it needs more cells, then cells are recruited from G_0 to enter the cell cycle. For example, during the digestion of food, the microvilli in the intestinal crypts shed about 80 million cells per minute.[5] The body needs to replace these cells. That is why these cells are a highly proliferating normal cell population.

The term *cell cycle* describes the journey of a cell to replicate or copy itself, resulting in two identical daughter cells. Early scientists knew what happened in the synthesis (S) phase and the mitosis (M) phase, but they did not know what happened in the periods between these phases, so they called them gaps (hence the G). G_1 is the time before the S phase, and G_2 is the time after the S phase and before the M phase. Cyclins, which are subunits of CDKs, regulate the cell's journey through the cell cycle. The movement of the cell through each phase of the cell cycle depends upon the synthesis of the correct cyclin. The cyclin binds to its CDK, and together they form an enzyme that activates other proteins via phosphorylation. While the CDK level stays about the same as the cell goes through the cell cycle, the cyclin level rises and falls, which is how the term *cyclin* was derived. The cyclins are degraded after mitosis so that the cell cycle can be shut off as a safety mechanism. When control of the cell cycle goes awry, as in cancer, chromosomes with mutations or damage can continue to go through the cell cycle, resulting in genetic instability. For example, normally the cell will divide into two daughter cells, each with 23 pairs of chromosomes. When the checkpoints of the cell cycle are ignored, as with cancer, cells can end up with fewer or more chromosomes (aneuploidy), or with gene rearrangement with parts of one chromosome ending up on another chromosome (translocation). Probably all cancer cells have mutations in the checkpoint genes and in the genes that control cell cycle progression.

G_0 Phase and Entrance into G_1

Once a cell is recruited into the cell cycle, it needs to make sure that the body can support new cells. The cell advances to the G_1 restriction point, and the cell then assesses if indeed the body needs more cells, if there is adequate nutrition to support the new cells (e.g., oxygen, glucose), if the cell is big enough, and if it has the resources to complete the replication (e.g., energy, proteins to make the membranes, organelles, DNA). If the answer is yes, then the cell proceeds to the S phase. This decision is irreversible once the cell begins to cycle. If the answer is no, the cell goes back into G_0.

The gene product is the protein that the gene codes for, and it is actually the protein that does the work of the gene. The protein product of the Rb TSG, pRb, regulates G_1 progression. In early G_1, pRb is in a hypophosphorylated state. It binds tightly to and represses (shuts off) the activity of the E2F family of transcription factors that need to be available to make the right genes expressed (turned on) when the cell gets to the S phase.

When the cell leaves G_0 and goes into G_1, CDK4 and CDK6 actively combine with D-cyclins (D1, D2, D3), which begin phosphorylation of the pRb; this lifts the hold on the E2F transcription factors so they can get the genes ready in the S phase. This process is critical for the cell to pass the restriction point.

A final check is made to see if there is any damage to the DNA; if so, the cell is not allowed to enter the S phase. If DNA damage has occurred, p53 accumulates in the cell, induces p21-mediated inhibition of cyclin D/CDK. When cyclin D/CDK complex is inhibited, the pRb is in a state of low phosphorylation and is tightly bound to the transcription factor E2F, which inhibits Rb.

Entrance into the S Phase

Once the cell gets the OK to pass into the S phase, the rest of the cell cycle is well programmed. Cyclin E picks up from cyclin D when pRb interacts with histone deacetylase proteins (HDACs), which are involved with chromatin remodeling.[6] Now that cyclin E is expressed, it complexes with CDK2 (CDK/cyclin E), keeping the pRb phosphorylated so the cell cycle can continue to progress. Next, cyclin A enters the picture and becomes the primary partner of CDK2 (CDK2/cyclin A). In order to set up replication of the chromosomes during the S phase, CDK2, which is now released from its cyclin, targets a protein Cdc6, which is necessary to start replication. It becomes phosphorylated (turned on) by CDK2/cyclin A and moves to the cytoplasm where it complexes with E2F.

The cell now replicates the chromosomes, and like a detective with a magnifying glass, the DNA damage checkpoint inspects the DNA to see if it is damaged. If so, progress is halted until it can be repaired.

Entrance into G_2

Cyclin A continues to G_2 but changes partners, now complexing with Cdc2 (cell division cycle 2, also known as CDK1).

The cell goes through the G_2 checkpoint; if DNA replication is not completed, the cell cannot enter the M phase.

If the replicated DNA is complete and there are no mistakes, then the cell is ready to begin mitosis. To pass through, cyclin B now replaces cyclin A and complexes with Cdc2.

Entrance into the M Phase

The cyclin B/Cdc2 complex phosphorylates proteins regulated during mitosis.[6]

Aurora kinases are very important enzymes that control chromatid segregation and make sure that the genetic material is correctly shared in each daughter cell. Aurora A functions during the first phase of mitosis (prophase), ensuring that the centrosomes make the mitotic spindle upon which the chromosomes line up. Aurora B helps the mitotic spindle attach to the centromere (the condensed and constricted area of a chromosome, like the waist, to which the spindle fiber is attached during mitosis). Aurora C's function is poorly understood. All or some may be mutated in cancer. See Chapter 4 for a discussion of aurora kinases as molecular targets.

Polo-like kinases (Plk1s) also are very active during the M phase. Plk1s help ensure the mitotic spindle is put together correctly and also can activate or inactivate CDK/cyclin complexes. They may be mutated in cancer.

The cell is checked to make sure the chromatids are assembled properly on the mitotic spindle, and if not, the cell cannot enter anaphase.

One group of proteins that can inhibit the CDKs by binding to them is the INK family (inhibitors of CDK4). This family includes p16^{INK4A}, which inhibits CDK4, and three others that bind to and inhibit CDK4 and CDK6: $p15^{INK4B}$, $p18^{INK4C}$, and $p19^{INK4D}$. These TSGs are often mutated in cancer, which allows the imperfect cell to continue through the cell cycle. Another family of proteins called CDK interacting protein/kinase inhibitory protein can bind to and inhibit many CDKs, but also may promote the activity of cyclin D-dependent kinases. Many tumors have subverted these inhibitory signals so that the progression through the cell cycle is not halted.[6–8]

Because the cell cycle is almost universally flawed in cancer, it presents many possible targets, and CDK inhibitors, DNA damage checkpoint kinase inhibitors, aurora kinase inhibitors, and Plk inhibitors are all being studied.[7]

The Multistage Model of Carcinogenesis

Cancer is a disease of mutations, and it is estimated that malignant transformation requires at least four separate mutations in key genes. Approximately 300 genes have been found mutated in cancer.[7] Malignant tumors are clonal; a group of cells with invasive and aggressive features are self-selected and then become invasive and metastasize. However, there is mounting evidence that cancer stem cells may play a key role in driving invasion and metastasis. Key genes that are mutated in cancer are proto-oncogenes, which then form oncogenes, TSGs, and DNA repair genes. In addition, often there are mutations in genes controlling the signaling cascade that can be turned on so that the message to divide and invade is continually sent. There is also increasing awareness that the tumor microenvironment ensures that the tumor has the necessary signals to grow, invade, and metastasize.

To review, normal cells obey very strict rules about how they behave, and they divide only when the body needs more cells. They respond to contact inhibition, so that the pressure of neighboring cells negates any stimulus to divide. It is almost as if the cells have an "area code" within which they must stay; if they leave the area, they will undergo programmed cell death or apoptosis. An exception to this is the neutrophil, which is able to migrate to areas of infection. Otherwise, normal cells stay where they are supposed to stay, grow only in one layer, and stop dividing when they touch their neighbors. Normally, when the cells do divide, they do it faithfully. If there are mutations in the DNA of the new cell, the DNA repair gene products try to excise or repair the mistake; if repair or excision is not possible, the cell is sent to programmed cell death, directed by *P53* gene and its protein product p53.

If there are mutations making this usual process ineffective, then cells with mutated genes accumulate and continue to divide, making more and more mutations. As billions of cells in the body are replaced every day, mistakes do occur. If the mutation is on or near a proto-oncogene, or a TSG, then the stage may be set for malignant transformation.

There are many mutations in DNA because so many cells are replaced daily. These mutations can be subtle alterations in the spelling of a gene, so that an incorrect protein is produced by the gene. This mutation can be harmless and is usually repaired by DNA repair genes. If the mutation is on or near a proto-oncogene, an oncogene can result, which can drive cell proliferation, new blood vessel formation, and other factors necessary for invasion and metastasis. Genetic mutations seen in cancer include subtle alterations such as small letter deletions, insertions, and single base pair substitution, such as a point mutation. They can involve:

1. Chromosome number changes such as aneuploidy or loss of heterozygosity (LOH; loss of normal function from one copy of the gene or allele when the other copy is already inactive)
2. Chromosome translocation wherein part of one chromosome ends up on another chromosome (if it lands near or on a proto-oncogene, it can result in an oncogene, as seen in Ph1-positive chronic myelogenous leukemia [CML], depicted in Figure 1-1)
3. Amplification of oncogenes (such as with HER2-positive breast cancer, where there are 5- to 100-fold more copies of a gene in a small region of a chromosome), or an amplicon that contains one or more genes that increase cell proliferation
4. Exogenous sequences such as a virus encoded in a cell's DNA that drives malignancy, such as HPV in cervical cancer, Epstein–Barr virus in Burkitt lymphoma, and hepatitis B, which leads to hepatocellular carcinoma

In cancer, there are mutations in the key genes that control the normal cell division scenario. A person has two copies of each gene, one from the mother and one from the father. People with a hereditary predisposition to cancer, such as familial polyposis coloni, inherit one copy of the damaged gene, but the other copy is usually normal. These people are considered *heterozygous* for the trait the gene encodes. Gene mutations that are inherited occur in the germ line; thus all the person's cells have this mutation. Through LOH, the normal gene mutates and the person loses its function so that now both genes are abnormal. Individuals without an inherited predisposition develop acquired mutations in somatic cells (i.e., the mutation occurs in regular cells, not germ line cells and is therefore not in all cells and cannot be inherited). In the course of these individuals' lives, first one, then the second copy is mutated, and the journey to malignancy begins.

Most mutations are not inherited. They occur through daily life, such as exposure to sun (ultraviolet light), the foods we eat, smoking (if we smoke), and aging, as well as through the wear and tear of normal cellular processes.

Proto-oncogenes drive cell division when the body needs cells. In malignancy, there are mutations in the proto-oncogene, forming an oncogene, which continues to send messages to the cell nucleus to divide, much like putting one's foot on a car's accelerator. Oncogenes are activated, or "turned on," so that they continue to send the message to the cell nucleus to divide, as if the accelerator pedal were pressed to the floor. When the oncogene is mutated, it matters where

Figure 1-1   Philadelphia chromosome: example of a reciprocal translocation and formation of an oncogene.

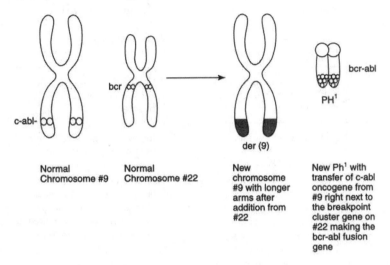

Normal Chromosome #9	Normal Chromosome #22	New chromosome #9 with longer arms after addition from #22	New Ph¹ with transfer of c-abl oncogene from #9 right next to the breakpoint cluster gene on #22 making the bcr-abl fusion gene

Wilkes and Barton Burke.[9] Reproduced with permission from the publisher.

on the chromosome the oncogene is positioned. Table 1-1 shows some examples of oncogenes. There are at least 100 oncogenes known at this time, and they fall within five major classes[10]:

1. *Growth factors*—These factors stimulate cell growth (e.g., c-sis overexpression results in the overproduction of PDGF).
2. *Growth factor receptors*, such as the EGFR1 (erbB1) and EGFR2 (HER2 or erbB2)—The receptor should be turned on when a growth factor binds to it, but when the gene is mutated, the receptor can be turned on indefinitely, constantly sending the message for cell division to the cell nucleus. The genes *erbB1* and *erbB2* can also be amplified, which means the cell has too many copies of the gene rather than the normal two copies, again resulting in many signals being sent to the nucleus of the cell for the cell to divide.
3. *Signal transducers*, such as ras and abl—These proteins help pass the message along to the cell nucleus. They are usually turned on or off based on the cell's need for signaling. When mutated, they stay on and constantly send messages to the cell nucleus to make the cell divide.
4. *Transcription factors*, such as myc—These factors are at the DNA level and direct the copying of the genes (recipes for protein[s]), which tell the cell to divide or other functions. They are normally turned on when needed, and off after they copy the gene's recipe for the protein so that no more proteins will be made. When mutated, these transcription factors can remain

Table 1-1   Selected Oncogenes

Oncogene	Function	Comments/Cancer Types
v-sis	Overexpresses and produces platelet-derived growth factor	Located on long arm chromosome 22; prostate
Erb1 (EGFR)	Increased cell proliferation, survival, angiogenesis, invasion, and metastases	Can be mutated or amplified; CRC, breast, lung, SCHNC, pancreatic
Erb2 (HER2)	Increased cell proliferation	Increased signaling or amplification; breast, gastric, lung
Ras	Increased cell proliferation	Pancreatic; K-ras colon; H-ras breast, melanoma, lung, kidney, bladder; NRAS ovarian, thyroid, melanoma, leukemia
Abl	Increased cell proliferation	CML
Myc	Increased cell proliferation, malignant transformation, remodeling of stroma	C-myc Burkitt lymphoma; N-myc neuroblastoma
Bcl2	Prevents apoptosis of abnormal cells	Lymphoma
BRAF	Involved in cell signaling; helps to regulate the MAPK signaling pathway, which is very important in cell growth and differentiation	Gastric, colon
RET	Its protein is a receptor tyrosine kinase that is important in communicating messages from outside the cell. It is essential in the development of normal kidneys and the nervous system. RET stands for "rearranged during transfection."	Thyroid, multiple endocrine neoplasia
MET	Makes receptor for hepatocyte growth factor (HGF)/scatter factor; important regulator of cell proliferation, motility, invation, and survival	Papillary renal cell cancer

on. Some transcription factors are activated when mutated in many cancers, and initiate and maintain the tumor phenotype (behavior) in remodeling the tumor microenvironment with inflammatory and other mediators.[4]

5. *Regulators of apoptosis* (programmed cell death), such as the gene *bcl-2*—When mutated, the gene becomes hyperactive and dominant, and prevents programmed cell death of abnormal cells.

TSGs halt cell growth when the body has the exact number of cells needed, again so cell birth equals cell death, and work much like the brakes on a car. In cancer, the TSGs are damaged, either through inactivation or through loss of the part of the chromosome that contains the TSG (locus). Unlike oncogenes, which are turned on and continue to send signals for growth, TSGs are turned off or inactivated so that they do not work. With first one copy of the TSG mutated, the brakes on cell division begin to fail, and when the second copy of the TSG is mutated or lost, the brakes really fail, so that cell division cannot be opposed. Table 1-2 shows examples of TSGs. Types of TSGs can be classified in terms of their function[10]:

* *Genes that control cell division*, such as the retinoblastoma gene (Rb1)—These genes are crucial for guarding the cell cycle from incompetent cells that should not pass through the cell cycle.
* *Genes that repair DNA*—These genes are crucial for "proofreading" the DNA strands after they have been replicated to identify any mistakes and to fix them by either excising the mistakes or correcting the misspelling (base pairs) in the DNA strand. People with hereditary nonpolyposis colon cancer (HNPCC) are born with one or more DNA repair genes that are mutated and cannot correct the errors in DNA.
* *Genes responsible for apoptosis*, such as p53—These genes are the guardians of the genome and the gene product that forces the irreparably mutated cell into programmed cell death (see Chapter 4). Many solid tumors have mutations in p53. Individuals with the Li-Fraumeni syndrome inherit p53 mutations and have a high risk for developing multiple cancers.

DNA is the building block of life and contains a person's complete genetic information (the "blueprint" for that individual), such as eye and hair color, as well as all the instructions to operate the billions of cells in the body. DNA is highly protected and is the only biomolecule in the body that is repaired, with all other defective biomolecules being replaced.[11] There are four general systems of DNA repair: (1) direct damage repair, (2) excision of the damaged DNA portion, with precise replacement of the correct sequence of nucleotides, (3) double-strand break repair, and (4) damage bypass. The excision of a damaged DNA portion and replacement of correct sequence can be subdivided into three types: (1) mismatch repair, (2) base excision repair, and (3) nucleotide excision repair.

Table 1-2   Tumor Suppressor Genes

Tumor Suppressor Gene	Function	Comments/Cancer Types
TP53	Transcription factor responsible for detecting irreparable DNA mutations and causing them to undergo apoptosis	Mutated in many solid tumors
RB1 (retinoblastoma)	Normally guardian of the genome; when mutated, the cell cycle is uncontrolled	Retinoblastoma, cervical
DNA Repair Genes *MLH1, MSH2,* or *MSH6*	Repair of DNA mutations	Hereditary nonpolyposis colon cancer (HNPCC)
BRCA1, BRCA2	DNA repair genes, act as tumor suppressor genes	Inherited susceptibility to breast (BRCA2), ovarian, or pancreatic
APC	Makes a protein that communicates with other proteins to control whether cell division occurs and to ensure that the correct number of chromosomes is present in the cell during cell division; helps verify adherence to neighboring cells and cell migration	CRC, gastric, pancreatic
ATM	Controls the rate of cell growth and coordinates the repair of damaged DNA by working with BRCA1 and other DNA repair genes	Leukemia, lymphoma, breast, ovarian
CDK4	Cyclin-dependent kinase that, together with CDK2, determines whether the cell will continue in cell division at the G1/S control point in the cell cycle	Melanoma
DCC	Helps regulate cell death and is important in axon guidance	Colorectal

Table 1-2   Tumor Suppressor Genes (continued)

Tumor Suppressor Gene	Function	Comments/Cancer Types
INK4A	Codes for 2 proteins (p), which help to control the cell cycle: p16 stops the cell cycle in the G1 phase, and p19^{ARF} stops p53 from being broken down	Melanoma
PTEN	Codes for the PTEN protein, which helps to regulate the cell cycle, thus preventing rapid cell growth and division	Breast, prostate, endometrial
VHL	Helps regulate the cell cycle, preventing rapid cell growth and division; works with other proteins to break down proteins when no longer needed, such as hypoxia-inducible factor (HIF), a key player in angiogenesis	Renal cell, pheochromocytoma, hemagioblastoma

In cancer, unfortunately, often the DNA repair genes are mutated so that cells with significant mutations can progress through the cell cycle and reproduce cells containing mutations. With each division, more mutated cells go through cell division, so that more cells with additional mutations are produced. Eventually a clone of cells with particularly aggressive behavior (phenotype) will be selected (selection of the fittest).

As mentioned, hereditary mutations in DNA repair genes often lead to malignancy, such as HNPCC, which is associated with mutations in the DNA mismatch repair (MMR) genes. The mutations prevent the gene from giving the correct recipe for making the repair protein. When MMR genes are unable to fix "spelling" errors in the DNA before mitosis, the spelling errors or "mismatches" accumulate, possibly leading to oncogenes or damaged TSGs.

If a person has a mutation in both copies of the MMR genes, such as mutations in both copies of the MSH2 or MLH1 gene (homozygous), then the person is at risk for not only developing colon and other cancer but also for leukemia, lymphoma, or neurofibromatosis (called CoLoN, for Colon tumors, and/or Leukemia, and/or Neuroblastomatosis) at an early age.[12]

Most patients (90%) with HNPCC colon cancers show a phenomenon called microsatellite instability (MSI), compared to only 15–20% of patients with sporadic colon cancers. Microsatellites are short, repeated sequences of DNA. Recall that the DNA sequences are made up of nucleotides that are represented by the four letters in DNA base pairing, A (adenine), T (thiamine), C (cytosine), G (guanine), where A always is matched with T, and C with G. The number of repeats at a single point in the DNA helix may differ among people in a given population, but in each individual, it has a constant length. For example, at a single place in the DNA strand (locus), one might have three AC repeats and another population may have four AC repeats at that same locus. But when an individual is born, he or she has a constant number of DNA repeats or microsatellites. Over time, there are mutations; this number can increase and sequences can be abnormally long or short.

In cancer, if there are more or less repeats of these DNA sequences in the microsatellite regions of DNA than in the DNA the person was born with, then MSI is indicated. When a laboratory does a test for MSI, the lab examines five different microsatellite regions of DNA. MSI-H(igh) is usually considered if microsatellite changes are found in two or more microsatellite regions; MSI-L(ow) is considered if changes are found in only one region, and MSS (stable) is considered if no changes are found. MSI-H is often the result of mutations in the DNA repair genes so that the mutations cannot be repaired. In HNPCC, MSI-H patients have a better prognosis than patients with sporadic colon cancer that is either MSS or MSI-L.[13] Additionally, there is evidence that 5-FU–based chemotherapy confers no benefit in patients with MSI-H colon cancer and may be harmful.[14]

Other well-known DNA repair genes that are mutated in cancer and that become targets for therapeutic intervention include BRCA1 and BRCA2, which are associated with the homologous recombination repair pathway and an increased risk for developing breast cancer. Both are TSGs. BRCA2 works to repair DNA double-strand breaks together with a molecule called RAD51. BRCA1 helps to repair DNA errors by interacting with other members of the DNA repair system and regulating the expression (turning on or off) of genes that are involved in the repair of DNA mistakes. If BRCA1 and/or BRCA2 are not functioning, then cells with abnormal chromosomes accumulate and continue to mutate, and malignant transformation can occur.[15] If BRCA1 and BRCA2 are not functioning, then a backup DNA repair process involves poly (ADP-ribose) polymerase (PARP) enzymes. PARP enzymes are needed to repair DNA following damage from internal or external stressors. PARP inhibitors selectively kill breast cancer cells with defective BRCA1 and BRCA2 repair genes. Normal cells with functional BRCA1 and BRCA2 are able to use a secondary, backup repair process to repair DNA damage, while BRCA1 and BRCA2 mutated malignant cells now have both pathways blocked.[16] See Chapter 4 for a discussion of PARP1 inhibitors.

It is known now that there are many different pathways to malignancy even within a tumor type, such as that observed in breast cancer and colon cancer. See Figure 1-2 for a sequence of mutations leading to malignant transformation in colon cancer. Figure 1-3 shows the development of metaplasia, dysplasia, carcinoma in situ, and finally invasive cancer and metastasis.

Figure 1-2 Mutations in colorectal cancer (CRC).

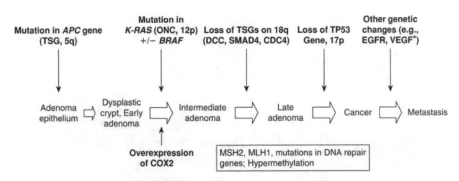

While a number of independent, different pathways are being identified, the following diagram highlights key mutations. In 85% of sporadic CRCs, the first mutation is the APC gene, while the remaining 15% have mutations in the mismatch repair genes, making them inactive. VEGF has been shown to occur early in the progression of CRC; however, VEGF expression correlates with invasiveness and metastasis. EGFR overexpression may occur early in tumor development and influence invasion; high EGFR expression in the primary tumor is associated with higher tumor stage.

TSG= tumor suppressor gene; ONC=oncogene; EGFR=epidermal growth factor receptor overexpression; VEGF=vascular endothelial growth factor; p= short arm of chromosome; q= long arm of chromosome.

Data from Deng Y, Kurland BF, Wang J, et al. High epidermal growth factor receptor expression in metastatic colorectal cancer lymph nodes may be more prognostic of poor survival than in primary tumor. *Am J Clin Oncol.* 2009;32(3):245-252; Fearon ER, Vogelstein B. A genetic model for colorectal tumorigenesis. *Cell* 1990;61:759–767; Hisamuddin IM, Yang VW. Molecular genetics of colorectal cancer: An overview. *Curr Colorectal Cancer Reports* 2006;2(2):53-59; Kabbinavar F, Hurwitz HI, Fehrenbacher L, et al. Phase II, randomized trial comparing bevacizumab plus fluorouracil (FU)/leucovorin (LV) with FU/LV alone in patients with metastatic colorectal cancer. *J Clin Oncol.* 2003;21:60-65; Walther A, Johnstone E, Swanton C, et al. Genetic prognostic and predictive markers in colorectal cancer. *Nature Rev Cancer* 2009;9:489-499.

Signaling Pathways

The message from the oncogene needs to reach the cell nucleus to tell the cell to divide, to ignore antigrowth and apoptotic signals, to make new blood vessels (angiogenesis), to invade, and to metastasize. The message is sent via a "bucket brigade" to signaling molecules, a process called signal transduction. Most of these bucket brigade proteins are protein kinases. The many areas along this pathway that can be targeted by new agents include the ligands, which bind to the cell's receptor and start sending the message (e.g., growth hormone), receptors on the cell surface, proteins that carry the message through the cell (intracellular second messengers), and the transcription factors that turn on genes in the DNA strand. This process results in a copy of the recipe for the protein that will tell the cell to divide, make blood vessels, and so forth.

Figure 1-3   Sequential mutations leading to cancer.

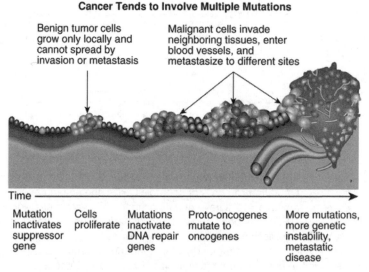

Cancer Tends to Involve Multiple Mutations

Benign tumor cells grow only locally and cannot spread by invasion or metastasis

Malignant cells invade neighboring tissues, enter blood vessels, and metastasize to different sites

Time →

| Mutation inactivates suppressor gene | Cells proliferate | Mutations inactivate DNA repair genes | Proto-oncogenes mutate to oncogenes | More mutations, more genetic instability, metastatic disease |

U. S. National Institutes of Health, National Cancer Institute. Cancer tends to involve multiple mutations. Slide 49 in Understanding cancer series. Available at http://www.cancer.gov/cancertopics/understanding-cancer/cancer/Slide49. Accessed December 4, 2009. Public domain.

Imagine walking into a dark room and turning on a light switch. There is an energy conversion as you raise the light switch and the light goes on. Similarly in a cell, there is a receptor on the outside cell membrane, and when a ligand attaches to it, it starts sending a signal to the cell nucleus. In most cases, the receptor has to grab a partner (dimerize) to start the message. Once the receptor is activated, the message in the cell passes through the membrane and into the inner part of the receptor, the RTK. Here the tyrosine kinase phosphorylates the message by adding phosphates to the side chain of other signaling molecules (e.g., serine/threonine or tyrosine residues of proteins) to pass the message along. At each point of the bucket brigade, there is an exchange of energy. This moves the message from molecule to molecule until it reaches the cell nucleus.

Important RTKs include epidermal growth factor (EGF), PDGF, VEGF, FGF, and hepatocyte growth factor (HGF). These molecules have inner and outer portions. The ligand binds to the external domain of the receptor; when it dimerizes, it activates the receptor and the message is sent to the inner portion of the receptor inside the cell. Here the tyrosine kinase activity happens, and a phosphate group is transferred sending the message "downstream" toward the cell nucleus. Inside the cell, there are many pathways, and some are redundant, so when blocking one pathway, the tumor cell can often figure out another way to send the message. Figure 1-2 shows some of the major signaling pathways that will be discussed here.

A ligand, such as EGF, binds to the EGFR on the outside of the cell; the receptor dimerizes, or "joins hands," with a neighboring receptor, either a EGFR receptor called homodimerization (the same), or another member of the family, such as HER2, 3, or 4, called heterodimerization. This dimerization starts the message through the cell membrane to the tyrosine kinase molecule just inside the membrane. Here, the addition of a phosphate group (phosphorylation) starts the message's journey from signaling messenger to messenger until it gets to the cell nucleus. The signaling molecules (proteins) that carry the message downstream to the nucleus include the mitogen-activated protein kinase (MAPK), which is very important in determining response to extracellular stimuli (mitogens) and in gene expression, mitosis, differentiation, and apoptosis; Akt (one of the most important kinases for cell survival, and important in cell metabolism, growth, and proliferation); and JNK (this is a type of MAPK that responds to stress stimuli). Akt is involved in the P13-kinase/Akt/mTOR pathway as well; mTOR (mammalian target of rapamycin) is like Grand Central Station, and it plays a key role in figuring out what to do when the cell receives input from multiple upstream receptors such as EGFR, IGF-1 and -2, and mitogens that are telling the cell to divide. It also senses whether the cell has sufficient nutrients and energy to do its work. If there is too little oxygen, it calls for the manufacture of blood vessels to bring oxygen to the cell and remove waste products. This is called a signal transduction cascade (see Figure 1-2). Once the message gets to the cell nucleus, it goes to the DNA strands and activates transcription factors that find the genes that need to be transcribed (the recipes for proteins copied onto mRNA that will take the recipe to the cook [ribosomes], which will make the protein). The genes that are transcribed code for proteins. These proteins will turn on the cell cycle (proliferation), and enable the cell to avoid apoptosis and ultimately to invade and metastasize.

Primary Tumor Formation

A series of mutations over time change a normal cell into a malignant one. Figure 1-3 shows the continuum of malignant transformation.[17] Initiation refers to the initial insult to the cell, causing a mutation in a proto-oncogene that results in an oncogene. Some cancers associated with altered oncogenes are CML (ABL1 is the oncogene), gastric cancer (BRAF), HER2-positive breast cancer (Erb-B2), and others, as shown in Table 1-1. Also, mutations can result from the loss of a TSG, such as APC in FAP.

Once initiation occurs, malignant transformation will continue if promotional factors drive additional mutations. This usually involves loss of more TSGs and their proteins, loss of DNA repair genes, and other factors. By this time, the cell acquires metaplastic cells, meaning one normal cell type is replaced by another normal type; for example, in an individual who smokes, the columnar cells lining the respiratory tree are replaced with stratified squamous epithelium. This process is reversible. If the person continues to smoke, the cells become dysplastic. Now they do not look like the parent tissue and are less differentiated and more primitive. This state is considered premalignant; if allowed, the cells will progress to a malignancy. In situ is a malignant cell that does not have invasive features. In contrast, certain cells in an invasive cancer are more aggressive and can invade through the basement membrane, invade locally, and disseminate to other parts of the body.

Transition to malignancy often occurs over years in solid tumors. For example, it may take 10 years for a tumor in the breast or lung to reach 1 cm in size. As the tumor cells double in number, the size of the tumor increases. When the tumor is larger than 1–2 mm (the size of a pen's tip), it needs to develop blood vessels to bring in oxygen and remove waste products. Much of the development of cancer is related to stimulation from the tumor microenvironment.

Inflammation and the Microenvironment

Areas of inflammation are infiltrated by phagocytic cells to clean up the debris: neutrophils and macrophages. These cells are then replaced by other cells including lymphocytes and later fibroblasts, endothelial cells, and adipocytes. All established tumors have these cells. The normal tissue cells respond to the chronic infection and co-evolve with the transformed malignant cell to allow tumor initiation and progression.[18] The pro-inflammatory immune cells that arrive to protect the normal tissue cells in the area of inflammation are tissue macrophages, mast cells, and dendritic cells.

As the tumor develops, normal fibroblasts undergo changes and become cancer-associated stromal fibroblasts (CAFs), which can help the tumor progress; they can also differentiate from tissue stem cells or migrate from the bone marrow.[8,18] This ability is thought to be due to epigenetic changes (which can be inherited and are not due to a change in DNA) that arise from the inflammatory condition. All fibroblasts express vimentin, but the CAFs also express α-smooth muscle actin, so they can move (also called myofibroblasts). The CAFs secrete soluble factors that bring in chemokines for angiogenesis, bring in more inflammatory cells, and directly support tumor growth and progression.

- Stromal-derived factor 1 (SDF-1) is a chemokine that attracts endothelial progenitor cells and activates MMP-9; it is also the ligand for CXCR4, a receptor for some viruses.
- TGFβ is increased; it can overproduce growth factors (e.g., HGF, also called Scatter factor) to promote metastasis. Chapter 2 further discusses HGF.

Mast cells are found in tissues and can induce angiogenesis. Mast cells can recruit endothelial cells, and they interact with the endothelial cells and other stromal cells. They also are responsible for activating MMP-9 and MMP-2, as well as proteases that can degrade the ECM to make a path for the blood vessels to travel, allowing the tumor to invade locally and to metastasize. Finally, by secreting FGF2, VEGF, TGFβ, and IL-8, they bring in and activate other bone marrow-derived cells.[8]

Dendritic cells (DCs) normally protect the body against invading pathogens; they are called the "sentinels of the immune system" and are the first responders to initiate the inflammatory response and then to bridge the innate resistance and adoptive immunity.[18] They can be conventional or plasmacytoid.

The conventional DCs can rapidly respond to an invading micro-organism by recognizing and taking up the micro-organism (i.e., presenting the antigen) and then secreting substances that call in the immune system. They can recognize the invaders because they have pattern recognition receptors (e.g., Toll-like receptors). They quickly mature and release cytokines, including IL-12, TNF, IL-6, IL-1, and type I interferons (IFNs). These cytokines then activate other bone marrow-derived cells as well as stromal cells in the tissue to bring in more inflammatory cells to the area of inflammation. IL-12 and IFN call for natural killer T cells, which produce both pro-inflammatory and anti-angiogenic factors.

The mature DCs then leave the tissue, migrating up the draining lymph vessels to the thymocyte-dependent (T-cell) area in the lymph nodes. There, they present the antigen of the invading pathogen to the memory T cells to see if they have been in the body before. The antigen is compared to the major histocompatibility antigens I and II, and CD8+ (cytotoxic T cells and suppressor T cells that can turn off the inflammatory response) and CD4+ (helper) T lymphocytes. Now, in cancer and in chronic inflammation, the DC cells are present, but they do not behave like normal DC cells because their phenotype has changed. Through communication with the microenvironment, probably via the anti-inflammatory cytokines IL-10, TGFβ, VEGF, and prostaglandins, they now do not mature and do not respond to the signals as they would in normal tissue. Immature DCs are found in tumors. However, rarely, mature, activated DCs may be found in tumor tissue, along with activated mature T cells; if found in the periphery, these DCs suggest that the immune system is functioning and conferring a positive prognostic factor.[19]

What about the second type of DCs, the plasmacytoid DCs? They are very different in appearance and function. Once activated, they may take on some of the antigen-presenting function, but in general they migrate via the bloodstream, rather than the lymphatic system, to the area of inflammation or infection. Once there, they secrete type I IFN and are especially important in directing resistance to viral infection. Finally, they are able to suppress the immune system by unclear mechanisms. When found rarely in breast cancer tissue, their appearance is independently associated with poor patient survival.[20]

Neutrophils are one of the few normal cells that can leave their home turf and travel through the blood or tissue without suffering programmed cell death. Neutrophils arrive at the area of inflammation early in the process, and they are also found in the tumor stroma or microenvironment. In the stroma, they express factors to begin the angiogenic process: MMP-9 and other cytokines. Neutrophils are able to communicate with their cousins the macrophages (cross-talk) and probably influence the development of TAMs. Eosinophils also play a role in regulating the inflammatory response, tissue repair, and remodeling of the microenvironment.

Both neutrophils and eosinophils probably release reactive oxygen species (ROS), as they are very toxic to pathogens; eosinophils additionally release leukotrienes and prostaglandins. ROS occur as a by-product of aerobic processes and include species such as superoxide, hydrogen peroxide, and hydroxyl radical. At low levels, ROS function in cell signaling, but at higher doses, they can damage RNA and DNA. ROS probably play a role in facilitating the genetic mutations that occur in the initiation of cancer cells but also in cancer promotion and progression. ROS act as signal transduction messengers, promoting either proliferation or death of cells. Cancer cells appear to be constantly under oxidative stress, and tumor-associated inflammation facilitates their survival and dissemination. However, anticancer therapies can target ROS to lead to cancer cell death.[21]

Macrophages are very important players in malignant transformation and progression.[22] Their role is paradoxical, as macrophages in large number can destroy tumors. However, when monocytes in the blood or their precursors are drawn to the tumor by tumor or stromal-secreted chemokines and are then changed to TAMs, the level is lower and these macrophages behave as tumor promoters. Chemokines are proteins that lure cells to a given area in the body; they can be CXC, which attracts neutrophils, or CC, which attracts monocytes, lymphocytes, basophils, and eosinophils.[23] TAMs are primarily recruited by CC chemokine ligand 2 (CCL2)/MCP1, as well as by macrophage–colony-stimulating factors (CSFs) and VEGF.[18] They help tumor growth and dissemination by (1) inducing new blood vessel formation (through secreting proangiogenic chemokines, VEGF, TNF, and FGF2); (2) producing tumor growth and survival chemokines; and (3) remodeling the stromal matrix so that local invasion and metastasis can occur (i.e., increasing the expression of MMPs, TGFβ, TNF, and chemokines).[18] Myeloid-derived immature cells (macrophages, granulocytes, DCs, etc.) play an emerging role in cancer and are referred to as myeloid-derived suppressor cells.

Together, in cancer-associated inflammation, unlike in acute inflammation, the macrophages and DCs behave in an immunosuppressive way, leaving the patient anergic. Therapeutic strategies include developing ways to halt the relationship between the tumor and the microenvironment, and turning the macrophages and DCs back to their behaviors (phenotype) in acute inflammation when they can kill tumor cells. Thus, macrophages and DCs are potential immunological targets.[18] While the new research advances have shed light on some processes, they have raised more questions such as the importance of tumor initiating cells, circulating tumor and/or stem cells.

INVASION AND METASTASIS

Invasion and metastasis are complex, and currently scientists are working very hard to understand and to identify the key targets in the process so that key molecules can be targeted. As previously discussed, approximately 90% of patients die from metastasis, not the primary tumor, and more than 80% of life-threatening cancers arise in epithelial cell-derived carcinomas.[8] Many changes that occur normally in embryogenesis to help the fertilized egg develop into a fetus, and which are then turned off, are called back into play in cancer. Examples include (1) the reemergence of telomerase, the enzyme that helps embryonic cells divide indefinitely (which is shut off after the fetus is formed), and (2) the transition from an epithelial appearance of the cell (phenotype) to one that has characteristics of a mesenchymal cell in a process called epithelial–mesenchymal transition (EMT) (Figure 1-4).

More than 80% of life-threatening cancers are epithelial in origin, offering an attractive picture of invasion and metastasis. To review, in the embryo, there are three main types of germ tissue, the endoderm (gives rise to the gastrointestinal [GI] and respiratory systems), the mesoderm (gives rise to connective tissue, blood, muscle, and bone), and the ectoderm (gives rise to skin and nervous tissue) (Figure 1-5).

The mesoderm contains mesenchymal cells that have the ability to differentiate (or specialize) into adult cells of the muscle, arteries, veins, bone cells, and phagocytic cells. These cells are loosely put together and can migrate to where they need to be. However, in the embryo, some of the other primitive cells need to move to a different area to make certain structures, like the spinal cord. The cells for the nervous system are in the ectoderm, or outer layer, where the epithelial cells are located. Here, the epithelial cells are tightly woven together into sheets and are also tightly tethered to the ECM that lies beneath

Figure 1-4   Epithelial–mesenchymal transition.

Mechanisms of EMT

(i) Polarized epithelial cells are rich with intact junctional proteins (cadherins, occludins and desmosomes)

(ii) Loss of cell-cell adhesion due to reduced junctional proteins causes epithelial cells to become isolated from its neighboring cells

(iii) Isolated epithelial cells begin to transform into mesenchymal cells, interact and degrade basement membrane proteins

(iv) Full blown mesenchymal cells acquire front-end and back-end polarity, become motile, interact with ECM to migrate

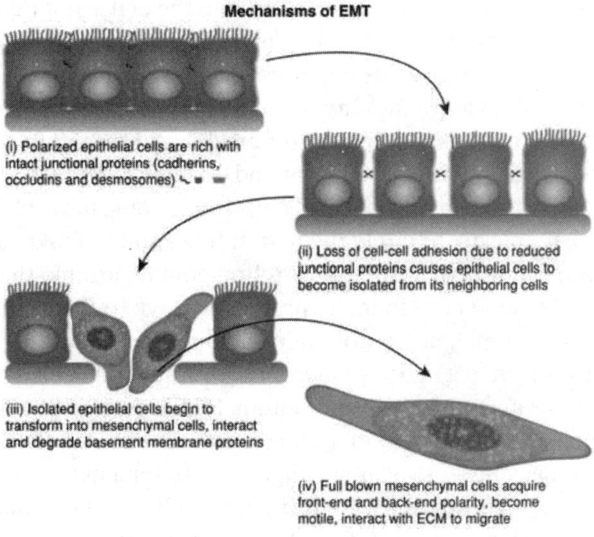

Reproduced with permission from Karger, AG. Figure from Newshad.[24]

Figure 1-5   Gastrulation in the embryo, with germ layers.

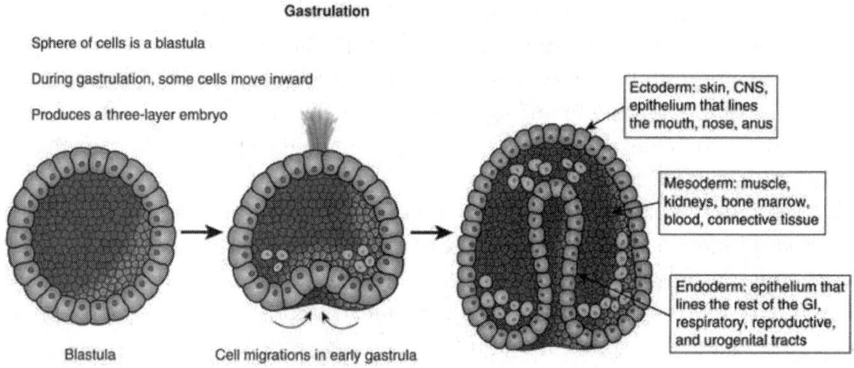

Data from The National Institutes of Health. Appendix A: Early Development. In *Stem cell information.* Available at http://stemcells.nih.gov/info/scireport/appendixa. Accessed November 4, 2009.

them by tight junctions (adherens junctions, containing E-cadherin, which links with catenins connected to the fibers within the cell cytoskeleton) so that they cannot move or migrate.

In order for the epithelial cells to move and form the vertebral column around the spinal cord and for the neural crest cells to move where they need to be in the embryo, the cells send messages. EMT comes into play by changing the epithelial cells into mesenchymal cells. Thus, the epithelial cell loses all its epithelial qualities, such as E-cadherin, which causes a loss of the catenins from the junctions, so the tight junctions fall apart and the cell is not tightly bound to its neighbor or to the underlying ECM). Furthermore, the cell develops filopodia so it can migrate, and it gains qualities of a mesenchymal cell, such as vimentin, myosin, and invasive motility. In addition, it changes polarity so it can migrate; where the epithelial cell has an apical–basal orientation (top to bottom), the new cell has mesenchymal front end–to back end polarity.[25] EMT then is used by the embryo to make epithelial cells into strong, movable cells, like fibroblasts and osteoblasts, to circle the neural tube, and to make an extracellular matrix of bone and cartilage of the vertebral column around the spinal cord. This process is also how cells in the neural crest move to their ultimate targets such as the cranial, spinal, and autonomic ganglia throughout the body.

Once the transition to a cell with mesenchymal qualities occurs, the cell still needs help to move away from the epithelium. MMPs—some of which are powerful enough enzymes to destroy all of a person's tissues and thus exist for the most part as pro-enzymes—appear and digest the basement membrane beneath the cell, forming a hole through which the new cell can move and invade the neighboring ECM. Here, collagen type I and fibronectin in the ECM help the mesenchymal cells move to where they are supposed to go.

Thus, in the embryo, mesenchymal cells can invade and move through the ECM. These cells are geared to move. Their front-to-back direction (polarity) allows them to have a pseudopodium (false foot) at the back end of the cell like strong tires on a four-wheel drive car; in the front where the engine would be, the Golgi apparatus (which stores and modifies proteins for distribution to other parts of the cell, and is normally found near the nucleus of the cell) sits and helps to make the membranes for the filopodia that will help to propel the cell along the ECM.[25] Filopodia are thin projections of cytoplasm that extend from the leading edge of migrating cells, contain actin, and attach to a point ahead of the cell in the ECM; they then pull the cell forward as the rear of the cell retracts.[26] Using both the filopodia and pseudopodia, the cell elongates and pulls itself through the hole in the epithelial basement membrane and into neighboring ECM where it continues to move forward. EMT is essential to remodel tissue in the embryo and in organogenesis so that the adult organs will develop correctly and be positioned in the appropriate place in the body. Key features of this transition to a mesenchymal cell are front–back end polarity, elongated morphology (shape), filopodia, and invasive motility.[25] TGFβ is an important driver of EMT in embryogenesis.[27] It also plays a very important role in cell proliferation and differentiation.

Finally, although genes regulating EMT are turned off after embryogenesis is completed, they are turned back on during wound healing, and probably during cancer metastasis. Genes can be turned on (so they are expressed) or off by epigenetic signals. These signals are not coded in DNA and are not therefore inherited as changes in DNA. Rather they involve the areas around the DNA, and they influence the genes that are coded in DNA (see Chapter 2). An example of this is back in the embryo: Once the cells have moved to where they need to be, they are able to differentiate or become the specialized cells needed to operate a specific organ, such as the thyroid gland; at this time, specific genes are turned on that allow the cells to work as specialized cells. This change is effected by turning on some genes and turning off others. Once the embryonic cells have migrated to their "new home," the cells need to shed the mesenchymal phenotype (behavior) and regain the epithelial qualities, a process called mesenchymal–epithelial transition (MET).

In using embryogenesis as a lens to view invasion and metastasis, it is believed the invasion–metastasis cascade involves six steps following establishment of a primary tumor and the identification of an aggressive clone of malignant cells[28]:

- Localized invasion of the basement membrane
- Intravasation into lymph or blood microvessels and interaction with formed blood cell elements such as platelets and lymphocytes
- Transportation through the circulation

- Arrest of the cells in the microvessels of specific organs, such as the lungs, bones, and liver
- Extravasation into the metastatic niche
- Colonization with formation of micrometastasis, dormancy, or formation of a macrometastasis

The larger the primary tumor becomes, the more likely it is to metastasize, and the larger the tumor is, the more metastatic cells that are shed.[29] As discussed earlier, epithelial cells exist in sheets of cells that are attached to one another; they lie above a basement membrane that is part of the ECM, to which they are also attached. The basement membrane lies above the stroma and is built with proteins secreted by both the epithelial cells and the stromal cells.[30] Benign neoplasms remain on the epithelial side of the basement membrane and do not invade, while malignant cells continue to proliferate, perpetuate mutations, and eventually evolve a clone of cells that acquire an invasive phenotype. These cells can then overcome the normal constraints such as cell-to-cell adhesion and anchorage dependency, and can invade the basement membrane and underlying stroma.

The question is whether there is a subpopulation of these cells that are analogous to stem cells, which have the ability to self-renew and also to acquire the invasive phenotype.[31] As the cell is transforming, it can also release angiogenic factors even before it goes through the basement membrane. When the cell degrades the basement membrane, it receives growth and survival factors attached to the basement membrane. Cells can travel one by one or together as a "finger" or "tongue" of cancer cells with a leading edge of cells that can degrade the matrix and lead the invasive cells to the nearest blood or lymph vessels.[30]

What gives the cancer cells the invasive qualities it needs to invade? The EMT process is already encoded in the genome. Similar to wound healing, the embryonic EMT process is reactivated by signals from the stroma or microenvironment to give the cells the ability to separate from neighboring cells and to acquire motility and invasiveness.[30] Polyak and Weinberg suggest EMT occurs as a result of specific growth factors, tumor–stromal interactions, and hypoxia.[32] Cross-talk between EMT-signaling and transcription factors allows the cells to be reprogrammed as mesenchymal cells, with stem-cell qualities.[32] Transcription factors are master regulator proteins that can turn on or off genes. Embryonic transcription factors that turn on genes to allow cells to leave their tissue home and to migrate are turned off at birth. However, it appears many are turned back on in metastasis to allow the EMT. These transformed cells are highly invasive and also resistant to anticancer treatment.

Normally, mesenchymal stem cells are recruited from the bone marrow to areas of inflammation or infection when they help the area to heal. A recent development suggests that in cancer, the mesenchymal stem cells are also recruited, and once they arrive at the newly formed tumor, they "teach" the cells how to become aggressive and metastasize.[33] In the lab, when breast cancer cells talk to the mesenchymal stem cells, the mesenchymal stem cells secrete CCL5 (chemokine 5, RANTES), which stimulates the cancer cells to move from the bloodstream into the lungs, where they lose their aggressive phenotype.[33]

During EMT, specific transcription factors that are highly expressed and that argue toward specialized stem cells alone will have the EMT-benefit of being highly aggressive and invasive. These factors are *TWIST1, FOXC2, SNAI1, ZEB2,* and *TWIST2,* in addition to vimentin and fibronectin, and levels have been found at the highest in CD44+/CD24– stem cell-like cells compared to the epithelial-differentiated cells, which are CD44–/CD24+ cells.[32] Interestingly, breast cancer CD44+/CD24– cells with these transcription factors tend to be highly invasive, metastatic, and associated with angiogenesis.[34] MicroRNA (miRNA) are involved in regulating the EMT process, as they regulate these EMT-inducing transcription factors.[32,35]

First, there are genetic changes, so the epithelial-derived cells can lose E-cadherin expression to allow them to become invasive through the silencing of E-cadherin, which otherwise would keep them bound to their neighbors in sheets of cells.[30] They now express N-cadherin, which allows the cells to be motile like mesenchymal cells. The CDH1 gene makes the instructions for making the protein E-cadherin, so it is repressed by promoter methylation in many cancers (which makes the gene inactive by reading frame mutations; see the epigenetics section in Chapter 2). Other cancers show loss or mutation of the gene (or in familial gastric cancers, there is a germ-line mutation of the CDH1 gene). N-cadherin binds loosely and weakly to stroma, so it can easily leave its home and, upon stimulation by the stroma, break through the basement membrane and invade locally. Vimentin, which is characteristic of a mesenchymal cell, is expressed, and the cell may start making fibronectin proteins.

EMT may be started by messages from the stroma only in the cells at the leading edge of the tumor mass that is breaking through the basement membrane, the stroma, and locally invading the tissue.[30] Messages to initiate EMT are sent from the reactive stroma: TGFβ, tumor necrosis factor α (TNFα), EGF, HGF, and IGF-1. TNFα is produced early in tumor formation and progression by the inflammatory macrophages; it activates the nuclear factor–kβ (NF–kβ) signaling pathway, which increases the production of inflammatory mediators. NF–kβ is a very important transcription factor that regulates the key genes of the innate and adoptive immune response, as well as genes controlling cell proliferation and survival; it is thought to be the link between inflammation and cancer.[36] If NF–kβ is blocked, EMT transformation is blocked.[30] TAMs also influence the invasive and metastatic behavior of cancer cells by promoting angiogenesis, inducing tumor growth, and enhancing tumor invasiveness and migration.[37]

EGF plays a very important role in helping the cell become invasive. In many cancers, the EGFR is overexpressed or the receptor gene amplified. EGF has been shown to help cells detach from the ECM, to become motile, to invade, and to metastasize.[38] In addition, EGF stimulates the secretion of colony-stimulating factor 1 (CSF1), which attracts and stimulates macrophages. In a reciprocal manner, CSF1 causes the macrophages to proliferate and also secrete more EGF to continue to activate the cancer cells via their EGF receptors. Finally, HGF, or scatter factor, is produced by the stromal cells to enhance the cells' ability to proliferate, move, invade, metastasize (scatter), and survive; it has a high affinity for the c-Met RTK (cognate receptor, as HGF is the only ligand for c-Met receptor) on epithelial cells.[30] For these reasons, inhibitors of c-Met RTK are being explored[39] (see Chapter 2).

In this setting, TGFβ promotes an aggressive phenotype, but under other circumstances, TGFβ suppresses cell proliferation and promotes apoptosis. In fact, in these cases, TGFβ stops the cell cycle at the G_1 phase to stop proliferation, induce differentiation of the cell, or promote apoptosis. It appears that the inactivation of the pRb pathway that occurs in many cancers makes cells lose the ability to respond to the antiproliferative and pro-apoptosis signals from TGFβ.[30] This growth factor tells the transformed cancer cells and neighboring stromal cells to proliferate, and to make more TGFβ, which acts on endothelial cells to make new blood vessels to support invasion. Finally, TGFβ changes the effector T-lymphocytes into regulatory cells (suppressor T cells), which then turn off the inflammatory reaction, thus preventing the effector cells from fighting the new cancer cells. Unfortunately, high levels of TGFβ in a tumor suggest a very aggressive cancer with poor prognosis.[30]

Some cancers, once they have undergone EMT, begin to produce their own TGFβ1, which ensures that the cells will keep their mesenchymal phenotype (autocrine production). It is no surprise then, that apparently TGFβ regulates the breast cancer stem cell phenotype.[34,40] In some cancers, there is also a mutation in the ras signaling pathway forming the raf oncoprotein, which can start the EMT transition on its own; the transformed cells are protected from the antiproliferative and pro-apoptotic effects of TGFβ by P13k, a protein in the Akt signaling pathway.[30] TGFβ is a powerful agent because most cells have receptors for TGFβ, allowing the cells to continue responding to it. In addition to proteases that are released to help degrade the basement membrane and ECF to permit the journey to and through the neighboring tissue, the transformed cell also takes on new cell surface integrins and growth factor receptors.

Other signals to proceed to EMT come from Wnt and Hedgehog signaling, and ligands of RTKs. Both the Wnt and Hedgehog signaling pathways are active during embryogenesis. Hedgehog gives the embryo direction in aligning organs. When activated, it leads to a decrease in E-cadherin and tight junctions. It is also important in angiogenesis and metastasis. Both pathways are potential targets for therapeutic drug development. See Chapter 2.

During the initial phase of invasion and metastasis, EMT requires these signals. It is possible, however, that when the metastatic cells have reached their metastatic destination, the cells revert back to their original epithelial phenotype (via the MET process).[30] However, once EMT has occurred, the new mesenchymal cells are indistinguishable from the mesenchymal cells in the stroma.[30]

Once the cancer cell takes on qualities that enable it to separate from the epithelial sheet of cells, with stimulation from the microenvironment, it can now move through the basement membrane into the stroma. However, the cell needs additional help to make it through the jungle of the ECM and succeeds by remodeling it. The major heavy deconstruction workers are the MMPs, which have the ability to digest all human cells. The MMPs are recruited by the stromal cells such as the macrophages, mast cells, and fibroblasts, and they dissolve the ECM in front of the advancing cancer cells. MT1-MMP (membrane type 1 MMP) is tethered to the cell's membrane; when activated, it is available to surface adhesion molecules such as cadherins and integrins. Other MMPs dissolve the cells in spaces around the cell so it has room to move. Cancer cells secrete two MMPs such as MMP-2. MMP-9, which dissolves collagens and laminin in the basement membrane and the ECM, is largely secreted by the macrophages, neutrophils, and fibroblasts at the invasive edge of the cancer cells.[30] The cancer cells that have undergone EMT now invade the underlying stroma and secrete laminin 2, which is cleaved by an MMP into the EGFR ligand, which shepherds the cancer cell, ensuring cell motility and survival.[30]

MMPs are dangerous, and in fact, may be able to drive malignant cells through all stages of malignant transformation, so they are tightly controlled in the body.[30] The soluble MMPs are synthesized as pro-enzymes that are inactive until activated by proteases, and they are controlled by tissue inhibitors of metalloproteinases. Urokinase plasminogen activator (uPA) is a non-MMP protease that is secreted by macrophages as a pro-enzyme and is tethered to the cell; it binds to its receptor (uPAR) on epithelial cells, thus activating itself, and it is able to degrade the ECM substrates around it. Plasminogen is one substrate cleaved by uPA; when it is activated, it cleaves and activates many of the MMPs.[30] In the laboratory, agents that block the uPA/uPAR complex can stop tumor growth and metastasis.[30] The invading cell develops small outpouchings of the cell surface (podosomes), which are able to degrade the ECM as the cell approaches it and continues to move through the path created by the MMPs. Women who overexpress the gene coding for MMP-3, stromelysin-1, develop hyperplasia that progresses to a primary tumor, invasion, and then metastasis.[41]

Now that the path is cleared, how do the cancer cells develop motility to move through the basement membrane and into the stroma? The cell is able to move by continually restructuring the actin cytoskeleton in different parts of the cell, pulling the cell forward, and then breaking the attachments to the ECM.[30] Similar to the embryo, lamellipodia (cytoplasmic feet) are made from reorganizing the actin filaments and are extended in the direction the cell wants to go. At the same time, proteases on the surface of the cell degrade the ECM that are in the way of the tumor tongue, or "leading edge," of cells that have been transformed. The cell then uses integrins like grappling hooks to pull the lamellipodia in the leading edge forward. The integrins that are holding the trailing edge (or end of the cell) break the attachment to the ECM so the cell can move forward. Filopodia are sticklike projections from the lamellipodia, which the cell uses to explore the territory ahead like a blind person with a cane.

Ras proteins called Rho proteins control the cell shape and motility.[30] P13k (phosphatidylinositol-3 kinase) is the most important motility effector. It establishes new adhesion points between the leading edge of the cell and the ECM and works with MMPs to coordinate the forward movement of the "leading edge" and remodeling of the ECM so it can move forward. The cell contracts, pulling the rear or "trailing edge" of the cell forward.

Now the cells need to circulate, either via the bloodstream or the lymph vessels. Tumor cells and the stromal cells may secrete VEGF-A, which binds to a VEGF receptor on the nearest blood vessel, and tells the endothelial cells to proliferate and migrate to the tumor. It calls in integrins to pull the new vessel to the tumor, as if by grappling hooks, and makes holes in the newly made tube, or C, which stimulates lymphangiogenesis. The leaky and poorly made blood vessels of tumors give ample opportunity for the cancer cells to enter the circulation between the endothelial cells in the newly developed blood vessel. A more comprehensive discussion of angiogenesis is found in Chapter 3 on antiangiogenic drugs. More tumor cells find their way into blood capillaries than lymph vessels because the lymph vessels are weak-walled and collapse if they are located within a tumor. In general, lymph vessels are found around the periphery of the tumor. Malignant cells drain into lymph nodes that are drained by the tissue where the tumor is located. Sentinel lymph node dissection provides an important way to evaluate whether the tumor has metastasized in breast cancer and thin melanoma.[42,43] However, in general, the aggressive clone of cancer cells embolizes into the bloodstream.[44]

Once through the stroma and neighboring tissue, the invasive cancer cells can intravasate through the blood vessel walls (or lymph vessel wall) and get into the circulation. Once in the circulation, however, most tumor cells die.[45] Some may not be successful in overcoming anchorage dependence, and having left their home, they undergo apoptosis. Others may be dependent upon the stromal stimulation factors they no longer receive or may die from the hydrodynamic shear forces of the capillaries. Still others cannot survive in hypoxic or acidic conditions.

If the tumor cell succeeds in entering a large vessel, it may reach the heart and lodge in the first set of capillaries it encounters—e.g., the lungs. Some cancer cells may attract a cloak of platelets that accompanies and protects them through the turbulent circulation, bringing them safely to a distant tissue capillary. With an internal diameter of more than 20 micrometers, cancer cells are usually much larger than the capillary circulation (internal diameter 3–8 micrometers); thus they become trapped in arterioles, which are larger.[30] It is possible that some cells pinch off their cytoplasm to make it through the capillaries or bypass the capillaries by getting into arteriolar–venule shunts. If the cells make it through the pulmonary capillaries, they are pumped through the heart, out the left ventricle, and into the systemic arterial circulation where they can lodge in any smaller vessel.[30]

While circulation patterns influence where the metastatic cells are deposited (for example, with colon cancer, the liver drains the GI tract, so that tumor cells quickly embolize via the blood supply that is going to the liver and lungs), there is very exciting research regarding where metastatic cells ultimately land.[45] Earlier research suggested that cells from a given primary tumor had programmed area codes that told the cell where to go. Clearly the microenvironment of the metastatic niche would need to have compatible adherent molecules so the tumor could attach to the host tissue and also provide growth factors for the particular tumor.[46] Andre et al. proposed that the primary tumor expresses chemokine receptors and that these can predict the site of women with axillary lymph node-positive breast cancer.[47] For example, CXCR4 was statistically associated with tumor progression in the liver, CCR6 was statistically associated with first metastasis to the pleura, CX3CR1 was associated with brain metastasis, and CCR7 with skin metastasis.

In the normal human, circulating leukocytes and stem cells know where they are going by using chemokines (chemo-attractants), which draw them to specific organs. The chemokines bind to guanine nucleotide-binding proteins (G-proteins), which are involved as second messengers in the signaling cascade. Once the chemokines bind to the leukocytes and stem cells, they start intracellular signaling cascades that tell the cells to migrate to the chemokine source. Similarly, Andre et al. understood that breast cancer cells have a receptor for leukocyte chemo attractant 4 (CXCR4) and chemokine receptor 7 (CCR7), and that these matched the chemokines that were expressed in common sites of metastasis: brain, liver, and lungs.[47] It now appears that miRNAs may in fact activate metastasis by acting on multiple signaling pathways.[35]

Once trapped in small vessels in distant tissue, the cell gets messages from the metastatic niche, and it either proliferates in the capillary and dissolves the vessel wall so that it can pass through the surrounding endothelial cells and pericytes and enter the tissue, or it uses its EMT qualities to invade through the vessel wall into the surrounding tissue.[45] Once through the vessel wall, the cell enters the tissue very slowly. Neutrophils use diapedesis so they can travel quickly (in less than a minute) from the blood vessels into tissues toward an area of infection or injury. Cancer cells, in contrast, use brute force to get through the vessel wall (taking upwards of a day) and may degrade parts of the endothelial wall.[30] It is believed that establishing a metastatic home or niche is the most inefficient step in metastasis. Once a distant home has been established, however, the cell may start proliferating or it may lie dormant, depending upon whether there are strong growth and survival signals from the microenvironment of the new niche.

It is possible that a premetastatic niche can be established prior to the arrival of the metastatic cell, much like getting the soil ready for the seed (i.e., the seed and soil hypothesis). Psaila and Lyden suggest that the niches form as a result of tumor-secreted factors and that the future success of the metastatic cell depends not only on the cell's qualities but also its interaction with the microenvironment.[22] The primary tumor secreted growth factors include VEGF-A, placental growth factor, TGFβ, and inflammatory chemokines, which bring in bone marrow-derived progenitor cells. Platelets provide stromal-derived growth factor 1 (SDF1), which acts as a magnet (chemotactic factor) drawing in the bone marrow-derived progenitor cells that have the CXC chemokine receptor 4 (CXC4) and metastatic tumor cells with this receptor.[45] The bone marrow-derived hematopoietic progenitor cells secrete TNFα, MMP9, and TGFβ. The mesenchymal stem cells from the bone marrow may turn into activated fibroblasts and then secrete fibronectin, which is an adhesion protein that will allow the metastatic cell to adhere to the ECM. Endothelial progenitor cells that came from the bone marrow provide new blood vessels and may turn the switch on to move from a micrometastasis to a macrometastasis.[22]

The cell must have adhesion molecules that allow it to attach to the newly found host tissue, and the microenvironment must make chemokines that not only attract the cells but also send out growth and survival signals.[22] As cells proliferate, they evolve a clone of cells that have an ability to live in this new environment. However, on biopsy, these cells are epithelial. Thus, possibly without the EMT signaling from the stroma, the cells lose their mesenchymal qualities and revert back to their epithelial characteristics (via MET).[30] Laboratory work shows that E-cadherin expression is turned back on, together with demethylation of the *CDH1* promoter, which can support MET, but this premise must still be rigorously tested.[22] Again, this hypothesis of MET remains to be validated. Colonization of the metastatic niche may or may not be successful. Growth factors stimulate the new cells to proliferate, and if there are adequate nutrients and if blood vessels as well as ongoing growth signals can be established, then the tumor continues to flourish. Bone marrow cells may be recruited and begin establishing a positive microenvironment for the tumor.[44] Also, the newly forming tumor may work collaboratively with host cells, such as breast cancer cells, which metastasize to bone. Here the breast cancer cells activate the bone-resorbing osteoclasts, which go on to form the osteolytic breast cancer lesions (see Chapter 4). However, if the bone-resorbing osteoclasts are not available, the cells lie dormant until activated at some later time.

Two additional advances that are beginning to help scientists and clinicians are the tumor mutational sequence signatures that predict metastasis in breast cancer, which is a template for other cancers, and expanding knowledge of miRNAs. Mutational gene signatures have helped scientists and clinicians better understand the different molecular types of disease, such as breast cancer, and the likelihood of a person's specific tumor to metastasize.[48] First, it was recognized that breast cancer is comprised of at least four different molecular types: basal-like cancers (ER, PR, HER2 negative, or triple negative), luminal-A (ER+, low grade), luminal-B (ER+ but may express low levels of hormone receptors, and may be high grade), and HER2+ (amplification and high expression of the ERBB2 gene, and others).[49,50] Subsequently, MammaPrint, a 70-gene signature identified from the patient's resected primary tumor, has been shown to be predictive of breast cancer recurrence (high or low risk) and is useful for clinicians planning adjuvant chemotherapy.[51] There are other, shorter gene signatures, and all are being prospectively studied in the Microarray in Node-Negative Disease May Avoid Chemotherapy trial.[52]

More recently, a 186-gene "invasiveness" gene signature (IGS) has been identified.[53] This model takes into account that perhaps only a small subclass of cancer cells has metastatic potential, those that are CD44+ and CD24 low expression, and that these cells share the ability to self-renew with stem cells. The genes are located in two signaling pathways: the Ikβ/NFkβ pathway in response to proinflammatory cytokines, and the RAS/MAPK pathway in response to proliferation factors.[54] Liu et al. found that the IGS was associated with risk of death and metastasis in patients with breast cancer (moderately differentiated ER+), lung cancer, and medulloblastoma.[53] However, because the cancer gene signatures do not appear to overlap, the question is raised as to whether the signature must reflect specific biologic qualities of the unstable cancer cell.[54] Clearly there is much work still to be done.

There is mounting evidence that miRNAs, small, noncoding RNA that regulate gene expression (among other functions), are also key players in all stages of malignancy. Noncoding miRNAs do not have an open reading frame and do not encode or carry a recipe for a protein.[35] However, they appear to have a very important regulatory role in cancer. They are very important in gene regulation and are found in abnormal levels in cancer. They can downregulate TSGs or cause oncogenes to be overexpressed. They bind to their target mRNA in such a way as to cause mRNA degradation, or they inhibit the translation of the mRNA, which has transcribed a gene and is taking the recipe to make a protein.[55]

Other recent developments include the finding that in one instance, the miRNA is activating another mRNA: miR-369-3 can upregulate TNFβ translation.[56] This finding suggests that as more is learned about the specific function of these miRNAs, they can become important targets in the war against cancer and metastasis.

EPIGENETICS

The appearance of a cell or phenotype is determined by which genes are expressed ("turned on" or transcribed), such as blue eyes in a blue-eyed person. Outside the DNA, genes in the DNA can be turned on or off by remodeling the chromatin (which is DNA plus proteins). The chromatin can be remodeled by two epigenetic processes. One way is by modifying the histones around which the DNA is coiled, and the second is by adding or removing methyl groups from specific genes in the DNA. Histones are structural proteins that pack the DNA into a tightly wound double helix or chromatin complex so that the DNA coils around the histones. Histones and methylation also are able to change the DNA so that once a cell has become specialized or differentiated, it cannot go back to being a stem cell. Histones do this by becoming modified, then becoming incorporated into the DNA strand, and finally altering the shape of the histones around the gene(s) that have brought about the differentiated state. It is now thought that histone modification may be influenced or mediated by small, noncoding RNAs (see Chapter 2).

First, because the DNA is wrapped around the histone proteins, the proteins are in close contact with the genes on the DNA strands. Normally, a cell controls the coiling and uncoiling of the DNA strand around the histones when it wants to turn a gene on (uncoil it) or turn it off (coil it). It does this by using histone acetylase to acetylate a section of the histone (lysine residues) to release the tension and loosen the chromatin or DNA so that it can open the DNA strands to be copied. If the chromatin structure is closed (i.e., if the DNA is so tightly coiled that the DNA cannot open to allow m-RNA to come close and copy or transcribe a gene), then that gene is essentially shut off or silenced. The cell closes the chromatin structure by using HDAC, which removes an acetyl group from the lysine residues and makes the DNA tightly coil or condense. There are four classes of HDACs. Some malignancies cause excessive HDACs, closing the chromatin or effectively silencing certain genes. When this process affects a TSG, the brakes are removed from cell division. If it affects a cell cycle protein that normally turns off the cell cycle, then again, the gene is silenced and the cell cycle is left in the "on" position, allowing any cell through to divide.

Another way to think of this is as a slinky toy (Figure 1-6). When the slinky is against a flat surface, the rings are closed. When the slinky moves, the rings at the top open. Similarly, the DNA strands need to pull apart like the open slinky

Figure 1-6   Histones are wrapped around DNA, and they influence gene expression like a slinky. When the slinky is open, it expresses the gene; when it is closed, the gene is turned off.

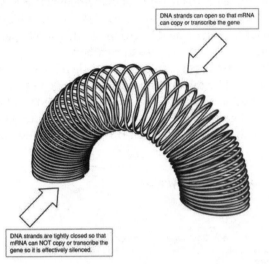

DNA strands can open so that mRNA can copy or transcribe the gene

DNA strands are tightly closed so that mRNA can NOT copy or transcribe the gene so it is effectively silenced.

Data from Wilkes GM. Drug essentials: Histone deacetylase inhibitors. *ONCOLOGY Nurse Edition* 2007;21(11):39–40; Garber K. Silence of the genes: Epigenetics arrives. *J Natl Cancer Inst.* 2002;94(11):793–795.

for mRNA to slip in and copy the gene sequence and to take this copy to the ribosome in the cytoplasm. If the DNA strands are tightly coiled and closed, like the end of the slinky on a flat surface, then mRNA cannot get in to transcribe the gene, and essentially the gene is shut off. The net effect is that the gene is not effective in producing proteins that will stop malignant cell division, even though the TSG is not mutated.

Cancer treatment has progressed in finding agents that inhibit HDACs. Inhibiting HDACs causes increased histone acetylation, resulting in uncoiling of the DNA from the tightly wound chromatin and in the ability of the TSGs to be transcribed or "turned on." This slight alteration in the transcription of a few genes results in cell cycle arrest, differentiation and/or apoptosis, and other lesser-known effects that cause cancer cell death.[57–59] Initially, investigators found that HDAC inhibitors can turn on the gene expression of p21, which regulates p53 activity, a very important TSG that is silenced in many solid tumors.[60] More recently, vorinostat (Zolinza), an HDAC inhibitor that inhibits class I (HDAC1, 2, 3) and class II (HDAC6) HDACs, was approved by the Food and Drug Administration (FDA) for treatment of patients with refractory cutaneous T-cell lymphoma.

The second way the cell can modify gene expression epigenetically is by modifying the amount of methylation in the DNA of the cell. This modification can be done in two ways, and each way involves different DNA sequences[61] (Figure 1-7). In the first of these, methyl groups are added to the DNA in areas that are normally unmethylated. These methyl groups are added at sites characteristically called CpG sites, which change cytosine to 5-methycytosine. The 5-methycytosine is then incorporated into the DNA strand because it behaves like cytosine alone. Areas of DNA that have many methyl groups or that are hypermethylated are silent, and the genes in this area are not transcribed.

Unfortunately, in cancer cells, these areas code for TSGs. DNA methylation patterns are influenced by the environment, and this can be inherited. In cancer, TSGs are often silenced, and CpG islands are often found with promoters of cancer-associated genes.[62,63] Hypermethylation leads to entry into the cell cycle, avoidance of apoptosis, defects in DNA repair, angiogenesis, and loss of

---

Figure 1-7   Comparison of methylation.

Cancer cell with CpG-island hypermethylation, closed chromatin so gene cannot be read or transcribed so tumor suppressor gene silenced

- Entry into cell cycle with cell proliferation
- Avoidance of apoptosis
- Defects in DNA repair genes so mutated cells complete the cell cycle
- Angiogenesis
- Loss of cell adhesion so cells can invade and metastasize

MALIGNANT TUMOR FORMATION

- Loss of imprinting
- Inappropriate cell-type expression
- Genome fragility

DNA Hypomethylation, now with open or relaxed chromatin formation

Normal tumor suppressor gene with open chromatin formation (expressed so it can be copied)

Data from Esteller.[62]

cell adhesion.[62] TSGs known to be hypermethylated and thus silenced in cancer include:

- MLH1—DNA mismatch repair, in colon, endometrium, and stomach, causing frameshift mutations
- BRCA1—DNA repair, transcription, in breast and ovary, causing double-strand breaks
- p16[INK4a]—Cyclin-dependent kinase inhibitor, in many cancers, allowing entrance into cell cycle
- p15[INK4b]—Cyclin-dependent kinase inhibitor in leukemia, allowing entrance into cell cycle
- p14[ARF] MDM2 (mouse double minute 2)—Inhibitor, in colon, stomach, and kidney cancers, causing degradation of p53 (the master policeman of the genome)

Cancer-associated hypermethylation of promoter regions of genes that protect against cancer is more common than cancer-associated hypomethylation that activates cancer genes involved in tumor formation, invasion, and metastasis. This second process of hypomethylation is less understood. In general, the DNA genome in cancer cells is hypomethylated compared to normal cells. In a study by Estécio et al. of colon cancer cells, those that showed MSI were hypermethylated compared to similar cells without MSI, which remained hypomethylated.[64] The areas in cancer cells that are hypomethylated are DNA sequences that are highly and moderately frequently repeated, which suggests an independent role in tumor formation and progression.[61] Cancer-associated hypomethylation appears to be related to loss of imprinting (certain genes are expressed based on the parent, such as expression of the gene in the copy or allele from the mother, such as CDKN1C, or from the father, such as IGF-2), inappropriate cell-type expression, genome fragility, and activation of sequences that lead to tumor formation. CDKN1C is a cyclin-dependent kinase inhibitor implicated in cancer,[65] and IGF-2 is implicated in the formation of neuroblastomas.[66] It also raises a flag of caution when hypomethylating drugs such as 5-azacytidine (Vidaza) are used therapeutically. Vidaza is FDA indicated for the treatment of patients with specific myelodysplastic subtypes or chronic myelomonocytic leukemia.

In addition, DNA methylation can also affect the length of the telomere, or the end of the chromosome, which is normally shortened with each cell division. After about 60–70 cell divisions, the chromosome is too short, and the cell is sent to programmed cell death, called senescence. In the embryo, and in up to 90% of malignant tumors, telomerase, the enzyme that lets the cell replace the snipped-off portion of the chromosome so that the length is not altered, is found in high amounts.[30,67] Telomeres are formed by repeated areas of guanine-rich sequences (TTAGGG DNA repeats). However, for the remaining tumors without telomerase, Blasco found that telomerase activity can be regulated by promoter methylation, and Vera et al.[68] showed that although telomeric DNA repeats cannot be methylated, the subtelomeric DNA repeats can.[69]

SUMMARY

While the process of initial tumorigenesis is well understood, the process of invasion and metastasis is not. This chapter reviews the sequential mutations necessary in malignant transformation, along with a discussion of epigenetic changes that affect the expression of TSGs, and key regulation of genes in the genome. The process of invasion and metastasis is described based on the current literature and suggests that there are specific cells within the tumor responsible for invasion and metastasis—tumor stem cell-like cells.

As the complex layers of tumor initiation, invasion, and metastasis are better understood, additional targets will be identified, and agents will be developed to address them. The cell cycle and a number of cell signaling pathways presented here will be discussed in more detail in Chapter 2, Targeted Cancer Therapy.

REFERENCES

1. Renan MJ. How many mutations are required for tumorigenesis? Implications from human cancer data. *Mol Carcinogenesis.* 1993;7:139-146.

2. Sporn MB. The war on cancer. *Lancet.* 1996;347:1377-1381.

3. Hanahan D, Weinberg RA. The hallmarks of cancer. *Cell.* 2000;100:57-90.

4. Mantovani A. Cancer-related inflammation: the seventh hallmark of cancer. In: *American Society of Clinical Oncology Educational Book.* ASCO; 2009:723-726.

5. Goodlad RA, Plumb JA, Wright NA. Simultaneous measurement of intestinal crypt cell production rate and water absorption. *Gut.* 1987;28(suppl):189-192.

6. Garrett MD. Cell cycle control and cancer. *Curr Science.* 2001;81(5):515-522.

7. Lapenna S, Giordano A. Cell cycle kinases as therapeutic targets for cancer. *Nat Rev Cancer.* 2009;8:547-566.

8. Weinberg RA. Mechanisms of malignant progression. *Carcinogenesis.* 2008;29(6):1092-1095.

9. Wilkes GM, Barton Burke M. *Oncology Nursing Drug Handbook 2009.* Sudbury, MA: Jones and Bartlett; 2009:430.

10. American Cancer Society. Oncogenes and tumor suppressor genes. http://www.cancer.org /docroot/ETO/content/ETO_1_4x_oncogenes_and_tumor_suppressor_genes.asp. Accessed September 9, 2009.

11. Wood RD, Mitchell M, Lindahl T. Human DNA repair genes, 2005. *Mutat Res.* 2005;577:275-283.

12. Bandipalliam P. Syndrome of early onset colon cancers, hematologic malignancies & features of neurofibromatosis in HNPCC families with homozygous mismatch repair gene mutations. *Fam Cancer.* 2005;4(4):323-333.

13. Popat S, Hubner R, Houlston RS. Systematic review of microsatellite instability and colorectal cancer prognosis. *J Clin Oncol.* 2005;23(3):609.

14. Watanabe T, Kanazawa T, Tada T, Kazama Y, Hata K, Nagawa H. Chemotherapy and survival in colorectal cancer patients with and without microsatellite instability: can MSI be a good prognostic marker? *Gastroenterology.* 2004;127(2):688.

15. Deng C-X, Wang R-H. Roles of BRCA1 in DNA damage repair: a link between development and cancer. *Hum Mol Genet.* 2003;12(1):113-123. doi:10.1093/hmg/ddg082.

16. Zaniolo K, Desnoyers S, Leclerc S, Guerin SL. Regulation of poly (ADP-ribose) polymerase-1 (PARP-1) gene expression through the post-translational modification of Sp1: a nuclear target protein of PARP-1. *BMC Mol Biol.* 2007;8:96.

17. Workman L. Cancer. In: Barton Burke M, Wilkes GM, eds. *Cancer Therapies.* Sudbury, MA: Jones and Bartlett; 2006.

18. Trinchieri G. Biology of cancer: inflammation. In: DeVita VT Jr, Lawrence TS, Rosenberg SA, eds. *Cancer: Principles and Practice.* 8th ed. Philadelphia: Lippincott Willliams & Wilkins; 2008:193, 195.

19. Galon J, Fridman WH, Pagès F. The adaptive immunological microenvironment in colorectal cancer: a novel perspective. *Cancer Res.* 2007;67:1883-1886.

20. Colonna M, Trinchieri G, Liu YJ. Plasmacytoid dendritic cells in immunity. *Nat Immunol.* 2004; 5:1219.

21. Manda G, Necchifor MT, Neagu TM. Reactive oxygen species, cancer and anti-cancer therapies. *Curr Chem Biol.* 2009;3:22-46.

22. Psaila B, Lyden D. The metastatic niche: adapting the foreign soil. *Nat Rev Cancer.* 2009;9:285-293.

23. Joyce JA, Pollard JW. Microenvironmental regulation of metastases. *Nat Rev Cancer.* 2009;9: 239-252.

24. Newshad AS. Complexity in interpreting embryonic epithelial-mesenchymal transition in response to transforming growth factor-β signaling. *Cells Tissues Organs.* 2007;185(1-3):131-145.

25. Hay ED. The mesenchymal cell, its role in the embryo, and the remarkable signaling mechanisms that create it. *Dev Dynamics.* 2005;233:706-720.

26. Mattila PK, Lappalainen P. Filopodia: molecular architechure and cellular functions. *Nat Rev Mol Cell Biol.* 2008;9(6):446-454.

27. Ahmed S, Nawshad A. Complexity in interpretation of embryonic epithelial-mesenchymal transition in response to transforming growth factor-β signaling. *Cells Tissues Organs.* 2007;185(1-3): 131-145.

28. Fidler IJ. The pathogenesis of cancer metastasis: the "seed and the soil" hypothesis revisited. *Nat Rev Cancer.* 2003;3:453-458.

29. Heimann R, Hellman S. Aging, progression and phenotype in breast cancer *J Clin Oncol.* 1998;16:2686-2692.

30. Weinberg, RA. *The Biology of Cancer.* New York: Garland Science, Taylor & Francis Group, LLC; 2007.

31. Visvader JE, Lindeman GJ. Cancer stem cells in solid tumors. *Nat Rev Cancer.* 2008;8:755-768.

32. Polyak K, Weinberg RA. Transitions between epithelial and mesenchymal states: acquisition of malignant and stem cell traits. *Nat Rev Cancer.* 2009;9:265-273.

33. Karnoub AE, Dsh AB, Vo AP, et al. Mesenchymal stem cells within tumor stroma promote breast cancer metastases. *Nature.* 2007;449:557-563.

34. Shipitsin M, Campbell LL, Argani P, et al. Molecular definition of breast tumor heterogeneity. *Cancer Cell.* 2007;11:259-273.

35. Nicoloso MS, Spizzo R, Shimizu M, Rossi S, Calin GA. MicroRNAs—the micro steering wheel of tumor metastases. *Nat Rev Cancer.* 2009;9:293-302.

36. Gilmore TD. Introduction to NF-κB: players, pathways, perspectives. *Oncogene.* 2006;25(51): 6680-6684. doi:10.1038/sj.onc.1209954.

37. Shih J-Y, Yuan A, Chen JJ-Y, Yang P-C.Tumor associated macrophage: its role in cancer invasion and metastasis. *J Cancer Molecules.* 2006;2(3):101-106.

38. Wilkins-Port, Ye Q, Mazukiewicz JE, Higgins PJ. TGF-β1+EGF-initiated invasive potential in transformed human keratinocytes is coupled to a plasmin/MMP-10/MMP-1-dependent collagen remodeling axis: Role for PAI-1. *Cancer Res.* 2009;69:4081.

39. Wang X, Le P, Liang C, et al. Potent and selective inhibitors of the Met (hepatocyte growth factor/scatter factor, HGF/SF receptor) tyrosine kinase block HGF/SF-induced tumor cell growth and invasion. *Mol Cancer Ther.* 2003;2:1085.

40. Mani SA, Guo W, Liao MJ, et al. The epithelial-mesenchymal transition generates cells with properties of stem cells. *Cell.* 2008;16:133(4):704-715.

41. Duffy MJ, Mcguire TM, Hill A, et al. Metalloproteinases: role in breast carcinogenesis, invasion, metastasis. *Breast Cancer Res.* 2000;2:252-257.

42. Mansel RE, Fallowfield L, Kissin M, et al. Randomized multicenter trial of sentinel node biopsy versus standard axillary treatment in operable breast cancer: the ALMANAC Trial. *J Natl Cancer Inst.* 2006;98:599-609.

43. Ranieri JM, Wagner JD, Wenck S, et al. The prognostic importance of sentinel lymph node biopsy in thin melanoma. *Ann Surg Oncol.* 2006;13(7):927-932.

44. Nguyen DX, Massague J. Genetic determinants of cancer metastases. *Nat Rev Genet.* 2007;8:341-352.

45. Chiang AC, Massague J. Molecular basis of metastasis. *N Engl J Med.* 2008;359(26):2814-2823.

46. Ring BZ, Ross DT. Predicting the sites of metastases. *Genome Biol.* 2005;6:241-244.

47. Andre F, Cabioglu N, Assi H, et al. Expression of chemokine receptors predicts the site of metastatic relapse in patients with axillary node positive primary breast cancer. *Ann Oncol.* 2006;17:945-951.

48. O'Shaughnessy JA. Molecular signatures predict outcomes of breast cancer. *N Engl J Med.* 2006;355(6):615-617.

49. Perou CM, Sørlie T, Eisen MB, et al. Molecular portraits of human breast tumors. *Nature.* 2000;406:747-752.

50. Sotiriou C, Pusztai L. Gene-expression signatures in breast cancer. *N Engl J Med.* 2009;360(8):790-800.

51. Mook S, Van't Veer LJ, Rutgers EJ, et al. Individualization of therapy using Mammaprint: from development to the MINDACT trial. *Cancer Genom Proteomics.* 2007;4(3):147-155.

52. Cardosa F, Van't Veer L, Rutgers E, Loi S, Mook S, Piccart-Gebhart MJ. Clinical application of the 70-gene profile: the MINDACT trial. *J Clin Oncol.* 2008;26:729-735.

53. Liu R, Wang X, Chen GY, et al. The prognostic role of gene signature from tumorigenic breast cancer cells. *N Engl J Med.* 2007;356(3):217-229.

54. Massague J. Sorting out breast-cancer gene signatures. *N Engl J Med.* 2007;356(3):294-297.

55. Negrini M, Calin GA. Breast cancer metastases: a microRNA story. *Breast Cancer Res.* 2008;10:303-307.

56. Vasudevan S, Tong Y, Steitz JA. Switching from repression to activation: microRNAs can up-regulate translation. *Science.* 2007;318:1931-1934.

57. Zaidi SK, Young DW, Javed A, et al. Nuclear microenvironments in biological control and cancer. *Nat Rev Cancer.* 2007;7:454-463.

58. Yoo CB, Jones PA. Epigenetic therapy of cancer: past, present and future. *Nat Rev Drug Discov.* 2006;5:37-50.

59. Marks PA, Rifkind RA, Richon VM, Breslow R, Miller T, Kelly WK. Histone deacetylases and cancer: causes and therapies. *Nat Rev Cancer.* 2001;1:194-202.

60. Richon VM, Sandhoff TW, Rifkind RA, Marks PA. Histone deacetylase inhibitor selectively induces p21WAF1 expression and gene-associated histone acetylation. *Proc Natl Acad Sci USA.* 2000;97:10014-10019.

61. Ehrlich M. DNA methylation in cancer: too much, but also too little. *Oncogene.* 2002;21(35): 5400-5413.

62. Esteller M. Cancer epigenomics: DNA methylation and histone modification maps. *Nat Rev Genet.* 2007;8:286-298.

63. Lin JC, Jeong S, Liang G, et al. Role of nuceosomal occupancy in the epigenetic silencing of the MLH1 CpG island. *Cancer Cell.* 2007;12:432-444.

64. Estécio MR, Gharibyan V, Shen L, et al. LINE-1 hypomethylation in cancer is highly variable and inversely correlated with microsatellite instability. *PLoS ONE.* 2007;2(5):e399. doi:10.1371 /journal.pone.0000399.

65. Larson PS, Schlechter BL, King C-L, et al. CDKN1C/p57[kip2] is a candidate tumor suppressor gene in human breast cancer. *BMC Cancer.* 2008;8:68.

66. Hedborg F, Igkssib R, Sandstedt B, Grimelius L, Hoehner JC, Pählman S. IGF2 expression is a marker for paraganglionic/SIF cell differentiation in neuroblastoma. *Am J Pathol.* 1995;146(4): 833-847.

67. Shay JW, Wright WE. Telomerase therapeutics for cancer: challenges and new directions. *Nat Rev Drug Discov.* 2006;5:577-584.

68. Blasco MA. The epigenetic regulation of mammalian telomeres. *Nat Rev Genet.* 2007;8:299-309.

69. Vera E, Canela A, Fraga MF, Esteller M, Blasco MA. Epigenetic regulation of telomeres in human cancer. *Oncogene.* 2008;27:6817-6833.

CHAPTER 2

Targeted Cancer Therapy: External and Internal Signaling Pathway Targets

Significant advances in cancer treatment have resulted from our improved understanding of the processes of malignant transformation and metastasis. The first targeted agent was tamoxifen (Nolvadex), which was approved by the Food and Drug Administration (FDA) in 1977 for the treatment of hormonally sensitive advanced breast cancer.[1] This drug was followed in 1997 by the monoclonal antibody (MAb) rituximab (Rituxan) for the treatment of lymphoma. Within the last decade, there has been a surge in the identification of cancer targets, and many drugs have been FDA approved. However, there are thousands of agents still being developed and tested, many of which are now in clinical trials; thus, the numbers will greatly increase. As more is learned about malignant transformation and metastasis, more targets and corresponding agents will be added to our armamentarium. We now know that cancer is a disease of the cell, the genes within a cell, and the networks within the cell. In addition, there are parallel studies in the best way to deploy these agents, such as intravenously (IV), orally (PO), or via nanoparticles.

Considering that proteins control all biologic processes, understanding their function can be daunting. Adjei and Hidalgo describe the amazingly complex, redundant communication pathways that tell cells what to do and that then, within the cell, carry out these instructions.[2] Outside the cell, cytokines, growth factors, and hormones are the bosses, acting as ligands that bind to their target receptors on the outside membrane of the cell. These molecules control cell proliferation, differentiation (once they differentiate, they cannot divide anymore), building of new blood vessels to feed the growing cells (angiogenesis), and cell death (apoptosis) or inactivity (senescence).[2] Once the growth factor or ligand binds to the receptor tyrosine kinase (RTK) on the outside of the cell, it sends the message to its key group of worker proteins in the cell—the tyrosine kinases or enzymes—which add a phosphate group (phosphorylate) to keep sending the message downstream toward the cell nucleus. Just like people, these proteins in the pathway need to talk to others outside their pathway team, and there is crosstalk among proteins in different pathways. Most astounding though, there are redundant pathways, so that if one pathway is blocked, another pathway emerges to take over signaling to carry the message to the nucleus. While this system is miraculous in human life, it is challenging to control and eradicate cancer that has developed. Flaws can occur in ligands, protein receptor kinases on

39

the outside of the cell, inner tyrosine kinases, or any of the secondary messenger protein kinases; or they can occur at the level of the gene, such as in the transcription and reading of the message. Thus, attractive targets appear at every level of communication.

Ma and Adjei suggest that one way to conceptualize the wide range of new biologic targets is to look at them by virtue of what they are and how they work[3]:

- Membrane-bound receptor kinases (e.g., human epidermal growth factor receptor [EGFR], human epidermal growth factor receptor-2 [HER2], hepatocyte growth factor [HGF/c-Met], insulin-like growth factor receptor [IGFR] pathways)
- Intracellular signaling kinases (e.g., src, P13k/Akt/mTOR, mitogen-activated protein kinase [MAPK], sonic hedgehog pathways)
- Epigenetic abnormalities (e.g., DNA methyltransferase, histone deacetylase [HDAC])
- Protein dynamics (e.g., heat shock protein [HSP]-90, ubiquitin–proteasome system)
- Tumor vasculature and microenvironment (e.g., angiogenesis with VEGF inhibitors and VEGFR inhibitors, hypoxia-inducible factor [HIF], endothelium such as vascular disrupting agents, integrins)

Figure 2-1 depicts the cellular signaling pathways involved in tumor cell proliferation, angiogenesis, and differentiation that are active targets for investigational or approved therapies. These include the membrane-bound EGFR, c-Met, and IGF-1 receptor (IGF-1R), which bring growth (mitogenic) signals from extracellular ligands, such as epidermal growth factor (EGF), HGF, and IGF, respectively, into the cell. The Ras/Raf/MEK/Erk (MAPK) and PI3k/Akt/mTOR pathways are major intracellular pathways that regulate many important signaling pathways within the cell. DNA methyltransferases (DNMTs) and HDACs are "epigenetic switches" that can influence or modulate the expression of oncogenes and tumor suppressor genes. The agents targeting the signaling proteins are indicated in boxes.

This chapter will review these agents in an outline format. Tumor vasculature and microenvironment will be discussed in Chapters 3 and 4, respectively.

Alternatively, the targets could be organized based on whether they are genetic or epigenetic and whether they are *growth-promoting pathways* such as EGFR/Ras/phosphatidylinositol 3-kinase (PI3K), *growth-inhibitory pathways* such as p53/Rb/P14^{ARF}, *apoptotic pathways* such as Bcl-2/Bax/Fas/FasL, and *DNA repair* and *immortalization genes*. The epigenetic pathways involve the modification of chromatin structures so that specific genes are expressed or not: *DNA methylation, histone and chromatin protein modification*, and *micro-RNA*.[4]

Today, only a fraction of the agents shown in Figure 2-1 are FDA approved. Agents that can be administered parenterally include MAbs (large molecules),

Figure 2-1   Novel targeted agents, and key signaling pathways to target.

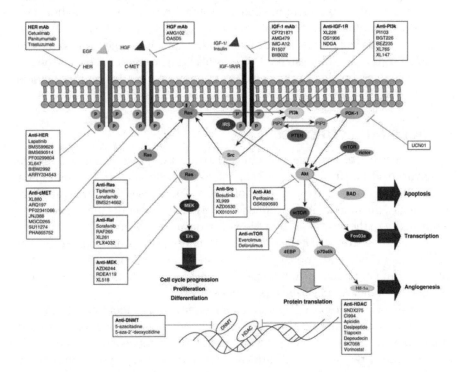

Courtesy of the publisher. Ma and Adjei.[3]

mammalian target of rapamycin (mTOR) inhibitors, demethylating agents, HDAC inhibitors; agents administered orally include small molecule tyrosine kinase inhibitors and protein kinase inhibitors. Anti-angiogenic agents will be discussed in Chapter 3. The end of this chapter addresses some of the pathways that are gaining great interest as promising targets: the HGF/c-Met pathway, the IGF pathway, the P13 signaling pathway, the sonic hedgehog (SHH) pathway, epigenetic approaches, and protein dynamics. Because these agents are different from those of chemotherapy, their toxicity raises new challenges for nurses and their patients and families. In addition, especially with the oral agents, it raises the challenge of prolonged adherence to oral therapy. Each of these classes of agents will be more fully discussed, along with currently FDA-approved drugs and selected investigational agents. The final chapters will discuss the challenges of adherence to oral agents, as well as drug interactions in the P450 microenzyme system.

The two main types of targeted therapy are MAbs and small molecule, oral, protein kinase inhibitors. The MAbs are able to bind specifically to their molecular target, most commonly membrane-bound receptors, and prevent ligand binding.

Because they are large molecules, they need to be administered IV. In addition, MAbs bring with them their ability to stimulate the immune system to kill the targeted cell, such as complement-mediated cytotoxicity, immune modulation, and in some cases, antibody-dependent cellular cytotoxicity (ADCC).[5] Small molecule protein kinase inhibitors on the other hand, are small enough to cross the cell membrane and can be administered PO. They also can be multitargeted and attack targets inside and outside of the cell (e.g., membrane-bound receptors outside the cell), as well as targets within the same family or class of protein kinases.[3]

MONOCLONAL ANTIBODIES

Because these drugs are large molecules, they must be given IV. They are made from hybridization (from a single cell, called a hybridoma) and recombinant DNA techniques to reduce the amount of murine (or mouse) protein in the MAb. Theoretically, the more human protein in the MAb, the lower the incidence of hypersensitivity to the mouse protein. However, during the process of humanizing the MAb, binding strength of the original MAb may be compromised.[6] MAbs can be all human (100%), all mouse (100% murine), some mouse (chimeric, 33% mouse), or mostly human (humanized, 10% mouse). Table 2-1 describes how the name of each MAb describes its composition.

All of the MAbs prepared against a single antigen are identical. The other important difference among MAbs is the immunoglobulin G (IgG) isotype used to make the MAb. IgG_1 MAbs have a potent ability to induce ADCC; once the Y portion of the MAb binds to the antigen like a "lock and key," the stem of the Y portion, the Fc portion, binds to immune effector cells such as natural killer

Table 2-1   Understanding Monoclonal Antibody Names (Example Trastuzumab)

Part of Name	Explanation
Syllable 1	Name unique to the product (e.g., tras)
Syllable 2	Target (e.g., tumor = tu)
Syllable 3	Source: o = mouse u = human i = chimeric (mouse and human)
Syllable 4	(e.g., mab = monoclonal antibody)
X and Z	Consonants to link syllables (tras-tu-z-u-mab)

Table 2-2 Relative Immunostimulatory Effects of Selected MAbs

	IgG_1	IgG_2	IgG_3	IgG_3
In vivo serum half-life	23 days	23 days	8 days	23 days
Function	Bind and activate host response	Bind with weak activation of host response	Bind and activate host response	Bind antigen
Complement activation	+	+/−	++	−
ADCC	++	+/−	++	+
Examples	cetuximab, rituximab, trastuzumab, bevacizumab	panitumumab	None, as half-life is too short	gemtuzumab ozogamicin (Mylotarg)

Note: + indicates positive immunostimulatory effect. The more + signs, the more powerful the immunostimulatory effect. − indicates absence of immunostimulatory effect.

Data from Adams and Weiner.[7,8]

(NK) cells, which can kill the cancer cells. In addition, MAbs can induce complement activation, which coats the antigen in complement so that it can effectively kill it, and theoretically can cause apoptosis of the antigen-bound cell just by binding to it. See Table 2-2 for relative immunostimulatory effects of anticancer MAbs. See Figures 2-2 and 2-3 for descriptions of MAb structure.

MAb therapy can cause hypersensitivity reactions and infusion reactions called cytokine release syndrome. Table 2-3 presents the National Cancer Institute (NCI) Common Toxicity Criteria of Adverse Events (CTCAE) of both these reactions. Although the cause may be different, the therapeutic intervention is similar.

Assessment of patients with hypersensitivity, anaphylactoid, and acute infusion reactions reveals similar findings. With a hypersensitivity reaction, a patient becomes sensitized to the antigen after the first exposure and makes immunoglobulin E (IgE) antibodies against the antigen. Upon the second exposure, the antigen binds to IgE, which is attached to previously sensitized basophils and mast cells, causing them to rupture and release histamine, leukotrienes, prostaglandins, and other substances.[10] Anaphylactoid reactions

Figure 2-2   Monoclonal antibody formation.

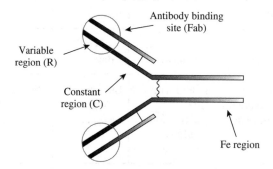

Barton Burke M, Wilkes GM. *Cancer Therapies*. Sudbury, MA: Jones and Bartlett; 2006:208.

Figure 2-3   Types of MAbs depend upon whether the antibody is made from human, mouse (murine), or both types of protein.

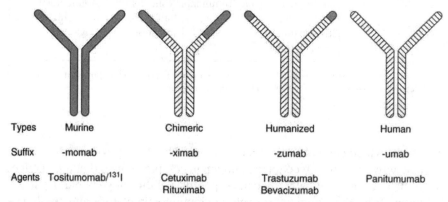

Types	Murine	Chimeric	Humanized	Human
Suffix	-momab	-ximab	-zumab	-umab
Agents	Tositumomab/^{131}I	Cetuximab Rituximab	Trastuzumab Bevacizumab	Panitumumab

A monoclonal antibody comes from a single clone of specially made MAbs. It is an immunoglobin that has an IgG backbone that binds to a specific antigen like a "lock and key" at the Fab region; this stimulates the immune system to attack the antigen at the Fc portion. It is considered a "Magic bullet" because MAbs target a single antigen. The MAb name ends in "mab."

Data from Brekke OH, Sandlie I. Therapeutic antibodies for human diseases at the dawn of the twenty-first century. *Nat Rev Drug Discov*. 2003;2(1):52-62.

occur upon first exposure to an antigen and are not IgE (immune) mediated. The antigen binds to the surface of the mast cells and basophils, causing them to rupture and to release inflammatory mediators (histamine, leukotrienes, prostaglandins), triggering the same signs and symptoms as occurs with true anaphylaxis. In contrast, the cytokine release syndrome occurs when administering an MAb and is related to the destruction of cells that release cytokines.

Table 2-3 National Cancer Institute (NCI) Common Toxicity Criteria of Adverse Events (CTCAE) for Hypersensitivity and Acute Infusion Reaction

Reaction	Grade 1	Grade 2	Grade 3	Grade 4	Grade 5
Hypersensitivity	Transient flushing, drug fever < 100.4°F (38°C)	Rash, flushing, urticaria, dyspnea, drug fever > 100.4°F (38°C)	Symptomatic bronchospasm +/– urticaria requiring IV meds, allergy-related edema, angioedema, hypotension	Anaphylaxis	Death
Acute infusion reaction (cytokine release syndrome)	Mild reaction; infusion interruption not indicated; intervention not indicated	Requires therapy or infusion interruption but responds promptly to symptomatic treatment (e.g., antihistamines, NSAIDs, opioids, IV fluids); prophylactic meds indicated for ≤ 24 hrs	Prolonged (i.e., not rapidly responsive to symptomatic meds and/or brief interruption of infusion) or recurrence of symptoms following initial improvement; hospitalization indicated for other clinical sequelae (e.g., renal impairment, pulmonary infiltrates)	Life-threatening reaction; pressor or ventilator support indicated	Death

Modified from NCI.[9]

These cytokines cause a systemic inflammatory response, with fever, hypotension, and rigors. If very severe, it is called a cytokine storm and may involve pulmonary edema.

Signs and symptoms of anaphylactoid or anaphylactic reactions include:

- Rapid onset of increased secretions from mucous membranes, leading to *increased pulmonary secretions* and *airway edema*
- Increased gastrointestinal (GI) secretions, leading to *nausea, vomiting, and diarrhea*
- Increased bronchial smooth muscle tone, leading to *stridor, wheezing, bronchospasm, laryngeal edema*, and *airway compromise*
- Decreased vascular smooth muscle tone, leading to *hypotension*
- Increased capillary permeability, leading to *hypotension*
- *Urticaria* and *pruritus* in the skin from histamine release
- Direct effects on the heart, causing *arrhythmias*

Symptoms usually appear within a few minutes up to 30–60 minutes.

Sampson et al. suggest that a diagnosis of anaphylaxis can be made if one of these three criteria are met[11]:

- Acute onset of illness affecting skin or mucosal tissue (e.g., hives, pruritus, flushing, swelling) together with dyspnea, bronchospasm, stridor, decreased pulmonary expiratory flow, hypoxia *or* hypotension, syncope, and other associated symptoms
- Rapid occurrence of two of the following after apparent drug exposure: skin/mucosal involvement in hives, pruritus/flush, swelling of lips/tongue/uvula; *or* compromised pulmonary function (e.g., dyspnea, bronchospasm, stridor, hypoxia); *or* hypotension with collapse, syncope, incontinence; *or* GI symptoms (e.g., abdominal pain, vomiting)
- Hypotension following exposure to a known allergen (occurring in minutes to hours), with systolic blood pressure (BP) < 90 mm Hg or a decrease of > 30% from baseline BP

Scarlet and Lenz identify the following signs and symptoms of an acute infusion reaction[12,13]:

- Neurologic: dizziness, headache, weakness, syncope, seizure
- Psychological: anxiety, feeling of "impending doom"
- Pulmonary: nasal congestion, rhinitis, sneezing, cough, dyspnea, oropharyngeal or laryngeal edema, bronchospasm, tachypnea, cyanosis, respiratory arrest
- Cardiovascular: tachycardia, hypotension, hypertension, arrhythmia, chest pain, ischemia or infarction, cardiac arrest
- Cutaneous: flushing, erythema, pruritus, urticaria, hives, angioedema, maculopapular rash, desquamation

- GI: nausea, vomiting, cramping, diarrhea
- Other: drug fever, rigors, chills, arthralgia, myalgia, flu-like symptoms

Key Points for Management

Non–life-threatening reactions can usually be managed by diphenhydramine 50 mg IV (for adults), acetaminophen, and, if needed, corticosteroid administration. Epinephrine may be needed if the patient is initially hypotensive and does not respond to fluid resuscitation (0.2–0.5 mL of a 1:1000 dilution, or 0.2–0.5 mg, given intramuscularly [IM] or subcutaneously [SQ], which can be repeated every 5 minutes as needed up to a 1-mg total dose). Most reactions resolve in 30 minutes to 2 hours after the infusion is stopped, and a steroid and antihistamine are administered.[14] Often the drug can be resumed at a slower (50%) infusion rate.

Life-threatening anaphylaxis requires deliberate planning. The nurse first stops the offending drug, then assesses the patient's airway, breathing, and circulation, as well as level of consciousness, which might indicate hypoxia. A code-cart should be readily available, along with IV bag, tubing, and supplies. The physician should be notified, and the patient's vital signs should be monitored closely. The patient should be in a recumbent position, or Trendelenburg if very hypotensive. The original IV tubing containing the drug should be changed so that 0.9% normal saline with new tubing is hung. If the patient is hypotensive, IV hydration should begin, and fluid should be administered as 1–2 liters at 5–10 mL/kg in the first 5 minutes.[10] Oxygen should be administered as needed if the patient is hypoxic or is desaturating based on oxygen saturation monitoring. If the patient does not respond to fluid resuscitation, or is profoundly hypotensive, 0.2–0.5 mL (1:1000 dilution) of epinephrine should be given IM (preferred) or SQ. This may be repeated every 10–15 minutes up to 1 mg/dose. If indicated, IV epinephrine can be given, but at a 1:10,000 dilution (10 μg/mL) or 1:100,000 dilution (1 μg/mL) at an initial rate of 1 μg/min, which can be increased to 2–10 μg/min.[14] Bronchodilators may be necessary if bronchospasm occurs, and an aerosolized beta-agonist such as nebulized albuterol 2.5–5 mg in 3 mL of saline may suffice. If the patient is receiving a beta-blocker, the response to epinephrine may be blunted. Administration of 1–5 mg of glucagon IV over 5 minutes, followed by a drip at 5–15 μg/min, may help the patient respond to the epinephrine. Corticosteroids are important adjuncts to prevent protracted or recurrent symptoms of anaphylaxis, such as methylprednisolone 0.5 mg/kg IV every 6 hours.[14]

MAbs can be naked, meaning they are unconjugated, and can kill cancer cells by first attaching to the cancer cell antigen, then (1) stimulating the immune system to kill the cell using complement-dependent cytotoxicity, (2) stimulating ADCC, or (3) interfering with the cell's complex signaling cascade, causing the cell to undergo apoptosis. MAbs can also be conjugated (attached) to a chemotherapy agent, such as gemtuzumab ozogamicin (Mylotarg), which brings the chemotherapy to the cell, where it is internalized and kills the cell. Or MAbs may be conjugated to a radioactive nucleotide, such as iodine-131 (^{131}I) tositumomab (Bexxar), which brings ^{131}I to the cell, thus killing the cell from a tiny, but lethal radiation dose. These agents are targeted, such as against a CD (cluster of differentiation) antigen on lymphocytes.

Drug: Alemtuzumab (Campath-1H, anti-CD52)

Indications: As a single agent, for the treatment of B-cell chronic lymphocytic leukemia (CLL)

Class: Humanized MAb directed against CD52

Mechanism of Action: Humanized MAb that targets the CD52 antigen present on the surface of most normal human lymphocyte cells, as well as malignant T-cell and B-cell malignant lymphocytes (lymphomas). Once the MAb binds with the CD52 antigen, it initiates ADCC and complement binding, which then lead to apoptosis and activation of normal T-cell cytotoxicity against the malignant cells. CD52 antigen is also present on a majority of monocytes, macrophages, NK cells, and a subpopulation of granulocytes, which explains the drug's potent immunosuppression during treatment and for 12 months afterward.

Pharmacokinetics: When given SQ or IV, pharmacokinetics appears similar, but the absorption is much slower with SQ administration. It takes a higher cumulative dose (an additional 6 weeks) to achieve a therapeutic level. The mean half-life is 11 hours after the first 30-mg dose, but steady-state plasma levels are not reached until week 6. Levels appear to correlate with the number of circulating CD52-positive cells. Drug clearance decreases with repeated dosing, as more leukemic cells are killed. Given SQ, CLL cells are cleared from the blood in 95% of patients in a median time of 21 days.[15] Host antibodies may develop 14–21 days after the first dose and theoretically can decrease lymphocyte killing.

Dosage and Administration:
- Premedicate with diphenhydramine 50 mg and acetaminophen 500–1000 mg 30 minutes prior to first infusion and each dose escalation.
- Administer trimethoprim/sulfamethoxazole DS twice daily, three times per week to prevent *Pneumocystis jiroveci* or *Pneumocystis carinii pneumonia* (PCP); continue for a minimum of 2 months after completion of therapy, or until CD+ count is ≥ 200 cells/μL, whichever occurs later.
- Administer famciclovir 250 mg twice daily or equivalent to prevent herpes infection; continue for a minimum of 2 months after completion of therapy, or until CD+ count is ≥ 200 cells/μL, whichever occurs later.
- Initial dose is 3-mg IV infusion over 2 hours, daily, with dose escalated to 10 mg daily when well tolerated (side effects are grade 2 or less).
- When dose of 10 mg is well tolerated, the dose is increased to 30 mg and becomes the maintenance dose given three times a week (e.g., Monday,

Wednesday, and Friday) for up to 12 weeks. Dose escalation to 30 mg usually takes 3–7 days.
- Dose modifications:
  - Withhold drug during serious infection or other serious adverse reactions until resolved.
  - Discontinue drug for autoimmune anemia or autoimmune thrombocytopenia.
  - If absolute neutrophil count (ANC) < 250 cells/μL and/or platelets ≤ 25,000 cells/μL:
    - 1st occurrence: Withhold drug and resume at 30 mg when ANC ≥ 500 cells/μL and platelet count ≥ 50,000 cells/μL.
    - 2nd occurrence: Withhold drug and resume at 10 mg when ANC ≥ 500 cells/μL and platelet count ≥ 50,000 cells/μL.
    - 3rd occurrence: Discontinue drug.
  - If ≥ 50% decrease from baseline in patients who started therapy with a baseline of ANC ≤ 250 cells/μL, and/or platelets ≤ 25,000 cells/μL:
    - First occurrence: Withhold drug and resume at 30 mg when counts return to baseline.
    - Second occurrence: Withhold drug and resume at 10 mg when counts return to baseline.
    - Third occurrence: Discontinue drug.
- SQ administration is better tolerated and results in similar efficacy.[15]
- Drug administration:
  1. Administer as an IV infusion over 2 hours. Do NOT give as IVP or IV bolus. Observe patient for infusion reactions.
  2. Escalate to recommended dose of 30 mg/day three times per week for 12 weeks.
  3. Premedicate with oral antihistamine and acetaminophen prior to dosing.
- Use personal protective equipment (PPE) when handling or administering drug.

Available as: 30 mg/1 mL single-use vial

Reconstitution and Preparation:
- Do not shake vial.
- Available in single-use vials containing 30-mg alemtuzumab in 1 mL of diluent.
- Draw up ordered dose, and use precise syringe. For a 3-mg dose, draw up 0.1 mL in a 1-mL syringe calibrated in 0.01 increments; for a 10-mg dose, withdraw 0.33 mL. For the 30-mg dose, withdraw 1.0 mL and dilute in 100 mL sterile 0.9% sodium chloride USP or 5% dextrose in water.
- Gently invert IV bag to mix. Use within 8 hours. Store at room temperature or refrigerated, and protect from light.

- Incompatible with polyvinylchloride IV bags (PVC) and PVC- or polyethylene-lined PVC administration sets. Do not administer any other drugs or add any drugs to the IV line.

Drug Interactions: Unknown

Black Box Warnings: Serious reactions, including fatal cytopenias, infusion reactions, and infections, can occur.
- Limit doses to 30 mg (single) and 90 mg (cumulative weekly); higher doses increase risk of pancytopenia.
- Escalate dose gradually, and monitor patients during infusion. Withhold therapy for grade 3 or 4 infusion reactions.
- Administer prophylaxis against *Pneumocystis jiroveci* or PCP and herpes virus infections.

Contraindications: None

Warnings and Precautions:
Cytopenias:
- Obtain complete blood counts (CBC) and platelet counts at weekly intervals during therapy and CD4 counts after therapy until recovery to ≥ 200 cells/μL.
- Discontinue for autoimmune or severe hematologic adverse reactions, as drug can cause hemolytic anemia, pure red cell aplasia, bone marrow aplasia, and hypoplasia. DO NOT exceed 30-mg dose or cumulative weekly doses greater than 90 mg per week, as this increases risk of cytopenias.

Infections:
- Campath induces severe and prolonged lymphopenia and increases risk of opportunistic infection. Administer PCP and herpes prophylaxis for a minimum of 2 months after drug therapy is completed, or until the CD4+ count is ≥ 200 cells/μL, whichever occurs later. In patients receiving alemtuzumab as initial therapy, recovery of CD4+ counts to ≥ 200 cells/μL occurred by 6 months posttreatment; at 2 months posttreatment, the median was 183 cells/μL, compared to ≥ 200 cells/μL in patients who had been previously treated. It may take more than 12 months for full recovery of CD4+ and CD8+ cells.
- Routinely monitor patients for cytomegalovirus (CMV) infection during treatment and for at least 2 months following completion of therapy. The incidence during clinical trials was 16% of previously untreated patients. Withhold alemtuzumab for serious infections and during antiviral treatment for CMV infection or confirmed CMV viremia. Administer therapeutic ganciclovir for confirmed CMV infection or viremia.
- Administer only irradiated blood products to avoid transfusion-associated graft versus host disease (TAGVHD).
- If a serious infection occurs, withhold treatment until infection resolves.

- Do not administer live viral vaccines (e.g., bacilllus Calmette-Guérin, measles, mumps, oral polio, rubella, varicella, yellow fever) to patients who have recently received Campath.

Infusion reactions:

- Can occur during or shortly after drug administration. Symptoms include fever, chills/rigors, nausea, hypotension, urticaria, dyspnea, rash, emesis, bronchospasm. Incidence is highest in the first week of treatment. Stop drug if signs and symptoms appear. Stop and hold drug if grade 3 or 4 infusion reactions occur.
- Additional symptoms that have occurred include syncope, pulmonary infiltrates, acute respiratory distress syndrome (ARDS), respiratory arrest, angioedema, anaphylactic shock.

Pregnancy: It is not known if the drug is fetotoxic. Women of childbearing age should avoid pregnancy by using effective contraception. If the woman becomes pregnant, the risks and benefits should be weighed, and treatment continued only if needed.

Avoid breastfeeding, as IgG antibodies are excreted in human milk. Discontinue nursing or the drug.

Adverse Reactions (**bold** indicates most common, occurring in > 25% of patients):

Cardiovascular: **Hypotension,** peripheral edema, hypertension, supraventricular tachycardia; rare congestive heart failure (CHF), cardiomyopathy, decreased left ventricular ejection fraction (LVEF)

Pulmonary: **Dyspnea, cough,** bronchitis, pneumonitis, pneumonia, pharyngitis, bronchospasm, rhinitis

Central nervous system (CNS)/neurologic: Insomnia, headache, dysesthesias, asthenia, dizziness, malaise, depression, tremor, somnolence, rare optic neuropathy

Dermatologic: Urticarial rash

Metabolic: Tumor lysis syndrome (TLS)

GI: **Nausea, vomiting, diarrhea,** anorexia, mucositis, abdominal pain, dyspepsia, constipation

Hematologic: **Neutropenia, thrombocytopenia, anemia,** rare aplastic anemia, fatal TAGVHD, fatal pancytopenia, marrow hypoplasia

Immune system: **Infections despite prophylaxis, CMV infection, other infections,** rare Goodpasture syndrome, Graves disease, Guillain-Barré syndrome, chronic inflammatory demyelinating polyradiculoneuropathy, serum sickness

Musculoskeletal: Skeletal pain, myalgias, back pain, chest pain

General: **Infusion reactions, rigors, fever, fatigue,** rare anaphylaxis

Nursing Discussion:

Increased risk for infusion reactions: Infusion reactions are common and require premedication to prevent. Hypotension occurs in 15%, rash in 30%, nausea in 47%, vomiting in 33%, drug-related fever in 83%, and rigors in 89% of patients. Infusion reactions usually resolve after 1 week of therapy. Subcutaneous dosing significantly reduces the risk of allergic reactions. Assess vital signs baseline and frequently during infusion, especially during dose escalation. Teach patient that reactions may occur and to tell the nurse or physician immediately. Administer premedication as ordered, usually acetaminophen and diphenhydramine. Provide adequate hydration (e.g., at least 500 mL before and after dose), as this seems to decrease the incidence of infusion reactions. Dose is begun low at 3 mg, then gradually increased based on patient tolerance to a 10-mg dose, then to a 30-mg dose. If the patient has a treatment break of 7 days or more, then it is necessary to reintroduce drug at the lower dose and gradually escalate. If reaction happens, stop infusion but keep main IV line open, notify physician, and, if rigors occur, give meperidine and any other medications ordered by physician. Expect the reaction to resolve in 20 minutes or so, and gradually resume infusion per physician order. Assess skin for integrity and presence of rash. Teach patient to report rash, and discuss management with physician. Teach patient that nausea may develop and to report it right away. Discuss antiemetic agent with physician, and administer as ordered.

Increased risk for infection, bleeding, and fatigue related to pancytopenia: All patients develop leukopenia, with approximately 85% developing *neutropenia* and 42% developing grade 3 or 4. Median time to onset is 31 days, with a median duration of 37 days. There is a dramatic fall in white blood cells (WBCs) during the first week. Because both T- and B-cell lymphocytes are destroyed, patients are at an increased risk for bacterial, viral, and other opportunistic infections. Most patients require prophylactic antimicrobials with/without antiviral therapy, especially heavily pretreated patients. Most common pulmonary infections are opportunistic: PCP, CMV pneumonia, and pulmonary aspergillosis. Commonly, there is reactivation of herpes simplex infections and development of oral candidiasis. *Thrombocytopenia* affects 72%, with 14% developing grades 3 or 4. Median time to thrombocytopenia is 9 days, with a median duration of 14 days. Incidence of *anemia* is 80%, with 12% grades 3 or 4. Median time to onset is 31 days, with a median duration of 8 days. Rarely, pancytopenia and marrow aplasia occur and may be fatal. The incidence of infections other than CMV is 50% in all patients. Assess baseline leukocyte, platelet, and Hgb/HCT and monitor before each treatment, during therapy, and more often as needed. Hold drug for ANC < 250/µL or platelets < 25,000/µL. See package insert for dose modifications. Baseline and prior to each treatment, assess risk for infection and integrity of skin and mucous membranes, pulmonary status, and ability to clear secretions, as well as history of past infections. Teach patient to self-administer prophylactic antibiotics, antiviral, and antifungal agents as ordered by physician. Ensure that patient has insurance or can purchase antimicrobial medications. Teach patient to self-administer oral antifungal agent if oral candidiasis develops. Teach patient to self-assess for signs/symptoms of infection, and to call the provider immediately or come to the emergency department if experiencing any of the following: temperature > 100.5°F and shaking chills, or rash, productive cough, burning during urination, or any signs/symptoms of infection or bleeding. Teach self-care strategies to minimize risk of infection and bleeding, including avoidance of over-the-counter (OTC) aspirin-containing medications.

Alteration in comfort related to pain, asthenia, headache, myalgia, dysesthesias: Pain is common. In clinical studies, 24% of patients experience skeletal pain, 13% asthenia, 13% peripheral edema, 10% back or chest pain, 9% malaise, 24% headache, 15% dysthesias, and 12% dizziness. Assess comfort and presence of peripheral edema, baseline and prior to each treatment. Teach patient that these side effects may occur and to report them. Teach patient local comfort measures, and discuss management plan with physician if ineffective.

Alteration in oxygenation (potential related to hypotension): Hypotension is common, affecting 32% of patients in clinical studies, while 11% had hypertension. Additionally, 11% of patients had sinus or supraventricular tachycardia. Assess baseline cardiac status, including BP and heart rate, noting rhythm and rate. Assess past medical history for arrhythmia and hypertension. If heart rate is irregular, document rhythm on electrocardiogram (ECG), monitor BP for evidence of decompensation, and discuss management with physician. If hypertension is noted, discuss management with physician. If hypotension is noted, assess patient tolerance and need for intervention; discuss management with physician.

Risk for TLS: Patients with a high tumor burden who are receiving their first treatment are at risk for TLS. Monitor baseline uric acid, renal function, and electrolytes. Ensure adequate hydration and urinary output, urinary alkalinization, and allopurinol to lower risk of hyperuricemia.

Drug: Rituximab (Rituxan)

Indications:
- Non-Hodgkin lymphoma (NHL): (1) relapsed or refractory, low-grade or follicular, CD20-positive, B-cell NHL; (2) previously untreated follicular, CD20-positive, B-cell NHL in combination with CVP chemotherapy; (3) Nonprogressing (including stable disease) low-grade, CD20-positive, B-cell NHL, as a single agent after first-line cyclophosphamide, vincristine, and prednisone (CVP) chemotherapy; (4) previously untreated diffuse large B-cell, CD20-positive NHL in combination with cyclophosphamide, doxorubicin, vincristine, and prednisone (CHOP) or other anthracycline-based chemotherapy regimens

- Rheumatoid arthritis (RA) in combination with methotrexate in adult patients with moderately to severely active RA who have inadequate response to one or more tumor necrosis factor (TNF) antagonist therapies

Class: Chimeric MAb directed against CD20

Mechanism of Action: Anti-CD20 antibody that is genetically engineered (chimeric) and directed against the CD20 antigen found on the surface of normal and malignant B-cell lymphocytes. The CD20 antigen is also present (expressed) on more than 90% of B-cell NHL cells but fortunately is not found on normal bone marrow stem cells, pre-B cells, normal plasma cells, or other normal tissues. A section of the rituximab (Fab domain) CD20 binds to the CD20 antigen on B lymphocytes; another section of the rituximab (Fc domain) calls together other immune effectors, resulting in lysis of the B lymphocyte.

Pharmacokinetics: Serum and half-life of the drug vary with dose and sequence; at 375 mg/m^2, the median serum half-life was 76.3 hours after the first infusion, as compared to 205 hours after the fourth infusion. Drug was detected in patient serum up to 3–6 months after completion of treatment.

Dosage and Administration:
- Premedicate prior to each infusion with acetaminophen and an antihistamine such as diphenhydramine.
- Relapsed or refractory, low-grade or follicular, CD20-positive, B-cell NHL: 375 mg/m^2 given as IV infusion weekly for 4 weeks or 8 doses.
- Retreatment for relapsed or refractory, low-grade, or follicular: 375 mg/m^2 once weekly for 4 doses. Diffuse large B-cell NHL in combination with CHOP chemotherapy.
- Previously untreated, follicular, CD20-positive, B-cell NHL: 375 mg/m^2 IV day 1 of each cycle of CVP chemotherapy for up to 8 infusions.
- Nonprogressing, low-grade, CD20-positive, B-cell NHL, after first-line CVP chemotherapy: Following completion of 6–8 cycles of CVP chemotherapy, administer 375 mg/m^2 once weekly for 4 doses at 6-month intervals to a maximum of 16 doses.
- Diffuse large B-cell NHL: Administer 375 mg/m^2 on day 1 of each cycle of chemotherapy for up to 8 infusions.
- RA in combination with methotrexate: two–1000 mg (NOT per meter squared) IV infusions separated by 2 weeks. Administer glucocorticoids (methylprednisolone 100 mg IV or equivalent) 30 minutes prior to each infusion to reduce incidence and severity of infusion reactions.
- As a component of Zevalin (ibritumomab tiuxetan) therapeutic regimen.
- Rituximab 250 mg/m^2 IV within 4 hours prior to the administration of indium-111 (^{111}In)-Zevalin, and within 4 hours prior to the administration of yttrium-90 (^{90}Y)-Zevalin.

- Rituximab and ^{111}In-Zevalin administration should precede rituximab and ^{90}Y-Zevalin by 7–9 days.

Available as: 100 mg/10 mL and 500 mg/50 mL solution in a single-use vial

Reconstitution and Preparation: Do not mix with or dilute with other drugs.
- Store at 2–8°C (36–46°F), and protect vials from direct sunlight.
- Aseptically, add ordered dose to 0.9% sodium chloride USP or 5% dextrose, resulting in a final concentration of 1–4 mg/mL; gently invert to mix, and inspect for presence of any particulate matter or discoloration.
- Drug is stable in infusion solution refrigerated at 2–8°C (36–46°F) for 24 hours, and, if refrigerated prior to being left at room temperature, for another 24 hours.

Administration: DO NOT GIVE AS AN INTRAVENOUS PUSH OR BOLUS.
- First infusion: Initial infusion rate should be 50 mg/hr; if no infusion-related problems occur, increase the infusion rate in 50 mg/hr increments every 30 minutes to a maximum of 400 mg/hr. If infusion reaction occurs, slow or stop the infusion depending on severity. May continue the infusion at half the previous rate once symptoms resolve.
- Second, third, and fourth infusions: If the patient tolerated the first infusion well, administer at initial rate of 100 mg/hr, and increase by 100-mg/hr increments every 30 minutes, to a maximum of 400 mg/hr as tolerated.
- RA patients: Administer glucocorticoids (methylprednisolone 100 mg IV or equivalent) 30 minutes prior to each infusion to reduce incidence and severity of infusion reactions.
- Fatal infusion reactions have rarely occurred within 24 hours of rituximab dose, characterized by hypoxemia, pulmonary infiltrates, ARDS, myocardial infarction (MI), ventricular fibrillation (VF), and shock.
- Drug has been associated with progressive leukoencephalopathy when used off-label in the treatment of patients with systemic lupus erythematosus (SLE).
- A rapid infusion of rituximab over 90 minutes, following demonstration of a safe first infusion, has been studied and shown to be safe. Of the dose, 20% is administered in the first 30 minutes, and the remaining 80% is administered over 60 minutes. In the study, 150 patients received the drug with corticosteroid-containing chemotherapy, and 56 patients received maintenance rituximab; no patient experienced grade 3 or 4 infusion reactions.[16] In an earlier study of 70 similar patients who received 319 rapid infusions with or without steroids, no patient had a grade 3 or 4 reaction, and only 3 patients developed grade 1 symptoms.[17]

Drug Interactions: There have been no formal drug interaction studies performed with rituximab. However, renal toxicity was seen with this drug in combination with cisplatin in clinical trials. Antihypertensive agents may potentiate hypotension if the patient experiences an infusion reaction.

Black Box Warnings: FATAL INFUSION REACTIONS, TLS, SEVERE MUCO-CUTANEOUS REACTIONS, and PROGRESSIVE MULTIFOCAL LEUKO-ENCEPHALOPATHY (PML)

- **Fatal infusion reactions** within 24 hours of Rituxan infusion can occur; approximately 80% of fatal reactions occurred with first infusion, with time of onset 30–120 minutes. Premedicate patients with acetaminophen and an antihistamine prior to starting the infusion. Monitor patients for signs and symptoms, including urticaria, hypotension, angioedema, hypoxia, bronchospasm, pulmonary infiltrates, ARDS, MI, VF, cardiogenic shock, or anaphylactic events. Stop the drug and institute medical management (glucocorticoids, epinephrine, bronchodilators, or oxygen) for infusion reactions as needed. If reaction is mild, and not severe, consider resuming infusion at a minimum 50% reduction of the infusion rate after symptoms have resolved. Discontinue rituximab infusion for severe reactions. Closely monitor patients with preexisting cardiac or pulmonary symptoms, those who experienced prior cardiopulmonary adverse reactions, and those with a high number of circulating malignant cells ($\geq 25,000/mm^3$), as the risk of cytokine release syndrome increases.
- **TLS** is a risk in patients with a sensitive, high tumor burden who have a rapid reduction in tumor volume leading to acute renal failure, hyperkalemia, hypocalcemia, hyperuricemia, or hyperphosphatemia, occurring 12–24 hours after the first infusion. Risk is increased in patients with a high circulating number of malignant cells ($\geq 25,000/mm^3$) or high tumor burden. Consider prophylaxis with allopurinol and aggressive hydration, correct electrolyte imbalances, monitor renal function and fluid balance, and give supportive care as needed, including dialysis.
- **Severe mucocutaneous reactions**, some with fatal outcomes (see Nursing Discussion section)
- PML resulting in death (see Nursing Discussion section)

Contraindications: None

Warnings:
- **TLS:** Administer prophylaxis and monitor renal function.
- **PML:** Monitor neurologic function. Discontinue rituximab.
- **Hepatitis B** reactivation with fulminant hepatitis: Sometimes fatal. Screen high-risk patients, and monitor hepatitis B virus carriers during and for several months after therapy. The median time to diagnosis of hepatitis is about 4 months after rituximab is started, and about 1 month

after the last dose. Discontinue rituximab and any concomitant chemotherapy in patients who develop viral hepatitis, and institute antiviral therapy. There are no safety data about resuming rituximab in these patients.

- **Other viral infections:** Serious viral infections can be exacerbated, reactivated, or initiated. Risk was highest for patients receiving rituximab in combination chemotherapy or as part of a stem cell transplant (SCT) program. Possible infections include CMV, herpes simplex virus (HSV), parvovirus B19, varicella zoster virus, West Nile virus, and hepatitis C. Infections can occur as late as 1 year after the discontinuation of rituximab, and some have reportedly caused death.

- **Cardiac arrhythmias** and angina can occur and can be life threatening. Monitor patients with, or with a history of, these conditions closely during and after all infusions. Discontinue infusions for serious or life-threatening cardiac arrhythmias.

- **Bowel obstruction and perforation:** Evaluate complaints of abdominal pain thoroughly, and institute appropriate treatment. Symptoms occurred with patients receiving rituximab plus chemotherapy early in the course of rituximab therapy. Mean time to documented GI perforation was 6 days (range 1–77 days) in patients with NHL.

- **Renal toxicity:** Severe, including possible fatal renal toxicity with rituximab administration to patients with hematologic malignances. Risk is increased in patients with high tumor burden ($\geq 25,000/\text{mm}^3$) or patients who experience TLS, and in patients with NHL who receive cisplatin together with rituximab in clinical trials (not approved). Consider discontinuing rituximab in patients with a rising serum creatinine or oliguria.

- **Do not administer live virus vaccines** prior to or during rituximab. For patients with RA receiving rituximab, review the vaccination status and follow Centers for Disease Control and Prevention guidelines for adult vaccination with non-live vaccines intended to prevent infectious disease prior to therapy. For patients with NHL, the benefits of a primary or booster vaccination should be weighed against the risks of delay in initiation of rituximab therapy.

- **Monitor CBC** at regular intervals for severe cytopenias. Rituximab binds to all CD20-positive B lymphocytes, both malignant and normal, so CBC and platelets should be assessed prior to each cycle and more frequently when cytopenias develop, which can extend for months after the treatment period.

- **RA patients:** (1) Concomitant use with biologic agents and disease-modifying antirheumatic drugs (DMARDs) other than methotrexate has not been well studied, except for the peripheral B-cell depletion following rituximab therapy. Observe patients closely for signs of infection if biologic agents and DMARDs are used together. (2) RA patients who have not had prior inadequate response to TNF antagonists should not receive rituximab, as effects have not been studied. (3) Retreatment in patients with RA: Safety and efficacy have not been well studied, but a limited number of patients have done so (2–5 courses, with 2 infusions per course; most received additional courses 24 weeks after the previous course, and none were treated sooner than 16 weeks).

Adverse Reactions (**bold** indicates most common, occurring in > 25% of patients):

Cardiovascular: Peripheral edema, hypotension, hypertension, rare arrhythmia, angina

Pulmonary: Increased cough, rhinitis, bronchospasm, dyspnea, sinusitis

CNS/neurologic: Dizziness, anxiety, rare PML

Dermatologic: Flushing, night sweats, rash, pruritus, urticaria, rare Stevens-Johnson syndrome, lichenoid dermatitis, toxic epidermal necrolysis, severe mucocutaneous reactions

Metabolic: Hyperglycemia, lactate dehydrogenase increase, TLS if not prevented in newly diagnosed patients

GI: Abdominal pain, throat irritation, nausea, diarrhea, vomiting, rare GI perforation, rare fulminant hepatitis, hepatic failure

Hematologic: **Lymphopenia**, leucopenia, neutropenia, thrombocytopenia, anemia

Immune system: **Infection**

Renal: TLS with renal failure if not prevented in patients receiving their first therapy

Musculoskeletal: Pain, myalgia, arthralgia

General: **Infusion reactions** (70% incidence first infusion: fever, chills/rigors, nausea, pruritus, angioedema, hypotension, headache, bronchospasm, urticaria, rash, vomiting, myalgia, dizziness, hypertension), fever, chills, asthenia

Nursing Discussion:

Risk for infusion reactions: Infusion-related reactions occur within 30 minutes to 2 hours of the beginning of the first infusion. Fever and chills/rigors affect most patients during the initial infusion. Other infusion-related symptoms include nausea, urticaria, fatigue, headache, pruritus, bronchospasm, dyspnea, sensation of swelling of tongue and throat, hypotension, flushing, and pain at disease site. Infusion-related reactions generally resolve by slowing or interrupting the drug infusion, and/or with symptomatic treatment (e.g., IV saline, acetaminophen, diphenhydramine). Premedications often reduce the severity and/or occurrence of these reactions. In patients who receive retreatment after having completed at least one course of drug therapy, reactions that were reported include fever, chills, asthenia, pruritus, and infusion-related events (i.e., fever, chills, pain, and throat irritation). The incidence of abdominal pain, anemia, dyspnea, hypotension, and neutropenia is higher in patients with bulky tumors > 10 cm. Discuss with physician or midlevel practitioner the use of premedications such as acetaminophen and an antihistamine before drug therapy. Ensure that medications necessary for the management of severe infusion reactions are readily available (e.g., epinephrine, antihistamines, corticosteroids). Assess baseline vital signs and monitor frequently during the infusion. Follow infusion rate guide (see Drug Administration section) for first and subsequent infusions. Slow or stop the infusion if severe infusion-related reactions occur. Monitor vital signs, and notify physician. Be prepared to provide emergency support as necessary (including IV saline, epinephrine, antihistamines, bronchodilators). If/when symptoms resolve, resume the infusion at 50% of the rate of the previous infusion, as directed by the physician.

Risk for TLS: Patients with high tumor burden receiving rituximab for the first time are at risk for rapid tumor lysis. TLS occurs as a result of rapid release of intracellular contents into the bloodstream. The risk of TLS appears higher in patients with a high number of circulating lymphocytes (e.g., > 25,000/mm^3). For first infusion, expect patient orders to include hydration at 150 mL/hr with or without alkalinization, oral allopurinol, strict monitoring of I/O, and daily weight and body balance determination. Monitor baseline and daily blood, urea, nitrogen (BUN), creatinine, K+, phosphorus, uric acid, and calcium. Monitor for renal, cardiac, and neuromuscular signs/symptoms; hyperkalemia; hyperphosphatemia; hypomagnesemia; hypocalcemia; and elevated uric acid.

Increased risk for infection related to bone marrow depression: B-cell lymphocytes are reduced in 70–80% of patients, together with a decrease in immunoglobulins in some patients. Bacterial infections that occurred in these patients were not associated with neutropenia, and 9% were severe, involving sepsis due to listeria, staphylococcus, and polymicrobials; posttreatment infections included rare sepsis and viral infections (herpes simplex and herpes zoster). Leukopenia occurs in 11% of patients, thrombocytopenia in 8%, and neutropenia in 7%. Serious bone marrow suppression was uncommon and may occur up to 30 days following treatment. Disorders include severe neutropenia, thrombocytopenia, and severe anemia. Rarely, transient aplastic anemia or hemolytic anemia may occur. Incidence of neutropenia, anemia, and abdominal pain was higher, as was the severity, in patients with bulky tumors > 10 cm. Monitor CBC and platelets baseline and regularly during treatment. If the patient develops cytopenia, monitor more frequently. Assess for signs/symptoms of infection, bleeding, fatigue, and chest pain prior to each treatment. Teach patient to self-assess for these, including taking temperature, and instruct to report them immediately. Transfuse red cells and platelets as ordered.

Risk for mucocutaneous reactions: Severe skin reactions have rarely occurred and, in some cases, ended in death of patient. Skin abnormalities include paraneoplastic pemphigus (uncommon autoimmune disorder, may be related to underlying malignancy), Stevens-Johnson syndrome (may be caused by HSV or other infectious disorder), lichenoid dermatitis, vesiculobullous dermatitis, and toxic epidermal necrolysis. Onset is 1–13 weeks following rituximab exposure. Assess baseline skin and mucous membrane integrity. Teach patient that rarely skin and mucous membrane reactions may occur, and to report any changes right away. Manufacturer recommends stopping rituximab therapy and obtaining skin biopsy to determine cause. Discuss with physician. Teach patient local care strategies depending upon symptoms.

Risk for PML: Although rare, PML may occur. It is a JC virus infection in an immunosuppressed patient. It occurs more frequently in patients receiving rituximab who have hematologic malignancies or autoimmune diseases. Risk is increased if patients are also receiving chemotherapy as part of a hematopoietic stem cell transplant (HSCT) program. PML was usually diagnosed within 12 months of the last rituximab dose. Assess patients for any changes in neurologic function, such as confusion, difficulty concentrating or doing tasks, or seizures. Discuss with physician evaluation of PML using brain magnetic resonance imaging (MRI) and referral to a neurologist or licensed practitioner. Rituximab should be discontinued during the workup, and consider discontinuance or a reduction in any concomitant chemotherapy or immunosuppressive therapy if the patient develops PML.

Drug: ^{90}Y-Ibritumomab Tiuxetan (Zevalin)

Indications: FDA indicated for the treatment of patients with relapsed or refractory low-grade, follicular, or transformed B-cell NHL, including patients refractory to rituximab

Class: Conjugated murine MAb, directed against CD20 B-cell lymphocytes, with chelated radioisotope ^{90}Y (yttrium-90)

Mechanism of Action: Ibritumomab tiuxetan is an MAb that targets the cell surface antigen CD20, which is found on the surface of normal and malignant B-cell lymphocytes. The CD20 antigen is also present (expressed) on more than 90% of B-cell NHL cells but fortunately is not found on normal bone marrow stem cells, pre-B cells, or other normal tissues. The complex is made up of a murine anti-CD20 MAb conjugated to the linker-chelator tiuxetan, which then securely chelates the radioisotope ^{90}Y. The complex attaches to the CD20 receptor, and the radioisotope then delivers high–beta-energy waves to the malignant cell, causing cell death. The isotope delivers high energy with a short half-life of 64 hours. It appears that if the malignant cells are pretreated with an anti-CD20 antibody (e.g., rituximab), this clears malignant and normal B lymphocytes from the blood, and ^{90}Y-ibritumomab tiuxetan is better able to target the lymphomatous B lymphocytes. ^{111}In-ibritumomab tiuxetan is used as an imaging and dosimetry agent so that an accurate and safe therapeutic dose can be determined.

Pharmacokinetics: ^{90}Y has a half-life of 64 hours and effective half-life in the blood of 28 hours; its median biologic half-life is 47 hours and median area under the curve (AUC) is 25 hours.

Dosage/Administration: There are two separate parts. The first dose is determination with ^{111}In (gamma emitter), which is used to determine biodistribution on day 1. This dose is followed by the therapeutic dose. Rituximab is given prior to the radionucleotide on both days to clear CD20 cells from the peripheral blood so that the tumors will take up the radiolabeled MAb.

- **Day 1:** Administer rituximab 250 mg/m^2 IV. Within 4 hours after rituximab infusion, administer 5 mCi ^{111}In-Zevalin IV.
- **Day 7, 8, or 9:**
  - Administer rituximab 250 mg/m^2 IV infusion.
  - If platelets $\geq$ 150,000/mm^3: Within 4 hours after rituximab infusion, administer 0.4 mCi/kg ^{90}Y-Zevalin IV.
  - If platelets 100,000–149,000/mm^3: Within 4 hours after rituximab infusion, administer 0.3 mCi/kg ^{90}Y-Zevalin IV.
- Each dose is validated by the radioactivity calibration system immediately before administration.[18]

Available as: 3.2 mg per 2 mL, single-use vial

Reconstitution and Preparation: See package insert. Must be prepared by a licensed radionuclear pharmacy by certified personnel.

Drug Interactions: Increased bone marrow suppression if combined with other myelosuppressive drugs or drugs interfering with blood clotting

Black Box Warnings:
- **Serious infusion reactions**, some fatal, may occur within 24 hours of rituximab infusion and are associated with hypoxia, pulmonary infiltrates, ARDS, MI, VF, or cardiogenic shock. Most (80%) occur with the first infusion. Discontinue rituximab, ^{111}In-Zevalin, and ^{90}Y-Zevalin infusions if the patient develops a severe infusion reaction.
- **Prolonged and severe cytopenias** occur in most patients. Do not give to patients with $\geq$ 25% lymphoma bone marrow involvement and/or impaired bone marrow reserve.
- **Severe cutaneous and mucocutaneous reactions**, some fatal, have been reported with the Zevalin therapeutic regimen. Discontinue rituximab, ^{111}In-Zevalin, and ^{90}Y-Zevalin infusions if the patient develops a severe mucocutaneous reaction.

- **Dosing:** Do not administer ^{90}Y-Zevalin to patients with altered biodistribution. Do not exceed 32 mCi (1184 MBq) of ^{90}Y-Zevalin.

Contraindications: None

Warnings and Precautions:

- **Infusion reactions:** Immediately stop and permanently discontinue rituximab, ^{111}In-Zevalin, and ^{90}Y-Zevalin for serious infusion reactions. Rituximab can cause severe, sometimes fatal infusion reactions, which typically occur with the first infusion, within 30 to 120 minutes of starting the infusion. Signs and symptoms of severe infusion reactions may include urticaria, hypotension, angioedema, hypoxia, bronchospasm, pulmonary infiltrates, ARDS, MI, VF, and cardiogenic shock. Temporarily slow or interrupt the rituximab infusion for less severe reactions. Immediately stop rituximab, ^{111}In-Zevalin, and ^{90}Y-Zevalin infusion for severe infusion reactions.

- **Prolonged and severe cytopenias:** Do not administer Zevalin to patients with ≥ 25% lymphoma marrow involvement or impaired bone marrow reserve. Cytopenias are delayed in onset and have prolonged duration, sometimes lasting > 12 weeks after drug dose. Incidence of severe nuetropenia and thrombocytopenia are greater in patients with mild baseline thrombocytopenia (100,000–149,000/mm^3) compared to patients with normal pretreatment counts. Monitor patients for cytopenias and complications such as febrile neutropenia and hemorrhage for up to 3 months after drug dose. Teach patient to avoid drugs that interfere with platelet or coagulation after therapeutic drug dose.

- **Severe cutaneous and mucocutaneous reactions:** Erythema multiforme, Stevens-Johnson syndrome, toxic epidermal necrolysis, bullous dermatitis, and exfoliative dermatitis, some fatal, have been reported. Time to onset after drug dose is a few days to 4 months. Discontinue rituximab, ^{111}In-Zevalin, and ^{90}Y-Zevalin infusions if patients develop severe cutaneous or mucocutaneous reactions.

- **Secondary acute myelogenous leukemia or myelodysplastic syndrome (MDS)** occurs in 5.2% of patients. Median time to diagnosis is 1.9 years following therapeutic dose, but cumulative incidence continues to increase.

- **Embryofetal toxicity:** May cause fetal harm when administered to a pregnant woman. Teach patient to avoid pregnancy and to use effective contraception.

- **Extravasation:** Monitor for extravasation, and terminate infusion if extravasation occurs. Resume infusion in another limb.

- **Immunization:** Do not administer live viral vaccines to patients who recently received Zevalin.

- **Laboratory monitoring:** Obtain CBCs and platelet counts at least weekly.

Adverse Reactions (**bold** indicates most common, occurring in > 25% of patients):

Cardiovascular: Hypotension, peripheral edema, rare angina, MI, VF

Pulmonary: Dyspnea, increased cough, rhinitis, bronchospasm, rare ARDS

CNS/neurologic: **Asthenia**, headache, dizziness

Dermatologic: Pruritus, rash, flushing, rare erythema multiforme, Stevens-Johnson syndrome, toxic epidermal necrolysis, bullous dermatitis, and exfoliative dermatitis

GI: **Nausea**, vomiting, diarrhea, anorexia, abdominal pain or enlargement, constipation, throat irritation

Hematologic: **Thrombocytopenia**, **neutropenia**, **anemia**, ecchymosis

Musculoskeletal: Back pain, arthralgia, myalgia

General: Hypersensitivity, rare secondary malignancy or MDS, infection, chills, fever

Nursing Discussion:
Agent has been shown to clear circulating lymphoma cells with the bcl-2 translocation (bcl-2 [t(14:18)])[19] and predicted response to therapy (80% response rate if these cells are cleared from circulation vs. 20% if the cells are not cleared).

After treatment, there is rapid reduction in malignant and normal B-cell lymphocytes, with circulating B cells undetectable for the first 12 weeks, followed by recovery of normal B cells starting in the sixth month after therapy.

Patient's own circulating antibodies stay within normal range after therapy.

Rarely, patient may develop an antiantibody response (human antichimeric antibody/human antimouse antibody).

Risk for anaphylaxis and hypersensitivity reactions: Rare but potentially life-threatening reaction may occur. Mouse antibodies are used that are foreign and may stimulate anaphylaxis. Rare, fatal anaphylactic reactions have occurred within 24 hours of rituximab dose. Of the reactions, 80% occur during the first rituximab infusion, and within 30–120 minutes of the infusion. Severe infusion reactions include pulmonary infiltrates, ARDS, MI, VF, and cardiogenic shock. Assess baseline temperature and vital signs. Administer premedications prior to rituximab as ordered, usually acetaminophen and diphenhydramine. Initiate infusion at 50 mg/hr, and increase in 50-mg/hr increments every 30 minutes to a maximum of 400 mg/hr. If patient develops discomfort, slow infusion; stop infusion if reaction is severe. Once symptoms have improved, resume rate at 50% of previous rate. Have emergency equipment and medications nearby, including epinephrine and corticosteroids. Assess patient for signs/symptoms, including generalized flushing and urticaria leading to pallor, cyanosis, bronchospasm, hypotension, and unconsciousness. Teach patient to report signs/symptoms, including sense of doom and tickle in throat. If signs/symptoms occur, stop infusion immediately, assess vital signs, and notify physician. Physician may prescribe epinephrine 0.3 mL (1:1000) IM if hypotensive. Oxygen, antihistamines, and corticosteroids may also be used.

Increased risk for bleeding and infection: Neutropenia is common, with 77% incidence, 25–32% of grade 4 neutropenia, with a median nadir of 900–1100/mm^3. Thrombocytopenia incidence is 95%, with a median platelet nadir of 49,500/mm^3. Anemia incidence is 61%, with a median nadir for red blood cells (RBCs) 9.9 g/dL hemoglobin. Nadir occurred around 7–9 weeks after treatment, and duration of cytopenias was 22–35 days. Chills and fever were common, affecting 27.5% and 21.6%, respectively, of patients in one study. There appears to be increased hematologic toxicity in patients with bone marrow involvement by tumor, as expected. Rare fatal cerebral hemorrhage and severe infections occur. Drug contraindicated in patients with > 25% hypocellular bone marrow or history of failed stem cell collection. Assess baseline CBC and platelet count, and monitor closely during and after therapy at least weekly for the first 12 weeks after treatment. Assess risk for increased hematologic toxicity—e.g., whether bone marrow involvement by tumor. Inform patient that blood counts will fall. Teach patient self-care measures, including self-assessment for signs/symptoms of infection, bleeding, fatigue, and anemia; self-care strategies to minimize risk for infection (e.g., avoiding crowds and proximity to people with colds), bleeding (e.g., avoid aspirin-containing OTC medicines), and fatigue (e.g., alternating rest and activity periods); and what/where to report fever, bleeding, signs/symptoms of infection. Most studies show that few patients developed severe infections, and there were few if any deaths from treatment-related infections. Transfuse RBCs and platelets as ordered.

Risk of radiation exposure: ^{90}Y-Zevalin is a beta-emitter; thus, patients should protect others from exposure to their body secretions (i.e., saliva, stool, blood, urine). Teach patient the importance of specific radiation precautions, beginning at the start of treatment and continuing for 1 week after treatment is completed: use condom during sexual intercourse, refrain from deep kissing, avoid transfer of body fluids, wash hands thoroughly after using the toilet, and continue effective contraception for 12 months following completion of treatment.

Drug: Gemtuzumab Ozogamicin for Injection (Mylotarg)

Indications: Treatment of patients with CD33-positive acute myeloid leukemia in first relapse who are 60 years of age or older and who are not considered candidates for other cytotoxic chemotherapy. The safety and efficacy of Mylotarg in patients with poor performance status and organ dysfunction has not been established.

Class: Humanized, conjugated MAb directed against CD33 antigen; conjugated with cytotoxic antibiotic

Mechanism of Action: Drug is composed of a recombinant humanized Ig4 kappa antibody conjugated with a cytotoxic antitumor antibiotic, calicheamicin. The antibody portion of the drug binds to the CD33 antigen found on the cell surface of leukemic blast and immature normal cells in the myeloid cell line but not the pluripotent stem cell. The CD33 antigen is expressed in more than 80% of patients with acute myeloid leukemia. Of the amino acids used, 98.3% are of human origin, while the remainder are derived from murine antibody. Once the MAb binds to the CD33 antibody, the complex is brought inside the cell; calicheamicin is released inside lysosomes within the myeloid cell and then binds to DNA, resulting in DNA double-strand breaks and cell death.

Pharmacokinetics: Drug is rapidly bound to CD33-positive tumor cells in the peripheral blood (within 30 minutes of dose). Following first dose, terminal half-lives of total and unconjugated calicheamicin are 45 and 100 hours; after the second dose 14 days later, the terminal half-life of total calicheamicin is 60 hours, and the area under the concentration–time curve is double that following the first treatment. The cytotoxic drug calicheamicin derivative is hydrolyzed to release it from the MAb and forms many metabolites.

Dosage and Administration:
- Administer 9 mg/m^2 as a 2-hour IV infusion for two doses separated by 14 days. Full bone marrow recovery is not necessary prior to the second dose. DO NOT give by IVP or IV bolus.
- Administer via in-line, low–protein-binding filter (e.g., 0.22 μm or 1.2 μm polyether sulfone, such as Supor, or 1.2 μm acrylic copolymer hydrophilic filter [Versapor], or 0.8 μm cellulose mixed).
- Premedicate 1 hour before the drug is given with diphenhydramine 50 mg PO and acetaminophen 650–1000 mg PO, with acetaminophen repeated every 4 hours as needed.
- WBCs should be < 30,000 cells/mm^3 to minimize infusion reaction; the patient may need to be leukapheresed or cytoreduced with other chemotherapy (e.g., hydroxyurea).
- Patients with high tumor burden, or first treatment, should receive TLS prophylaxis.
- Monitor vital signs and oxygen saturation during the 2-hour infusion, and for 4 hours after infusion.
- Wear PPE when handling the drug.

Available as: 5-mg single-dose vial as a sterile, preservative-free lyophilized powder for injection

Reconstitution and Preparation:

- Protect from direct and indirect sunlight and unshielded fluorescent light during preparation and administration of drug (fluorescent light must be turned off in biological safety cabinet during preparation).
- Allow refrigerated vials to come to room temperature.
- Reconstitute 5-mg vial with 5 mL sterile water for injection USP using sterile syringes. Gently swirl the vial to dissolve. Final concentration is 1 mg/mL. While in the amber vial, the reconstituted solution can be refrigerated (2–8°C, 36–46°F) and protected from light for up to 8 hours.
- Withdraw ordered dose and inject into 100-mL bag of 0.9% normal saline injection, then place the bag inside a ultraviolet-protectant bag. Use the medication immediately.

Drug Interactions: None known, but may interact with drugs metabolized by the P450 microenzyme system

Black Box Warnings:
- Mylotarg should be administered under the supervision of physicians experienced in the treatment of acute leukemia and in facilities equipped to monitor and treat leukemia patients.
- There are no controlled trials demonstrating efficacy and safety using Mylotarg in combination with other chemotherapeutic agents. Therefore, Mylotarg should be used only as single-agent chemotherapy and not in combination chemotherapy regimens outside clinical trials.
- Severe myelosuppression occurs when Mylotarg is used at recommended doses.
- **HYPERSENSITIVITY REACTIONS INCLUDING ANAPHYLAXIS, INFUSION REACTIONS, PULMONARY EVENTS may occur.**
- Mylotarg administration can result in severe hypersensitivity reactions (including anaphylaxis) and other infusion-related reactions that may include severe pulmonary events. Infrequently, hypersensitivity reactions and pulmonary events have been fatal. In most cases, infusion-related symptoms occurred during the infusion or within 24 hours of administration of Mylotarg and resolved.
- Mylotarg infusion should be interrupted for patients experiencing dyspnea or clinically significant hypotension.
- Patients should be monitored until signs and symptoms completely resolve.
- Discontinuation of Mylotarg treatment should be strongly considered for patients who develop anaphylaxis, pulmonary edema, or ARDS.
- Because patients with high peripheral blast counts may be at greater risk for pulmonary events and TLS, physicians should consider leukoreduction with hydroxyurea or leukapheresis to reduce the peripheral WBC count to below 30,000/µL prior to administration of Mylotarg.
- **HEPATOTOXICITY:**

- Hepatotoxicity, including severe hepatic veno-occlusive disease (VOD), has been reported in association with the use of Mylotarg as a single agent, as part of a combination chemotherapy regimen, and in patients without a history of liver disease or HSCT.
- Patients who receive Mylotarg either before or after HSCT, patients with underlying hepatic disease or abnormal liver function, and patients receiving Mylotarg in combinations with other chemotherapy are at increased risk for developing VOD, including severe VOD. Death from liver failure and from VOD has been reported in patients who received Mylotarg.
- Physicians should monitor their patients carefully for symptoms of hepatotoxicity, particularly VOD. These symptoms can include rapid weight gain, right upper quadrant (RUQ) pain, hepatomegaly, ascites, and elevations in bilirubin and/or liver enzymes. However, careful monitoring may not identify all patients at risk or prevent the complications of hepatotoxicity.

Contraindications: None

Warnings:

- **Myelosuppression:** All patients will develop severe myelosuppression requiring careful and systematic assessment, and treatment of infections that arise.
- **Hypersensitivity, including anaphylaxis:** Most infusion reactions or hypersensitivity reactions occur during or immediately after the infusion reaction. Interrupt the drug if patient develops dyspnea or hypotension, and discontinue the drug if patient develops anaphylaxis, pulmonary edema, or ARDS. The risk is increased in patients with high peripheral blast counts, so patients should receive leukoreduction (hydroxyurea or leukapheresis) prior to receiving the drug.
- **Infusion reactions:** Postinfusion complex of fever/chills, and less commonly hypotension and dyspnea during the first 24 hours after drug dose may occur. Symptoms usually occur after the end of the 2-hr infusion and resolve in 2–4 hours with acetaminophen, diphenhydramine, and hydration. Grade 3 or 4 events include chills, fever, hypotension, hypertension, hyperglycemia, hypoxia, and dyspnea. Premedicate patient with diphenhydramine 50 mg PO and acetaminophen 650–1000 mg PO, with acetaminophen repeated every 4 hours, for two doses, as needed. Monitor patient's vital signs during the infusion and for 4 hours after the infusion ends.
- **Pulmonary events:** Severe pulmonary events that can be fatal have rarely occurred. Signs and symptoms are dyspnea, pulmonary infiltrates, pleural effusions, noncardiogenic pulmonary edema, pulmonary insufficiency,

hypoxia, ARDS. The risk is increased in patients with peripheral WBC counts > 30,000/mm^3 prior to the administration of the drug.

- **Hepatotoxicity:** Severe hepatotoxicity, including VOD, may occur either with a single-agent regimen or with a combination regimen, and may occur in patients without a history of liver disease or SCT. Patients at increased risk are those who receive Mylotarg either before or after SCT, patients with underlying hepatic disease or abnormal liver function tests (LFTs), and patients receiving the drug in combination with chemotherapy (not recommended). Patients who receive SCT before Mylotarg had a 22% risk of developing VOD, compared to 1% in patients who had not been transplanted. Patients who received SCT after Mylotarg also were at higher risk (15%) of developing VOD than those without SCT (1%). Assess for, and closely monitor patients who develop rapid weight gain, RUQ pain, hepatomegaly, ascites, and increased bilirubin and/or liver enzyme levels.
- **Use in patients with hepatic impairment:** Drug has not been studied in patients with bilirubin > 2 mg/dL. Extreme caution should be used in treating these patients.
- **TLS:** Prophylax with hydration and allopurinol, and assess electrolytes, phosphate, uric acid, and renal function studies closely prior to the first dose in patients with high tumor burden; leukoreduce patients with peripheral WBC count > 30,000/mm^3.
- **Pregnancy:** Drug causes double-stranded breaks in DNA and can be fetotoxic and embryotoxic. Teach women of childbearing age to avoid pregnancy while receiving the drug and to use effective birth control.

Adverse Reactions (**bold** indicates most common, occurring in > 25% of patients):

Cardiovascular: Hypotension, hypertension, peripheral edema, tachycardia

Pulmonary: **Dyspnea**, pharyngitis, rhinitis, cough, rare pulmonary edema, ARDS, pulmonary infiltrates, pleural effusions

CNS/neurologic: **Headache**, dizziness, depression, insomnia, anxiety

Dermatologic: Pruritus, rash, petechiae, cutaneous herpes simplex infection

Metabolic: **Hypokalemia**, hyperglycemia, hypocalcemia, hypophosphatemia, hypomagnesemia

GI: **Nausea**, **vomiting**, **abdominal pain**, **stomatitis**, **anorexia**, constipation, dyspepsia, increased aspartate aminotransferase (AST), hepatotoxicity, rare VOD, rare fatal hepatotoxicity

Hematologic: **Severe thrombocytopenia**, **neutropenia**, **anemia**, **epistaxis**, hemorrhage, eccymosis

Musculoskeletal: Back pain, myalgia

Renal: Risk of TLS with renal failure

General: Fever, chills, infection, anaphylaxis, infusion reactions (which are generally mild to moderate, occurring during or right after the drug dose and resolving in 2–4 hours)

Nursing Discussion:

Increased risk for acute infusion-related events: Patients often experience an infusion syndrome during or after the infusion characterized by chills (62%), fever (61%), nausea (38%), vomiting (32%), headache (12%), hypotension (11%), hypertension (6%), hypoxia (6%), dyspnea (4%), and hyperglycemia (2%). Rarely, severe pulmonary complications can occur, including ARDS. Syndrome may occur any time within 24 hours after administration and resolves about 2–4 hours later with supportive therapy of acetaminophen, diphenhydramine, and IV fluids. Hypotension can be severe especially if WBC count > 30,000 cells/mm^3 before treatment. Patients are less likely to experience this syndrome when receiving the second treatment. Premedicate patient as ordered with acetaminophen and diphenhydramine, and consider corticosteroids 1 hour before drug therapy. If TLS is possible, give hydration and allopurinol as ordered. Monitor vital signs and oxygen saturation every 15–30 minutes during the infusion and for at least 2 hours but up to 24 hours depending on the patient's response after the infusion has finished. Ensure that medications necessary for the management of hypersensitivity/anaphylaxis are readily available (e.g., epinephrine, antihistamines, corticosteroids). Assess baseline vital signs and monitor frequently during the infusion, and for 4 hours after infusion; keep IV line patent. Monitor vital signs, and notify physician of abnormalities. Be prepared to provide emergency support as necessary (including IV saline, epinephrine, antihistamines, and bronchodilators).

Increased risk for infection and bleeding related to bone marrow depression: Severe (grade 3 or 4) neutropenia occurs in 98% of patients, with recovery of an ANC of 500 cells/μL by day 40 (after first dose) in those patients who respond. During treatment phase, 28% developed grades 3 and 4 infections, with 16% experiencing sepsis and 7% pneumonia. Twenty-two percent of patients developed herpes simplex infection. Thrombocytopenia is common, with 99% of patients developing grades 3 and 4. For those responding to treatment, platelet recovery (25,000/ μL) occurs by day 39 after first day of drug. Twenty-three percent of patients required platelet transfusions. During treatment phase, bleeding occurred in 15% of patients (grades 3 and 4). These episodes included epistaxis (3%), cerebral hemorrhage (2%), disseminated intravascular coagulation (2%), intracranial hemorrhage (2%), and hematuria (1%). Anemia also was common, with 47% of patients developing grades 3 and 4 anemia, and 26% of patients requiring transfusions. Monitor CBC and platelets baseline and regularly during treatment. Assess for signs/symptoms of infection, bleeding, and fatigue baseline, between treatment, and prior to each treatment. Teach patient to self-assess for these, including taking temperature, and instruct to report them immediately. Teach patient measures to minimize infection, bleeding, and fatigue, including avoiding crowds and not taking OTC medications that contain aspirin. Transfuse RBCs and platelets as ordered. Teach patient strategies to conserve energy and minimize fatigue.

Increased risk for TLS: Patients with high tumor burden receiving the first dose of Mylotarg are at risk for developing rapid tumor lysis. TLS occurs as a result of rapid release of intracellular contents of the lysed CD33 cells into the bloodstream, such as protein (uric acid and phosphates) and potassium; as uric acid, it is insoluble and can overwhelm the kidneys causing acute tubular necrosis and renal failure. The risk of TLS appears higher in patients with a high number of circulating CD33 lymphocytes (e.g., > 30,000/mm^3). For first infusion, expect patient orders to include hydration at 150 mL/hr with or without alkalinization, oral allopurinol, strict monitoring of intake/output, daily weight, and body balance determination. Monitor baseline and daily BUN, creatinine, K+, phosphorus, uric acid, and calcium. Monitor for renal, cardiac, and neuromuscular signs/symptoms.

Increased risk for alteration in nutrition related to nausea, vomiting, mucositis, and hepatotoxicity: Nausea is common, affecting 70% of patients, with 63% developing vomiting. Stomatitis affected 35% of patients, with 4% having grades 3 or 4 toxicity. Transient increases in LFTs occurred and were usually reversible. In clinical studies, 23% of patients developed grades 3 or 4 hyperbilirubinemia, 9% in levels of alanine aminotransferase (ALT), and 17% in levels of AST. In clinical studies, there were deaths reported: One patient died with liver failure as part of multisystem failure related to TLS, another patient died of persistent jaundice and hepatosplenomegaly 5 months after treatment, and 4 (of 27) patients died of VOD following SCT after Mylotarg administration. Assess nutritional status, integrity of oral mucosa, and liver function studies baseline and regularly after treatment. Administer antiemetic medications prior to chemotherapy to prevent nausea/vomiting, and teach patient self-administration of antiemetics after discharge if drug is given on an outpatient basis. Teach patient to report persistent or continued nausea and/or vomiting. Assess efficacy and discuss change in antiemetic drug with physician if regimen ineffective. Teach patient to assess oral mucosa regularly, use oral hygiene regimen, and report signs/symptoms of stomatitis. If patient develops stomatitis, teach patient self-administration of oral analgesics and antifungals, as ordered and appropriate. Monitor LFTs, and discuss any abnormalities with physician.

Drug: Ipilimumab (investigational)

Indications: Being studied in patients with malignant melanoma, renal cell, ovarian, prostate, and pancreatic cancers. Also being studied alone and in combination with cytokines (e.g., IL-2), chemotherapy (e.g., dacarbazine), or vaccines

Class: Anticytotoxic T-lymphocyte antigen-4 (CTLA-4); human MAb

Mechanism of Action: CTLA-4 is an antigen expressed on human activated T-lymphocytes that is believed to be very important in regulating the body's immune response; it has an affinity for B7 costimulatory molecules, which determine how the T-lymphocyte will interact with antigen-presenting cells. T-lymphocytes are important in immune surveillance to distinguish between self and nonself antigens. CTLA-4 downregulates (turns off) T-lymphocytes after the invading antigen has been removed so that the immune system does not injure normal tissue. Ipilimumab is a fully human MAb that binds (blocks) the antigen (CTLA-4) so that it enhances the activation of the cytotoxic T-lymphocytes (sustaining an active attack against cancer cells and allowing T-cell replication and differentiation) and at the same time blocks B7-1 and B7-2 costimulatory pathways (blocks the activity of this off switch so the activated T-lymphocytes keep working).

Pharmacokinetics: Unknown. Long half-life of 2–4 weeks.

Dosage and Administration: Per protocol. For example, in treatment of metastatic melanoma, 10 mg/kg IV infusion, and in the adjuvant setting, 3 mg/kg every 8 weeks for 12 months. Response may take 12 weeks or longer of treatment, and responses have been documented up to 3 months after drug is stopped. Patients may have short-term progression followed by delayed regression with a prolonged duration of clinical response or stable disease.[20]

Available as: Per protocol

Reconstitution and Preparation: Per protocol

Administration: Per protocol. IV infusion may be associated with infusion reactions, such as chest pain, flushed/red face, back pain. Stop infusion and assess response. Administer ordered antihistamines (H_1 and H_2) and corticosteroid.

Drug Interactions: Unknown

Warnings: Increased T-lymphocyte activation and resulting inflammation are responsible for the major toxicities: dermatitis, enterocolitis and hypophysitis (rare). Rarely, inflammation of the eyes (uveitis), pituitary, thyroid, kidneys (nephritis), lungs (alveolitis), and adrenal glands can occur, as can aseptic meningitis and arthritis. Grade 3 or 4 events are largely reversible with high-dose steroid therapy.[20]

Adverse Reactions (**bold** indicates most common, occurring in > 25% of patients):

Pulmonary: Rare alveolitis

CNS/neurologic: Rare uveitis, inflammation of pituitary gland

Dermatologic: **Dermatitis**

Metabolic: Rare inflammation of thyroid and adrenal glands with alterations in cortisol, adrenocorticotropic hormone (ACTH), testosterone, TSH, free T_4 levels

GI: Elevated LFTs (must distinguish between liver metastases and immune hepatitis), rare enterocolitis

Genitourinary: Rare hypophysitis, nephritis

Nursing Discussion:

Increased risk for dermatitis: Dermatitis is the most common side effect, often associated with pruritus. Biopsy may show T-lymphocyte infiltrates. Assess baseline skin integrity and presence of abnormalities, and monitor during therapy. Teach patient that dermatitis may occur and to manage it with nonsteroidal topical lotions. Assess need for antipruritic medications such as diphenhydramine and hydroxyzine and oral steroids.

Increased risk for enterocolitis: Incidence is approximately 17% and manifests initially as diarrhea. Rarely, enterocolitis can result in bowel perforation. Check protocol for guidance. Diarrhea grades 1 and 2 are generally treated with diphenhydramine. Most protocols require patient admission for more than three diarrhea stools in 24 hours and treatment with IV fluids and nothing by mouth status. Expect endoscopy and colonoscopy to be performed, with biopsies. If enterocolitis is found, high-dose IV corticosteroids are initiated. Once symptoms have resolved, patient resumes nutrition with a progressive graft-vs-host diet (i.e., low in fat, fiber, and lactulose), and IV steroids are converted to oral. Patients are discharged home on an oral steroid, dose taper over at least 1 month.[20] If the patient is refractory to high-dose parenteral steroids, infliximab (Remicade, a chimeric MAb targeting tumor necrosis factor alpha [TNFα]) as a single dose may be prescribed.[21] This treatment requires tuberculosis (TB) testing, as it can reactivate dormant TB. Teach patient to report signs and symptoms of diarrhea, both when three episodes occur in 24 hours and when fewer than three episodes per 24 hours do not resolve. Teach patient to go to the emergency department or call 911 if severe abdominal pain, with or without vomiting and constipation, occurs, as the patient needs to be evaluated for bowel perforation right away, although this is a rare event. If bowel perforation occurs, anticipate and prepare patient for immediate surgical intervention.

Increased risk for changes in metabolism related to hypophysitis: Uncommon but significant because symptoms are vague initially (e.g., fatigue, headaches, low thyroid-stimulating hormone (TSH) and serum cortisol levels) and if untreated, dysfunction of the hypophysis (such as pituitary enlargement) is far reaching (e.g., severe headaches, severe fatigue, memory loss, loss of libido).[22] Monitor baseline and periodic blood tests for TSH and cortisol levels during treatment. Ensure that patient has a baseline MRI to evaluate any increased size of the pituitary gland. Assess activity and comfort levels baseline and at each visit. Teach patient to report onset of worsening fatigue, headaches, and changes in mental status. If hypophysitis is suspected, discuss evaluation with physician or nurse practitioner/physician's assistant: MRI to compare size of pituitary baseline, cortisol, ACTH, TSH, and free T_4 levels. If the diagnosis of hypophysitis is confirmed, teach patient about, and administer ordered high-dose steroids and hormonal replacement as needed (e.g., thyroid hormone, testosterone for male patients). Expect that most patients will continue on low-dose hydrocortisone to protect the pituitary gland.[22]

Increased risk for immune hepatitis: Uncommon, but may occur, characterized by increasing LFTs. Assess baseline LFTs and monitor during therapy as ordered. If increasing LFTs and/or bilirubin, check labs every 3 days or per protocol until stable or decreasing and then weekly. Hold drug per protocol. If LFTs continue to rise and immune hepatitis suspected, follow protocol, or anticipate physician will admit patient with daily lab assessment, and order IV steroids to reduce inflammation. If this treatment is ineffective, mycophenolate mofetil, tacrolimus, or infliximab may be tried.[20]

MEMBRANE-BOUND RECEPTOR KINASES (E.G., EGFR, HER2, HGF/C-MET, IGFR PATHWAYS)

Targeting the EGFR Pathway—EGFR and Its Inhibitors

The EGFR or HER family contains four receptors that are very important in normal cell growth. Ligand binding and dimerization lead to activation of the HER, which leads to growth proliferation, survival with a decrease of apoptosis, cellular migration, and angiogenesis.[23] In cancer, when the HER family receptors are overexpressed (extra receptors on the outside membrane of the cell) or amplified (extra gene copies in the DNA of the cell), as they are in many epithelial solid tumors, tumor development and metastasis result. Thus, EGFR and HER2 are both called oncogenes. It is thought that even as early as the formation of benign hyperplasia, HER family members play an active role, and it is well known that they play powerful roles in tumor invasion and metastasis. Thus, it appears that HER family activation can be involved in all aspects of breast tumor development.[24] The family is also called the ErbB family. The four members of the family are EGFR (erbB1), HER2/*neu* (erbB2), HER3 (erbB3), and HER4 (erbB4). HER2/*neu* is overexpressed in approximately 20–25% of women with breast cancer, and EGFR is overexpressed in many solid tumors, including[25]:

- Squamous cell cancer of the head and neck: 80–100%
- Renal cell cancer: 50–90%
- Non–small cell lung cancer (NSCLC): 40–80%
- Breast cancer: 40–80%
- Ovarian cancer: 35–70%
- Colorectal cancer (CRC): 25–77%
- Glioblastoma: 40–50%
- Gastric cancer: 40%
- Pancreatic cancer: 40–50%

When overexpressed, HER2/*neu* and EGFR are activated to produce a signaling cascade resulting in an aggressive cancer phenotype (behavior). We have discussed how important the EGFR is in cell proliferation and cell survival. EGFR stimulates the release of VEGF to build new blood vessels that support tumor cell proliferation. It also stimulates the release of metalloproteinases (MMPs) to make a pathway for the new blood vessel to migrate to the tumor. MMPs also help aggressive malignant cells invade and metastasize.

The EGFR Pathway

Both EGFR and HER2, when overexpressed or when the gene is amplified with extra copies of the gene, confer very aggressive tumor behavior (see Figure 2-4). Interestingly, there is some suggestion that HER4 overexpression is associated with an improved rather than worsened prognosis.[26] As mentioned, a ligand is a protein or growth factor outside the cell that binds to the receptor on the cell membrane or outer covering. EGFR stimulation by its ligands EGF or transforming growth factor beta initiate a signaling cascade, bringing the message to the nucleus to turn on the cell cycle for cell proliferation, to release VEGF to make new blood vessels (angiogenesis), to release matrix MMPs to make the path for the blood vessels to get to the tumor, to invade locally, and then to metastasize. Amphiregulin is also a ligand for EGFR. HER2 has no known ligands. Betacellulin, epiregulin, and heparin-binding EGF-like growth factor bind to EGFR and HER4. Neuregulins 1–4 (NRGs 1–4, heregulins) bind either EGFR, HER3, or HER4; NRGs 3 and 4 bind to HER4 alone; and NRGs 1 and 2 bind to both HER3 and HER4.[27] Normally the body is very careful to limit the amount of ligand so that it is released only when the body needs more cells. Cancer cells, unfortunately, are able to make ligand growth factors that continue to turn on the tumor cell growth and division, as well as other factors.

When the ligand binds to the receptor, it actually causes the receptor shape to change, which allows the receptor now to dimerize (or "join hands") with a neighboring receptor in the same family. For example, a ligand such as EGF binds to an EGFR on the outside of the cell; the receptor dimerizes with a neighboring receptor, either a EGFR receptor (called homodimerization) or another member of the family, such as HER2, 3, or 4 (called heterodimerization). Because each of the family members can partner together, there are many combinations possible, and these can overlap.[28] In addition, this allows for diverse signaling and amplification of the HER family signaling.[27] This dimerization activates the receptor and starts the message through the cell membrane to the tyrosine kinase molecule just inside the membrane. Here, the exchange of a phosphate group (phosphorylation) starts the message's journey like a bucket brigade from one signaling messenger (also called a second messenger) to another until it gets to the cell nucleus. The signaling molecules (proteins) that carry the message downstream to the

Figure 2-4 Antibody-dependent cellular cytotoxicity.

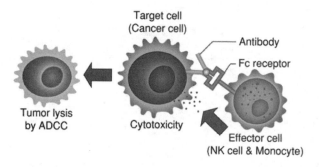

Data from Carter P. Improving the efficacy of antibody-based cancer therapies. *Nat Rev Cancer* 2001;1:118-129; Eureka Therapeutics, http://www.eurekainc.com.cn/technology.html. Accessed November 5, 2009.

nucleus include a pathway that stretches from just inside the membrane (called ras) through the MAPK (which is important in determining response to extracellular stimuli [mitogens] and in gene expression, mitosis, differentiation, and apoptosis), to Akt (one of the most important kinases for cell survival and also important in cell metabolism, growth, and proliferation), and JNK (a type of MAPK that responds to stress stimuli). This process is shown in Figure 2-5.

EGFR also talks to the ras pathway, which allows another message to be sent to the cell nucleus to divide and allows other functions. If the ras pathway is not mutated (i.e., KRAS is a wild-type or normal gene), then turning off the EGFR will also silence the ras pathway as shown in Figure 2-6. If, however, KRAS is mutated, then turning off EGFR will not silence KRAS, and it will continue to send its own messages to the cell nucleus. In approximately 30% of patients with CRC, KRAS is mutated.[29] In these patients, epidermal growth factor receptor inhibitors (EGFRIs) are not effective, which has been consistently shown in numerous studies of patients with advanced CRC.[30–32] Figure 2-7 depicts the importance of the EGFR signaling pathway in cell survival.

Akt is involved in the P13-kinase/Akt/mTOR pathway as well; mTOR is like Grand Central Station; it plays a key role in figuring out what to do when the cell receives input from multiple upstream receptors such as EGFR, IGF-1 and -2, and mitogens that are telling the cell to divide. It also senses whether the cell has sufficient nutrients and energy to do the work of making more cells; if there is too little oxygen, it calls for the manufacture of blood vessels to bring oxygen to the cell and remove waste products, called angiogenesis. This process is called a signal transduction cascade (see Figure 2-5). Once the message reaches the cell nucleus, it goes to the DNA strands and activates transcription factors that find the genes that need to be transcribed (the recipes for proteins copied onto mRNA that

Figure 2-5   Multiple signaling pathways.

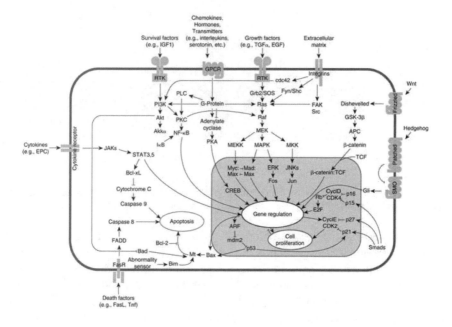

Figure 2-6   Schematic of KRAS signaling in colorectal cancer.

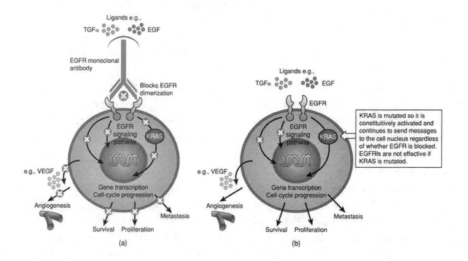

Figure modified from http://www.kras-info.com. Used with permission.

Figure 2-7   EGFR signaling cascade.

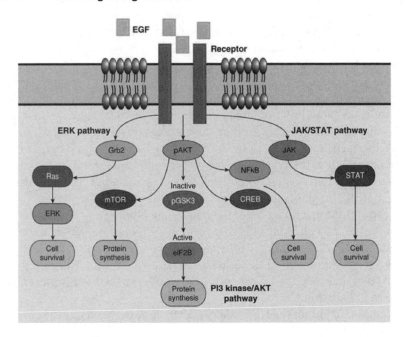

Image courtesy of abcam.[33]

will take the recipe to the cook [ribosomes], which will make the protein). The genes that are transcribed code for proteins that will turn the cell cycle: proliferation, avoidance of apoptosis, cell survival, and ultimately invasion (cell adhesion and migration) and metastasis.

Thus, overexpression of HER (too many receptors) can be stimulated by ligand binding, leading to increased intracellular signal transduction, resulting in tumor growth, invasion, and metastasis. However, receptors can turn themselves on when genetic mutations occur in the HERs, so they do not need a ligand to bind to the receptor. It is called an autocrine loop when the cancer cell both has HERs overexpressed and makes its own ligand.[34]

We have seen how important EGFR is in cell proliferation and survival. HER2 overexpression or amplification of the HER2 gene confers an aggressive cancer phenotype (behavior) as well. HER2 overexpression is defined as an increased number of receptors on the outside of the cell, determined by immunohistochemistry (IHC). Amplification (i.e., having extra copies of the HER2 gene in the DNA of the cell) is determined by fluorescence in situ hybridization (FISH) or chromogenic in situ hybridization. Because HER2 does not have a ligand, the receptor remains in an open conformation so that it can dimerize with other members of the HER (EGFR) family.[34] Once dimerization occurs, the receptors are very close to each other; thus, they can activate each other so that the tyrosine kinases inside the cell membrane now will send the messages downstream to the nucleus via the signaling proteins (bucket brigade).

In the past, the roles of HER3 and HER4 were unclear, other than their function in dimerizing with EGFR or HER2 after the ligand (growth factor) binded to the receptor. Now, however, it appears that although HER3 is an "inactive kinase"—that is, it cannot start sending the message on its own—once it partners with EGFR or HER2, it sends a powerful message turning the cell into a very malignant one.[35] When HER2 is blocked by a tyrosine kinase inhibitor, eventually, the tumor becomes resistant to it or may not respond at all. This reaction may be due to HER3 prosurvival signaling.[36] HER4 looks like EGFR, in that it is a protein receptor kinase with an outer ligand-binding domain and a tyrosine kinase domain inside the cell.[37] Ligands that turn on HER4 are heregulin, neuregulin, epiregulin, and betacellulin.[34] There are many less HER4 receptors on the outside of the cell compared to the other HER family members. In healthy breast tissue, HER4 may help the breast cells in becoming specialized (differentiated) as well as in lactation.[37]

Strategies to turn off the HER family activity in cancer cells can approach the tumor at four levels[35]:

- Ligand binding
- Receptor dimerization
- Tyrosine kinase domain activation
- Downstream signaling molecules

Clearly, each of these specific receptors can be blocked outside the cell at the level of the receptor (e.g., extracellular domain), either by blocking the receptor so that the ligand cannot bind to it or by decreasing the activity of the receptor. In addition, the drug could bind to the ligand so it is unavailable to bind to the receptor, except for HER2, which does not appear to have a ligand or require a ligand to change the shape of the receptor to open, as it is already open.[34] MAbs are perfect for this type of targeting, as they can be made to target individual receptors. They are large molecules, so they must be given parenterally. In addition, many are made in such a way that they call in the immune system to help attack and kill the cancer cell. Any of these ways will stop the message from being sent to the tyrosine kinases so that the signaling cascade (proteins in the bucket brigade) is not turned on.

The receptor can also be targeted from inside the cell membrane at the level of the tyrosine kinase. If phosphorylation is blocked, the message cannot be sent downstream to the rest of the bucket-brigade proteins, so the message is not sent to the cell nucleus. These agents could be single- or multitargeted, and attack both this tyrosine kinase as well as others. Small molecule tyrosine kinase inhibitors can block the phosphorylation. These agents can be given orally as pills.

By preventing the signal transduction, the message would not be sent to the nucleus. Unfortunately, there are many redundant pathways, so with the many tumor cell divisions, eventually a clone of cells is produced that allows the tumor cell to escape control, often via alternate pathways. Thus, some of the multi-targeted kinase inhibitors may need to be used for each step, or major steps, of the signaling pathway.

Individualized or tailored therapy is emerging, especially in the treatment of EGFR- or HER2-positive tumors. In CRC, patients are now tested to see if the tumor has a wild-type or normal *KRAS* gene, or if it is mutated. *KRAS* is mutated, so silencing EGFR does not silence KRAS, and the message still gets to the cell nucleus, driving proliferation, metastasis, etc. EGFRIs are not effective if KRAS is mutated. See Figure 2-6 to better understand why mutated KRAS tumors will not respond to EGFR inhibitors. American Society of Clinical Oncologists (ASCO) as well as the National Comprehensive Cancer Network (NCCN) guidelines recommend that all patients have KRAS testing and be shown to be KRAS wild-type before receiving either of the EGFR inhibitors cetuximab or panitumumab.[38,39] After studies demonstrated that only patients with wild-type KRAS benefited from EGFRI MAbs, other scientists explored whether there were other factors that influenced whether a patient responded to EGFRIs. B-raf is also in the ras–MAPK signaling pathway, so if KRAS is not mutated but B-raf is, then in this small percentage of patients (10–14%), EGFRIs also are ineffective[40] (see Figure 2-6).

Similarly, HER2 testing is carried out on all invasive breast cancer tissue.[39] Studies have shown marked success in improving disease-free and overall survival in patients with HER2-positive breast cancer who receive adjuvant trastuzumab, an MAb that blocks HER2 signaling.[41]

The following ligands turn on the EGFR in addition to EGF[42]:

- Heparin-binding EGF-like growth factor
- Transforming growth factor-α
- Amphiregulin
- Epiregulin
- Neuregulin 1–4

EGFR activation is also important for human innate immunity in skin. EGFR signaling can also turn on other receptors or can be activated by cross-phosphorylation; thus, cross-talk among signaling pathways is very important. Mutations to EGFR can result in uncontrolled cell division where the message to divide is constantly sent to the cell nucleus. Therefore, EGFR mutation is called an oncogene.

The EGFR can be turned off by blocking it outside the cell at the ligand-binding site on the receptor by large molecule MAbs or just inside the cell at the site of the tyrosine kinase using small-molecule tyrosine kinase inhibitors. MAbs that have been developed to block EGFR outside the cell include the designer MAb cetuximab (Erbitux) and panitumumab (Vectibix). The advantage of MAbs is that they also can mobilize the immune system. In addition to direct blockade of the receptor-binding site, the MAb can theoretically stimulate complement-mediated cytotoxicity, immune modulation, and in some cases, ADCC, which all can kill cancer cells. See Table 2-3 and Figure 2-4, which show these mechanisms. Small molecules (oral agents) that have been FDA improved are erlotinib (Tarceva), gefitinib (Iressa), and lapatinib (Tykerb, which also blocks HER2/*neu*), which block the tyrosine kinase phosphorylation that occurs just inside the cell.

There are three EGFRI class-related toxicities, related to the normal function of EGFR in tissue and cell repair and to the replacement (proliferation) of cells that have died. The side effects are skin toxicities, including skin, hair, nails, and eyelids; diarrhea; interstitial lung disease. These effects will be discussed as a group prior to discussion of each drug.

Skin Rash, and Disturbances of Skin Appendages, with Risk for Infection

The incidence of rash/desquamation in CRC clinical trials was 89%, dry skin 49%, pruritus 40%, and nail changes 21%.[43] To better understand the pathology underlying the cutaneous side effects of EGFRIs, it is important to recall the role of EGFR in skin formation and repair. The normal skin and skin appendages depend upon EGFR activation for repair and replacement of cells. EGFR is highly expressed in the epidermis, the hair follicles, sebaceous glands, periungual tissue, conjunctival epithelium, corneal epithelium, skin of the eyelids, and eyelash follicles. It is also found in the nail plates, especially of the thumbs and great toes. When EGFR is blocked, toxicity is seen in the skin and skin appendages.[44] The normal skin has an outer keratinized layer of epidermis, called the stratum corneum, that protects the body and preserves water balance by keeping body water inside the body. It is continually replaced as it is used by keratinocytes that migrate into the epidermis from the basement membrane. As they migrate, the young keratinocytes differentiate into adult cells, but both the ability to migrate and the ability to differentiate depend upon activation of EGFR and, consequently, being released from the basement membrane to migrate. It takes the keratinocytes about 14 days to make the journey from the basement membrane to the stratum corneum.[44] Figure 2-8 shows where the EGFR receptors are in relation to the skin layers.

When EGFR is blocked, the migrating keratinocytes stop. Because they do not belong in the epidermis, they undergo apoptosis. Neutrophils that are patrolling the

Figure 2-8   Anatomy and location of EGFR receptors in the skin.

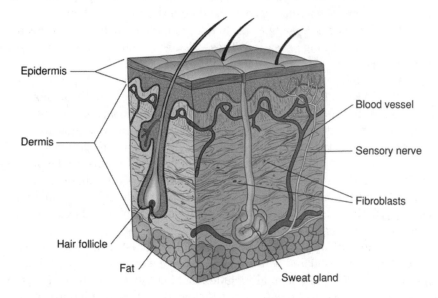

Courtesy of the National Institutes of Health Image Bank.[45] Public domain.

area recognize that these dead keratinocytes do not belong, and they begin an inflammatory response that brings in more neutrophils, monocytes, and lymphocytes. As the neutrophils begin to engulf the dead keratinocytes, they themselves are destroyed. The dead neutrophils develop into pus, and this sterile inflammatory reaction results in the papulopustular rash that is characteristic of EGFR rash. In addition, without the new keratinocytes to replace those on the stratum corneum, the skin loses its ability to conserve water and becomes dry and flaky.

Initially, the first week following the initial dose of the EGFRI, the patient feels tightness and tenderness of sun-exposed body parts, especially the face. The area becomes erythematous and may be slightly edematous, all typical of an inflammatory response. It looks like a sunburn. The papulopustular rash begins to appear following this and peaks in 14–21 days. By week 4–6, crusting appears over the papulopustular rash. This crusting is the drying of purulent debris, including the dead neutrophils, keratinocyte debris, fibrin, and serum.[44] At about week 6–7 after the initial dose of EGFRI, the papulopustules and crusting have cleared, and the skin now becomes excessively dry (xerosis) and itchy (pruritus). Telangiectasias often appear in the papulopustular sites, and, as the skin appendages also depend upon EGFR activation, blockade results in the formation of changes in hair and nails. Changes in the hair depend upon the location on the body, with scalp hair thinning (reversible alopecia) and hair on the face becoming excessive (hypertrichosis), with thick eyebrows and long eyelashes (trichomegaly). The long eyelashes can become misdirected and enter the eye, causing irritation of the conjunctiva. In addition, the conjunctiva can become dry and cause a burning sensation. These changes occur after 7–10 weeks to many months.[46]

In about 4–8 weeks after the initial EGFRI dose, paronychia (periungual inflammation) begins to occur, with the development of crusted cuts along the nail folds in about 16% of patients.[44] Fissures on the fingers and nail changes also occur and may not develop until 2–4 months after the drug was first started.

There is a correlation between rash, intensity of rash, and response, so although rash may be bothersome to patients, it suggests a response to therapy and a surrogate marker for efficacy.[31,47,48] The nurse plays a very important role in helping the patient minimize the distress associated with rash and skin effects, ensuring that the patient does not require dose adjustments and can maximize benefit from the drug.

Nursing assessment and management: EGFRI rash is more frequent and severe than rash associated with the oral tyrosine kinase inhibitors. Initial patient and family teaching should include teaching the patient that rash is expected and that there are specific things the patient can do to minimize distress and prevent infection. These measures include using skin moisturizers frequently during the day to prevent dryness and cracking of the skin, which can lead to infection; drinking 2–3 liters of fluids throughout the day to remain hydrated; avoiding sun exposure if possible, or using sunscreen SPF-15 or higher (preferably a zinc- or titanium-based) and wearing a hat and clothing to cover exposed body parts; and not scratching the skin, talking to the provider about anti-itch medicine, or wearing white cotton gloves at night to protect the skin. The sterile inflammatory rash is not infected, and it is critical that the patient prevent infection until the rash and crusting resolve; skin infection can rarely lead to sepsis and death.[49] Thus, the challenge is to help patients remain on therapy without dose reduction if possible to derive maximal benefit from the prescribed therapy. It is important to teach the patient and family that the rash is not acne and that it will go away.

The nurse, together with the physician/nurse practitioner/physician's assistant, can develop a plan to minimize skin rash. The baseline teaching for skin maintenance should be continued throughout treatment: frequent application of thick, alcohol-free emollient cream on clean skin, sunscreen SPF-15 or higher (preferably containing zinc oxide or titanium dioxide),[46] avoidance of sunlight if possible (as cetuximab is a radiosensitizer), and remaining well hydrated. Therapy is aimed at reducing the inflammatory response and promoting skin integrity so that infection does not occur. The most recent U.S. EGFRI rash consensus statement was published in May 2007.[46] It was followed in 2009 by the

Canadian practice guideline.[50] In clinical trials, the NCI-CTCAE version 3.0 was used to grade rash, but it did not reflect the impact of the rash on the patient; for instance, a patient could have a grade 1 rash confined to the face, but if it caused body image distortion, the patient might choose to end treatment. While not prospectively validated, the consensus groups developed a more user-friendly grading system, with corresponding treatment recommendations[46,50]:

- **Mild (grade 1):** Generally localized, minimally symptomatic, does not impact activities of daily living (ADLs), and there is no infection. *Treatment*: Continue dose of the EGFRI at current dose, and monitor for change(s) in severity. Either no treatment or topical hydrocortisone 1% or 2.5% cream, and/or clindamycin 1% gel (may use topical clindamycin 2% plus hydrocortisone 1% in lotion base) applied twice daily to affected areas until resolution of rash. Reassess in 2 weeks, and if worse or no improvement, proceed to next step.
- **Moderate (grade 2):** Generalized, mild symptoms (e.g., pruritus, tenderness), minimal impact on ADLs, no sign of superinfection. *Treatment*: Continue current dose of EGFRI, and monitor for change(s). Continue skin treatment with hydrocortisone 2.5% cream or clindamycin 1% gel, PLUS doxycycline 100 mg twice daily or minocycline 100 mg twice daily for a minimum of 4 weeks. Continue as long as rash is symptomatic.
  - *Scalp rash or lesions:* Topical lotion clindamycin 2% plus triamcinolone acetonide 0.1% in equal parts of propylene glycol and water until resolved.
- **Severe (grade 3):** Generalized, severe symptoms (e.g., painful, intolerable), significant impact on ADLs, and potential for infection. *Treatment*: Cetuximab, hold treatment for 1 week; panitumumab, hold treatment until toxicity improves to ≤ grade 2. Continue prior skin therapy (hydrocortisone 2.5% cream or clindamycin 1% gel PLUS doxycycline 100 mg twice daily or minocycline 100 mg twice daily), PLUS Medrol dose pack OR apply topical clindamycin 2% plus hydrocortisone 1% in lotion base twice daily to affected areas until improves to grade 1 or 2 PLUS doxycycline or minocycline 100 mg twice daily for a minimum of 4 weeks and continuing for the duration of treatment as long as rash is symptomatic. If improvement, dose reescalate according to manufacturer's package insert; if no improvement or worsening, discontinue MAb permanently.
  - *Scalp lesions:* Clindamycin powder 2% in amcinonide lotion twice daily.

The agents used are anti-inflammatory in nature. Tetracycline analogues such as doxycycline and minocycline have demonstrated anti-inflammatory properties in the skin.[51] Local application of hydrocortisone cream is also anti-inflammatory. Clindamycin ointment offers comfort rather than antimicrobial function. Unfortunately, it is drying, so metronidazole 0.75% cream provides similar effects with less toxicity.[52] Other studies that have established much of the current evidence base are:

- Skin and Eye Reactions to Inhibitors of EGFR and kinaseS (SERIES) retrospective study showed combination oral tetracyclines (doxycycline or minocycline), topical calcineurin inhibitors (pimecrolimus, tacrolimus), and corticosteroids twice daily was effective in the majority of patients. In 43 patients, with mean age of 60 years, 60% received erlotinib and 40% cetuximab; 51% of patients had reduction of severity by 2 grade levels, 42% had reduction of 1 grade level, 7% had no change in grade.[53]

- A randomized, controlled double-blind study compared prophylactic oral minocycline, topical tazarotene, or both, in 48 patients receiving cetuximab (starting day 1 of cetuximab therapy and continuing 8 weeks). Total facial lesion count (weeks 1–4) and moderate to severe itch (week 4) significantly lower in minocycline group; rash global severity was less, but not significantly. Topical tazarotene showed no benefit and is not recommended.[54]

- A randomized, controlled double-blind study assessed the role of tetracycline in preventing rash in 61 patients receiving EGFRI therapy (tetracycline 500 mg PO twice daily vs. placebo). Tetracycline did not prevent rash but significantly reduced severity, with higher quality of life (i.e., less skin burning, stinging, irritation, being bothered by rash).[55]

- A single-center, prospective, crossover study evaluated the effectiveness of Regenecare (MPM Medical, Inc., Irving, TX), which contains lidocaine (HCl 2% topical anesthetic), collagen to promote tissue formation, aloe vera, and sodium alginate to absorb exudates. Patients ($N = 13$) had a significant decrease in itch but not pain when compared with no treatment.[56]

- An observational study of urea cream containing 0.1% K_1 vitamin (Reconval K_1) followed 30 patients receiving cream when rash developed. Six patients had grade 3, 18 patients had grade 2, and 6 patients had grade 1. Rash improved (median 8 days) and decreased one or more grades (median 18 days). Conclusion: Vitamin K may restore EGFR function in skin.[57]

Recently, Lacouture announced the findings of the STEPP trial, a prospective trial of preventive care compared to reactive treatment of EGFRI rash.[58] Ninety-five patients were enrolled and randomized to receive either preemptive care (doxycycline 100 mg PO twice daily, para-amino benzoic acid-free, sun protection > SPF-15 UVA/UVB, 1% hydrocortisone cream starting the day before first treatment with panitumumab and continuing daily throughout therapy for 6 weeks), or reactive care when rash occurred. Patient's quality of life as well as rash occurrence and intensity were measured. The authors found that the prophylactic treatment was well tolerated and resulted in a 50% reduction in incidence of grade 2 or higher skin toxicity, less grade 3 or higher skin toxicity, and improved quality of life compared to the reactive group (as reported by patients). Also, there was no difference in median overall survival between groups.[58] This is the first evidence that beginning skin treatments prior to starting therapy has an effect in decreasing severity.

Nurses are called upon to offer recommendations for skin emollients and other OTC products that can ameliorate skin problems. Eaby et al.[59] and others[50,60,61] recommend the following practical tips, and although the evidence needs to be established, they are reasonable approaches:

- Dry skin:
    - Emollients: Vanicream (Pharmaceutical Specialties, Inc), Eucerin (Beiersdorf AG), Aquaphor (Beiersdorf AG), Aveeno (Johnson & Johnson, Inc), Cutemol (Summers Lab). Creams are more effective than lotions. When kept in the refrigerator, they can provide added symptom benefit.
    - Remain hydrated: Avoid long, hot showers, and instead use lukewarm water and mild soap, ensuring that genital, rectal, and skin-fold areas are cleaned thoroughly. Apply moisturizer within 15 minutes of showering or bathing.
    - Avoid laundry detergent with strong perfume, acne medications, and greasy ointments.
    - Wash skin with liquid cleanser such as Neutrogena, Dove, or Ivory soap; use hypoallergenic makeup such as DermaBlend.
    - Oatmeal baths can be soothing and may be anti-inflammatory.
    - Use sun protection, as sun will exacerbate the rash severity.
    - Other topical agents: Sarna Ultra cream, Regenecare
    - Scalp care: Capex shampoo, Olux foam
- Xerosis/pruritus: Rehydrate, provide barrier and remove dryness with emollients such as Vaseline Intensive Care, Neutrogena Norwegian Formula hand cream, Sarna Ultra cream, Eucerin, and Aveeno.
- Prevent/relieve itch:
    - Use antihistamines (e.g., hydroxyzine) to relieve H_1-mediated pruritus.
    - Pregabalin (Lyrica) may decrease itching (75–100 mg PO two–three times per day).
    - Gabapentin could be cheaper alternative to pregabalin.
    - Cool compresses may increase comfort.
    - Exfoliate: ammonium lactate 12% ± urea 40%
- Xerotic dermatitis: topical corticosteroid (hydrocortisone 2% or alclometasone 0.05%) and urea 20% cream
- Crusting:
    - Keratolytics remove crusts and thin as well as loosen the skin on and around the crusts. They may be irritating, so require caution. Examples are lactic acid 12% ± urea 40%, salicylic acid, urea products such as ammonium lactate (AmLactin, Lac-Hydrin).

- If severe, try topical corticosteroid and urea 20% cream.
- Emollients (Cetaphil, Sarna Ultra cream)
- Nail problems:
  - Keep finger- and toenails clean and trimmed. Avoid biting of the nails, pushing back cuticles, tearing skin around the nail bed, and applying artificial nails.
  - Avoid tight-fitting shoes.
  - Wear gloves when washing dishes or using chemical cleaning agents.
  - Moisturize hands and feet frequently. Consider applying petroleum jelly around nails periodically during the day; at night, apply a thick coat to hands and feet, and cover hands and feet with white cotton gloves and socks.
  - Paronychial inflammation: Discuss with provider to obtain culture and sensitivity (C&S), and begin doxycycline 100 mg PO twice daily or minocycline 100 mg PO twice daily, and use flurandrenolide (Cordran) tape over paronychial area. Assess after 4 weeks; if improving, continue regimen and add topical mupirocin 2% cream in nail folds; if not improving, discuss with provider drug dose modification and nail avulsion.[44]
- Teach patient to avoid trauma because once the skin integrity is breached, infection may occur.
- If pyogenic, granuloma-like lesions occur with excessive granulation tissue, discuss these options with provider: weekly applications of silver nitrate, antiseptic soaks, and cushioning of the area.[62]
- If bacterial superinfection suspected, discuss oral antibiotics with provider.
- Fissures: Seal with cyanoacrylate, apply urea 40% cream twice daily, and reassess in 4 weeks.
- Mucosal dryness:
  - Use saline nasal spray followed by petroleum jelly if nosebleeds develop.
  - Use personal lubricant for sexual intercourse.

The patient should be referred to a dermatologist for the following:
- Skin lesions that are severe and that do not improve within 1–2 weeks
- Appearance of blistering, necrosis, petechiae, or purpura
- Multiple hair, nail, and skin issues, or a lesion that does not "look right"

When a patient is receiving EGFRI together with radiation therapy (RT), the management of rash that may be radiation dermatitis or EGFRI rash, becomes more difficult. Consensus guidelines have been developed.[63] The main goal is to minimize the need to change the RT dose and/or EGFRI, which might result in undertreatment of the patient. In general, the guidelines recommend the following:

- Establish that the skin reaction is not due to a drug reaction (excluding the EGFRI).

- Follow established institutional guidelines for care of the irradiated skin, and reinforce techniques for hygiene so that the irradiated area is kept clean and the risk of infection is minimized. Patients should be taught to wash the area with a gentle cleanser and dry with a soft, clean towel. Soap can irritate the skin, so a pH-neutral synthetic detergent is preferable.
- Topical treatment approaches depend upon the location. Drying pastes may be useful within skin folds to help dry the area of skin reaction; gels can help in seborrhoeic areas; creams can be useful in areas outside skin folds and seborrheic areas; hydrophilic dressings should be used in moist areas to absorb wound exudates and help skin to heal. Avoid greasy topical skin products.
- Do not apply topical moisturizers, gels, emulsion, or dressings shortly before RT, as they may cause a bolus effect, giving an increased dose to the epidermis. Teach patients to gently clean and dry the radiation field before each RT treatment. Topical moisturizers and dressings should be applied after the RT treatment to minimize the risk of the bolus effect the next day.
- Corticosteroid topical ointment, if used, should be time-limited. Pain relief should be considered in the context of other pain-relieving interventions— for instance, if the patient also has pain from mucositis.
- Teach patients to avoid sun exposure when possible, using soft clothing to cover the area when outside; to avoid skin irritants such as perfumes, deodorants, alcohol-based-lotions; and to avoid scratching the affected skin.
- **Grade 1 radiation dermatitis (faint erythema or dry desquamation):** General measures (above bullets). Topical moisturizers may be used after the RT session; if an antibiotic cream is needed, consider triclosan- or chlorhexidine-based cream. Manage EGFRI rash outside the treatment field as any EGFRI rash, but do not give doxycycline or minocycline, which are radiation sensitizers.
- **Grade 2 (moderate to brisk erythema, patchy, moist desquamation, mostly confined to skin folds and creases; moderate edema):** Keep irradiated field clean, even if ulcerated. If no clinical infection, use drying gels, possibly mixed with antiseptic (e.g., chlorhexidine-based), OR anti-inflammatory emulsion (e.g., trolamine), OR hyaluronic acid cream, OR hydrophilic dressings applied after RT to the clean, irradiated area; zinc oxide paste (remove before each treatment); OR silver sulfadiazine or beta-glucan cream applied after RT or in the evening after cleaning the affected area. *If infection is suspected,* discuss with physician C&S of site and use of appropriate topical antibiotic. Assess blood counts, especially the ANC if receiving concomitant chemotherapy. Assess blood cultures if there are signs/symptoms of sepsis and/or fever. **Skin reactions should be assessed at least once a week.**

- **Grade 3 (moist desquamation other than skin folds and creases; bleeding induced by minor trauma or abrasion):** Same as grade 2
- **Grade 4 (skin necrosis of ulceration of full thickness of dermis; spontaneous bleeding from involved site):** Verify that correct RT dose and distribution are being delivered; involve skin/wound care nurse specialist or dermatologist as needed.
- **In summary, when radiation dermatitis and EGFRI rash occur together in the irradiated field, the management depends upon the grade. For grade 1, follow EGFRI rash guidelines. For grades 2 and higher, follow recommendations for RT dermatitis.**

Ocular toxicities are related to the adverse skin effects as well. The reported incidence is 7–15%, but it is probably closer to 33% of patients who will develop these problems, which occur after a few months of treatment.[64] As mentioned, the EGFR is located in cells of the skin of the eyelids, and eyelash follicles. Basti separates EGFRI-related issues into two broad categories: changes in the eyelids and changes in the tear film.[64]

Changes in the eyelids include the skin of eyelid, lid margin, lashes, meibomian glands. The first condition seen is *squamous blepharitis*, an acute skin reaction of the eyelids in which the edge of the eyelid is covered with small white scales. This condition is treated with fluorometholone (0.1%) ophthalmic ointment (skin and eyelid margin) twice daily for 1 week (never > 2 weeks); because it is a steroid, the patient needs an ophthalmologist referral for examination within 4 weeks of initiating topical agent to measure intraocular pressure. The second eye condition a patient might develop is *trichomegaly*, involving elongated eyebrow hairs and eyelashes that may become misdirected into the eyeball, causing irritation. Teach the patient that these changes may occur, are reversible after the drug is stopped, and NOT to cut the eyelashes. If the eye is irritated by a misdirected eyelash, the patient should make an appointment with the ophthalmologist to have the eyelash directed outside of the eyeball. The third eye condition is *meibomitis*, or inflammation of the meibomian glands, causing symptoms of a burning sensation in the eye and mild redness, with perhaps mucous discharge; it may occur only in the morning upon awakening. The meibomian glands normally make sebum, which is discharged through tiny holes in the glands that open on the edge of the eyelid. Teach the patient to perform lid scrubs and to apply warm compresses to the eyelid for at least 5 minutes twice daily. If the meibomitis is severe and does not improve, discuss with the patient's provider oral doxycycline 50 mg PO twice daily for 2 weeks, followed by 4 weeks at 50 mg daily.[64]

Changes in the tear film refer, more specifically, to the dysfunctional tear syndrome (DTS). This condition may occur along with any of the other conditions already mentioned.[64] Symptoms include fluctuating or mild decreases in vision, transient eye pain, burning or foreign body sensation in the eye, and eye fatigue. For mild symptoms, teach the patient to apply supplemental tears (e.g., Refresh

Tears or Systane Lubricant Eye Drops) 4–6 times daily. If the symptoms do not improve, or if they worsen, refer to ophthalmologist for evaluation and management.

Other uncommon ocular problems that may arise and require referral to an ophthalmologist are iridocyclitis (sensitivity to light, sustained eye pain, decrease in vision) and corneal epithelial defect (significant eye pain, sensitivity to light).

Nurses need to teach patients to assess for any changes in their eyes or eye function and to report such symptoms as eyelid and eye irritation, oily secretions, dryness, burning sensation in the eye, crusty skin, growth of eyelashes, and fluctuation in vision. Nurses are able to manage simple changes in the eyelids and DTS. If symptoms do not improve, the patient should be referred to an ophthalmologist. The nurse should refer patients with any of the following symptoms to an ophthalmologist right away[64]:

- Sustained eye pain
- Vision loss
- Severe eye redness
- Sensitivity to light
- Significant decrease in vision
- No response within 1 week of beginning treatment for squamous blepharitis, meibomitis, or DTS
- Any patient receiving topical steroid (e.g., fluorometholone ophthalmic ointment)

In summary, the nursing role in patient education and management of EGFRI skin effects is significant and can encourage a patient who is responding to treatment to continue treatment. In addition, the nurse must use excellent assessment skills to identify early changes, to recommend appropriate management strategies, and to evaluate the response to the plan and need for plan revision.

Diarrhea is a class effect of EGFRIs. EGFR is important in repair of injured cells, as well as intestinal cell restitution, proliferation, and maturation.[65] As the digested food is propelled along the gut, its digestion causes constant injury to the cells lining the gut. When EGFR is blocked, these cells cannot be repaired, and diarrhea results. Diarrhea was a dose-limiting toxicity for the tyrosine kinase inhibitors erlotinib and gefitinib clinical trials; it is less common or severe with the MAbs cetuximab and panitumumab. The incidence of diarrhea with erlotinib is 54%, with diarrhea starting on day 12 after beginning therapy. The incidence with cetuximab is 19–39%; however, when cetuximab is combined with irinotecan chemotherapy, diarrhea related to irinotecan is increased and can be severe.

Diarrhea usually occurs within the first 3 weeks of treatment, with stool that is characteristically watery without blood or mucus. Diarrhea responds well to OTC loperamide and, if severe, to high-dose loperamide (4 mg [2 tablets] followed by 2 mg [1 tablet] every 2 hours until no bowel movements for 12 hours.[66] Treatment is based on that of chemotherapy-induced diarrhea until prospective studies can be done, such as Benson et al.[67]

The nurse should assess the patient's baseline bowel elimination status and teach the patient to report the onset of diarrhea. Review with the patient current drug profile, and eliminate any laxatives or cathartics. Teach the patient to self-administer loperamide if diarrhea occurs and to call if diarrhea persists after 24 hours. At that point, increase the loperamide regimen to high dose. At each visit, review with the patient any changes in bowel pattern (e.g., frequency, character, or presence of blood or mucus in the stool) and ability to maintain hydration and electrolyte balance. Teach the patient to increase oral fluids to 2–3 L/day, drinking one glass of fluid each hour; to self-administer antidiarrheal medications; and to report diarrhea that persists longer than 24 hours, the presence of blood or mucus in the stool, inability to take oral fluids, and abdominal pain and/or fever. If the patient has continued diarrhea and is unable to take oral fluids or has abdominal pain and/or fever, the patient must be seen, and parenteral fluids and other antidiarrheal medication must be given. Fortunately, refractory diarrhea is a rare occurrence with EGFRIs. Modifying diet can help control diarrhea as well, so it is important to teach the patient to avoid lactose-containing products; to increase soluble fiber (e.g., psyllium, Benefiber); to decrease insoluble fiber (e.g., raw fruit and vegetables, nuts, popcorn); to avoid greasy, fatty, and/or spicy foods; to avoid or limit caffeine to < 2–3 servings per day; and to eat small but frequent meals during the day.[68]

The NCI-CTCAE version 3.0 criteria for diarrhea is shown in Table 2-4.

Increased risk for development of interstitial lung disease (ILD) is also a class effect of EGFRIs. EGFR activation is necessary for the repair of injured cells in the lungs, such as occurs with chronic obstructive pulmonary disease. The mechanism is poorly understood, but EGFRs appear to be essential for repair of pulmonary damage.[70] Patients with prior pulmonary damage are at increased risk for developing ILD, such as patients with prior or concurrent RT, chemotherapy that causes ILD (e.g., gemcitabine), preexisting pulmonary fibrosis, or lung cancer, or patients living in Japan. Symptoms may occur suddenly or late, such as 5 days to 9 months, with a median onset of 42 days.[71] Diagnosis is made by high-resolution chest computerized tomography scan, with identification of patchy, ground-glass opacity bilaterally, and increased interstitial markings consistent with ILD.[70–72] Additional testing that may be done includes pulmonary function tests, arterial blood gases, and bronchoscopy with bronchoalveolar lavage. However, a definitive diagnosis is made by lung biopsy.

Assess the patient for, and teach the patient to report, symptoms of dyspnea and worsening shortness of breath right away. Occasionally, simply by stopping the drug, symptoms may remit.[73] Usual treatment includes high-dose corticosteroids (e.g., methylprednisolone), oxygen therapy, antibiotics, bronchodilators, and hospitalization as needed.[74,75]

Table 2-4   Common Toxicity Criteria of Adverse Events (CTCAE) Diarrhea Grading Scale

Grade 1	Grade 2	Grade 3	Grade 4
Increase of < 4 stools/day over baseline; mild increase in ostomy output compared with baseline	Increase of 4–6 stools/day over baseline; IV fluids indicated < 24 hours; moderate increase in ostomy output compared to baseline; not interfering with ADLs	Increase of 7 stools/day over baseline; incontinence; IV fluids indicated for > 24 hours; hospitalization; severe increase in ostomy output compared with baseline; interferes with ADLs	Life-threatening consequences (e.g., hemodynamic collapse)

Data from National Cancer Institute.[69]

MAbs Targeted Against EGFR

Because EGFR plays an important role in colorectal cancers, MAbs against EGFR first demonstrated activity in this tumor type. The first MAb, cetuximab (Erbitux), is a chimeric MAb with an IgG_1 backbone that may help explain the differences in response compared to the second MAb, panitumumab (Vectibix), which has an IgG_2 backbone.

Drug: Cetuximab (Erbitux, IMC-C225)

Indications: Cetuximab (Erbitux) is FDA approved for the treatment of patients with:
- Advanced CRC:
  - As a single agent in patients who have progressed after both irinotecan- and oxaliplatin-based regimens, or in patients intolerant to irinotecan-based regimens
  - In combination with irinotecan, in patients refractory to irinotecan-based chemotherapy

- Squamous cell cancer of the head and neck (SCCHN):
  - With locally or regionally advanced disease, in combination with RT
  - Recurrent or metastatic disease, progressing after cisplatin-based therapy

Effective only in patients with KRAS wild-type gene, without B-raf mutation.

Class: MAb EGFR inhibitor

Mechanism of Action: Cetuximab competitively inhibits the binding of EGF and other ligands to the EGF receptor on both normal and cancer cells, thus blocking activation of receptor-related kinases so that the stimulatory message to the cell nucleus is not sent. In addition, the EGFR is pulled into the cell so it can no longer be stimulated. This inhibits cell growth, induces apoptosis so the cell dies, and decreases the production of VEGF and MMPs. In the lab, cetuximab can mediate ADCC against tumor types. The drug is synergistic when combined with RT or with irinotecan, compared to radiation or chemotherapy alone.

Pharmacokinetics: Steady state achieved by the third weekly infusion. Mean half-life of cetuximab is 112 hours (range 63–230 hours). Female patients with CRC had a 25% lower clearance of the drug compared to males, but no dose adjustments need to be made, as they had a similar safety profile.

Dosage and Administration:
- Wear PPE (to ensure safe handling).
- Premedicate with an H_1 antagonist, such as diphenhydramine 50 mg 30–60 minutes prior to cetuximab.
- Administer through a low-binding 0.22 micron in-line filter over a rate not to exceed infusion rate of 10 mg/min. Administer within 6 hours of initial vial puncture (in a hood), or within 1 hour if punctured outside of a hood. Solution is stable 12 hours refrigerated, or 8 hours at room temperature. Recommended infusion time: 120 minutes initial infusion, 60 minutes subsequent doses.
- Assess patient during infusion with vital signs and oxygen saturation monitoring every 15–30 minutes, especially during first infusion, although serious infusion reactions can occur later. Assess patients with a history of drug or mouse allergies very closely or at clinical sites in the "Bible Belt" geography.
- Assess patient for 1 hour after infusion; thus, if giving multiple drugs, give cetuximab first.
- Reduce infusion rate 50% for grade 1 or 2 infusion reaction (see Table 2-3).
- Discontinue drug for grade 3 or 4 infusion reaction (see Table 2-3).
- In patients with SCCHN receiving RT, initiate cetuximab 1 week prior to starting RT.
- Immediately interrupt and permanently discontinue drug for serious infusion reactions.

- Withhold infusion for severe, persistent acneform rash.
- **Dose reduce for recurrent, severe rash:**
  - First occurrence: Delay infusion 1–2 weeks; if improvement, continue 250 mg/m^2 dose; if no improvement, discontinue cetuximab.
  - Second occurrence: Delay infusion 1–2 weeks; if improvement, reduce dose to 200 mg/m^2; if no improvement, discontinue cetuximab.
  - Third occurrence: Delay infusion 1–2 weeks; if improvement, reduce dose to 150 mg/m^2; if no improvement, discontinue cetuximab.
  - Fourth occurrence: Discontinue cetuximab.
- Biweekly doses of 500 mg/m^2 offer similar pharmacokinetics and response rates to weekly dosing.[76]
- Cetuximab plus vinorelbine and cisplatin was shown superior to chemotherapy alone in the FLEX trial (First-Line Treatment for Patients with EGFR-EXpressing Advanced NSCLC), in that survival was 11.3 months as opposed to 10.1 months in the chemotherapy only arm.[77] Patient characteristics of responders with longest survival were: female, better performance status (ECOG 0), adenocarcinoma histology, never-smokers, Asian.[77]

Available as: 100 mg/50 mL single-use vials, and 200 mg/100 mL single-use vials

Reconstitution and Preparation: Store in refrigerator but do not freeze. Aseptically withdraw vial contents. Do not shake or dilute. Solution should be clear and colorless. **Infusion pump:** Inject calculated dose of solution into evacuated sterile container or bag. **Syringe pump:** Draw up one vial at a time, fill syringe, and administer; follow by remaining dose in another syringe.

Drug Interactions: None known

Black Box Warnings:
- Serious infusion reactions occur in approximately 3% of patients and may be fatal.
- Cardiopulmonary arrest and/or sudden death occurs in 2% of patients receiving cetuximab in combination with RT.

Contraindications: None. However:
- Administer cetuximab to a pregnant woman only if the potential benefit outweighs the risk to the fetus.
- Mothers should discontinue nursing during and for 60 days after treatment with cetuximab.
- Women of childbearing age should receive birth control counseling and use effective contraception measures during treatment and for 6 months following the last dose of cetuximab.

Warnings:

- Infusion reactions: Of severe reactions, 90% occurred with the first infusion. Immediately stop and permanently discontinue cetuximab for serious infusion reactions. Monitor patients closely following infusion.
- Cardiopulmonary arrest: Closely monitor serum electrolytes during and after cetuximab.
- Pulmonary toxicity: Interrupt therapy for acute onset or worsening of pulmonary symptoms.
- Dermatologic toxicity: Limit sun exposure. Monitor for inflammatory or infectious sequelae.

Adverse Reactions (**bold** indicates most common > 25%):

Cardiovascular: Peripheral edema (10%); when combined with RT, cardiac arrest and sudden death (2%; higher risk if preexisting cardiovascular disease, hypomagnesemia)

Pulmonary: **Dyspnea (48%)**, **cough (29%)**, interstitial lung disease (< 0.5%)

CNS/neurologic: **Headache (33%)**, **pain (51%)**, bone pain (15%), **insomnia (30%)**, anxiety (14%), depression (13%)

Dermatologic: **Rash (89%; 12% severe)**, **pruritus (40%)**, nail changes (21%), paronychia (16%), conjunctivitis (7%)

Metabolic: **Hypomagnesemia (50%; 10–15% severe)**

GI: **Diarrhea (39%; 22% grades 3 or 4)**, **constipation (46%)**, **nausea (39%)**, **vomiting (37%)**, **stomatitis (25%)**, mouth dryness (11%), anorexia (23%), weight loss (7%), dyspepsia (6%)

Hematologic: **Infection without neutropenia (35%)**, leucopenia (17% grades 3 or 4), mild anemia (10%)

Musculoskeletal: Back pain (10%)

General: Infusion reaction (20%), **fever (27%)**, chills (13%), asthenia, malaise, anaphylaxis (3%; see Nursing Discussion), fetal damage

Nursing Discussion:

Infusion Reactions: While severe infusion reactions, such as grade 3 symptomatic bronchospasm and grade 4 anaphylaxis, occur in only about 3% of patients overall, 90% of these occur during the first infusion. Usually, a patient becomes sensitized to the antigen after the first exposure, makes IgE antibodies against the antigen, and upon the second exposure, the antigen binds to IgE, which is attached to previously sensitized basophils and mast cells; this causes them to rupture, releasing histamine, leukotrienes, prostaglandins, and other substances.[78] Anaphylactoid reactions occur upon first exposure to an antigen and are not IgE (immune) mediated. The antigen binds to the surface of the mast cells and basophils, causing them to rupture and to release inflammatory mediators (histamine, leukotrienes, prostaglandins), triggering the same signs and symptoms that occur with true anaphylaxis, as discussed earlier in the chapter.

How, then, can we understand how 90% of the rare, but severe reactions occur during or after the first dose of cetuximab? Chung et al. found that these reactions were hypersensitivity reactions (HSRs), and anaphylaxis was related to IgE-specific antibodies the patients developed against the cetuximab molecule (Fab portion), even though the patients had yet to be exposed to the drug.[79] They studied 76 patients who received cetuximab, and of them, 25 had a HSR. Of these patients, 17 had antibodies against cetuximab. The incidence of antibodies against cetuximab was 20.8% in patients living in Tennessee, 6.1% in patients in northern California, and 0.6% in those living in Boston, MA. These findings correlated with nurse descriptions that there was a geographical high-risk area involving the "Bible Belt" of Tennessee, North Carolina, and Missouri compared to the Northeast, where the incidence was very uncommon. In addition, cytokine release syndrome is possible.

Thus, as recommended by the drug manufacturer, patients should receive premedication with an H_1 antagonist such as diphenhydramine, and despite the fact that most patients tolerate cetuximab infusion without incident, it is important to monitor the patient for 1 hour following infusion to ensure there is not a reaction.[43] In addition, the patient should be monitored closely during the infusion, especially the first infusion, although anaphylactic reactions can occur with subsequent cycles. If the patient develops any signs or symptoms of an infusion reaction or HSR, stop the infusion immediately, connect a new IV bag and tubing, assess the patient, and discuss the plan with the physician/nurse practitioner/physician's assistant. If it is a grade 1 or 2 infusion reaction, the drug can usually be restarted following resolution of the symptoms at 50% of the infusion rate. This rate should be the permanent rate for all future infusions. If the patient develops a severe, life-threatening reaction, the drug should be permanently discontinued and resuscitation measures implemented. Nursing assessment of the patient should be meticulous so that early signs and symptoms can be identified and possible complications avoided.

Risk for cardopulmonary arrest, possibly related to hypomagnesemia: Patients with low serum magnesium are at risk for torsades de pointes, cardiopulmonary arrest, and sudden cardiac death. Magnesium is necessary for the function of enzymes involved in transferring phosphate groups and all reactions involving adenosine triphosphate (ATP), the energy currency of the cell. It is involved in DNA replication and transcription and in membrane stabilization, nerve conduction, ion transport, and calcium channel activity.[80] Magnesium is initially excreted by the kidneys but is reabsorbed later by the distal renal tubules. EGFR is highly expressed in the kidneys, especially in the ascending limb of the loop of Henle, where 70% of filtered magnesium is reabsorbed. When the EGFR is blocked, magnesium is not reabsorbed and is therefore wasted, taking with it calcium and potassium. It is estimated that 55% of patients receiving cetuximab experience hypomagnesemia and that it is severe in 10–15% of patients. Risk factors for hypomagnesemia in patients receiving cetuximab are duration of treatment (the longer the treatment, the higher the risk), elderly, baseline low magnesium level, malabsorption syndromes, and patients on diuretics. Because magnesium is an intracellular ion, when it is low in the serum, it is very low in the cell and requires lengthy repletion to fill the cell before the serum level shows a rise. The NCI-CTCAE version 3.0 gives the following grading of hypomagnesemia. Oral magnesium supplements are usually not effective and often cause diarrhea. Saif and Fakih recommend the following repletion titration[81,82]:

- Grade 0: Within normal limits (WNL)
- Grade 1: < Lower limit of normal (LLN)–1.2 mg/dL; replete with 2 g IV weekly
- Grade 2: < 1.2 mg/dL–0.9 mg/dL; replete with 4 g IV weekly
- Grade 3: < 0.9 mg/dL–0.7 mg/dL; replete with 6–10 g IV daily to biweekly, and hold EGFRI until magnesium WNL; consider increase in subsequent intervals between treatment
- Grade 4: < 0.7 mg/dL; same as grade 3 repletion
- Grade 3 or 4: 6–10 g IV daily to biweekly, and hold EGFRI until magnesium WNL; consider increase in subsequent intervals between treatment
- If the magnesium level remains < 1.5 mg/dL at next visit, increase the dose of magnesium in 2-g increments or higher based on magnesium level correction and duration of EGFRI therapy, until the level is WNL.
- Consider initiating IV magnesium at higher doses for patients who are elderly (age ≥ 70 years) or have a history of cardiac arrhythmias or seizures.

Patients should have their serum magnesium assessed prior to each treatment, and the magnesium repletion should be begun early, as it is difficult to replete patients when their levels are low. Continue to monitor serum electrolytes including magnesium for 8 weeks after completing therapy.

Nursing assessment of patients with hypomagnesemia includes the neuromuscular system (e.g., muscular weakness, tremors, seizure, paresthesias, tetany, positive Chvostek and Trousseau signs, and vertical and horizontal nystagmus), ECG abnormalities (nonspecific T-wave changes, appearance of U wave, prolonged QT interval), and arrhythmias (premature ventricular contractions, torsades de pointes, ventricular tachycardia in crescendo and decrescendo pattern, and VF). Also, symptoms of accompanying hypocalcemia may be apparent before those of hypomagnesemia and hypokalemia.

When repleting magnesium, the following signs and symptoms indicate hypermagnesemia (magnesium > 4 g/dL): neurologic symptoms (muscular weakness, flaccid paralysis, ataxia, drowsiness, confusion, depressed reflexes);

flushing, seating, and vasodilation; hypotension and depression of cardiac function; hypothermia; and respiratory depression.

Risk for severe dermatologic reactions, with risk for infection: See prior discussion on nursing management of skin rash and skin appendage assessment and management (see p. 106 management of class effects).

Risk for nausea and vomiting: Drug has low to moderate risk of causing nausea and/or vomiting. Administer oral antiemetic 360 minutes prior to drug dose.

Reproductive risk: EGFR plays an important role in embryogenesis; thus, blocking this receptor in the fetus may result in altered fetal development. Teach patients of childbearing age to use effective contraception.

Drug: Panitumumab (Vectibix, ABX-EGF)

Indications: Panitumumab (Vectibix) is FDA approved for the treatment of patients with advanced CRC:
- As a single agent in patients who have progressed on or after fluoropyrimidine, oxaliplatin, and irinotecan chemotherapy regimens. While panitumumab increases progression-free survival compared to best supportive care, there is no evidence of increased survival.
- Not effective in tumors that have KRAS mutations in codon 12 or 13.
- Panitumumab is NOT indicated in combination with chemotherapy as the PACCE trial showed decreased overall survival and increased grade 3–5 adverse toxicity in the arm containing panitumumab compared to the arm with bevacizumab and chemotherapy alone.[83]

Class: MAb EGFR inhibitor

Mechanism of Action: Panitumumab competitively is an IgG_2 MAb that inhibits the binding of EGF and other ligands to the EGF receptor on both normal and cancer cells. This blocks activation of receptor-related kinases so that the stimulatory message to the cell nucleus is not sent. In addition, the EGFR is pulled into the cell so it can no longer be stimulated. This inhibits cell growth, induces apoptosis so the cell dies, and decreases the production of VEGF and MMPs.

Pharmacokinetics: Steady state achieved by the third weekly infusion. Elimination half-life is approximately 7.5 days.

Dosage and Administration:
- Wear PPE (to ensure safe handling).
- Administer 6.0 mg/kg every 2 weeks infused over 60 minutes (doses ≤ 1000 mg) or over 90 minutes (> 1000 mg).
- Administer via low-protein-binding 0.2 micron or 0.22 micron in-line filter.
- Do not give as IVP or IV bolus.

- Reduce the infusion rate by 50% for mild or moderate (grades 1 and 2; see Table 2-3) infusion reactions, and consider premedication with diphenhydramine prior to the next dose.
- Immediately interrupt and permanently discontinue drug for serious infusion reactions.
- Withhold infusion for severe or intolerable rash; may resume at 50% of dose if toxicity improves.
  - Hold panitumumab for grade 3 or 4 rash or if considered intolerable; if toxicity does not improve to ≤ grade 2 and the patient symptomatically improved after withholding no more than 2 doses, may resume panitumumab at 50% of original dose.
  - If toxicities recur, permanently discontinue panitumumab
  - If toxicities do not recur, may increase subsequent panitumumab dose by increments of 25% of original dose until the dose reaches 6 mg/kg (original dose).

Available as: 10 mg/mL vials in 100 mg/5 mL, 200 mg/10 mL, and 400 mg/20 mL single-use vials (preservative free).

Reconstitution and Preparation: Store in refrigerator but do not freeze. Aseptically withdraw ordered dose and add to 0.9% sodium chloride for injection USP to make a total volume of 100 mL; if dose is > 1000 mg, add to volume to make final solution of 150 mL. Do not exceed final concentration of 10 mg/mL. Do not shake IV bag to mix, but use gentle inversion. Use within 6 hours of preparation if left at room temperature, or within 24 hours if refrigerated at 2–8°C (36–46°F). DO NOT FREEZE. Discard any remaining drug.

Drug Interactions: Increased toxicity when combined with chemotherapy

Black Box Warnings:
- Dermatologic toxicities occur in 89% of patients, with 12% severe (grades 3 or 4).
- Severe infusion reactions occurred in approximately 1% of patients.

Contraindications: None

Warnings:
- Infusion reactions: Stop infusion if a severe infusion reaction occurs (e.g., anaphylaxis, bronchospasm, hypotension).
- Pulmonary toxicity: Interrupt therapy for acute onset or worsening of pulmonary symptoms; discontinue panitumumab if patient develops ILD, pneumonitis, or lung infiltrates.
- Dermatologic toxicity: Withhold or discontinue drug and monitor for inflammatory or infectious sequelae in patients with severe dermatologic toxicity. Limit sun exposure. Monitor for inflammatory or infectious sequelae.

- Electrolyte depletion/monitoring: Monitor electrolytes during and for 8 weeks after completion of panitumumab therapy; replete as necessary.
- Administer panitumumab to a pregnant woman only if the potential benefit outweighs the risk to the fetus. Physicians are encouraged to enroll pregnant patients in Amgen's Pregnancy Surveillance Program (1-800-772-6436).
- Mothers should discontinue nursing during and for 60 days after treatment with panitumumab.
- Women of childbearing age should receive birth control counseling and use effective contraception measures during treatment and for 6 months following the last dose of panitumumab. Mothers should not resume nursing after drug discontinuation for 2 or more months after the last dose, as IgG is known to be excreted in human milk.

Adverse Reactions (**bold** indicates most common > 25%):

Cardiovascular: Peripheral edema (12%)

Pulmonary: Cough (14%), ILD (< 0.5%)

CNS/neurologic: **Fatigue (26%)**, ocular toxicity (15%, including eyelash growth disorder 6%, conjunctivitis 4%, ocular hyperemia 3%, increased lacrimation 2%, eye or eyelid irritation 1%)

Dermatologic: **Rash (57%; severe in 7%), erythema (65%; severe in 5%), pruritus (57%), nail changes (29%), paronychia (25%), skin exfoliation (25%)**, rash (22%), skin fissures (20%), eye (15%), acne (13%), dry skin (10%), hair (9%), growth of eyelashes (6%)

Metabolic: **Hypomagnesemia (38%; severe in 4%)**

GI: **Abdominal pain (25%)**, diarrhea (21%; grades 3 or 4 in 2%), constipation (21%), nausea (23%), vomiting (19%), stomatitis (7%), mucosal inflammation (6%), mouth dryness (11%), anorexia (23%), weight loss (7%), dyspepsia (6%)

General: General deterioration (11%), infusion reaction (4%; severe in 1%, including anaphylaxis and potential fetal damage)

Nursing Discussion:

Infusion Reactions: While infusion reactions can occur in 4% of patients, severe reactions, such as grade 3 symptomatic bronchospasm and grade 4 anaphylaxis, occur in only about 1% of patients. Usually, a patient becomes sensitized to the antigen after the first exposure, makes IgE antibodies against the antigen, and upon the second exposure, the antigen binds to IgE, which is attached to previously sensitized basophils and mast cells; this causes them to rupture, releasing histamine, leukotrienes, prostaglandins, and other substances.[78] Anaphylactoid reactions occur upon first exposure to an antigen and are not IgE (immune) mediated. The antigen binds to the surface of the mast cells and basophils, causing them to rupture and to release inflammatory mediators (histamine, leukotrienes, prostaglandins), triggering the same signs and symptoms that occur with true anaphylaxis, as discussed earlier in the chapter. In addition, cytokine release syndrome is possible.

While unlikely to have infusion reactions, the patient should be monitored closely during the infusion, especially the first infusion, although anaphylactic reactions can occur with subsequent cycles. If the patient develops any signs or symptoms of an infusion reaction or HSR, stop the infusion immediately, connect a new IV bag and tubing, assess the patient, and discuss the plan with the physician/nurse practitioner/physician's assistant. If it is a grade 1 or 2 infusion reaction, the drug can usually be restarted following resolution of the symptoms at 50% of the infusion rate. This rate should be the permanent rate for all future infusions. If the patient develops a severe, life-threatening reaction, the drug should be permanently discontinued, and resuscitation measures should be implemented. Nursing assessment of the patient should be meticulous so that early signs and symptoms can be identified and possible complications avoided.

Hypomagnesemia and risk for torsades de pointes (sudden cardiac death): **Although this reaction has not been described for panitumumab, with low magnesium, calcium, and potassium, the patient is at risk for torsades de pointes, cardiopulmonary arrest, and sudden cardiac death.** Magnesium is necessary for the function of enzymes involved in transferring phosphate groups and all reactions involving ATP, the energy currency of the cell. It is involved in DNA replication and transcription and in membrane stabilization, nerve conduction, ion transport, and calcium channel activity.[80] Magnesium is initially excreted by the kidneys but is reabsorbed later by the distal renal tubules. EGFR is highly expressed in the kidneys, especially in the ascending limb of the loop of Henle, where 70% of filtered magnesium is reabsorbed. When the EGFR is blocked, magnesium is not reabsorbed and is therefore wasted, taking with it calcium and potassium. It is estimated that 55% of patients receiving monoclonal antibody EGFR inhibitors experience hypomagnesemia, and that it is severe in 10–15% of patients. Risk factors for hypomagnesemia in these patients are duration of treatment (the longer the treatment, the higher the risk), elderly, baseline low magnesium level, malabsorption syndromes, and patients on diuretics. Because magnesium is an intracellular ion, when it is low in the serum, it is very low in the cell and requires lengthy repletion to fill the cell before the serum level shows a rise. The NCI-CTCAE version 3.0 gives the following grading of hypomagnesemia. Oral magnesium supplements are usually not effective and often cause diarrhea. Saif and Fakih recommend the following repletion titration[81,82]:

- Grade 0: WNL
- Grade 1: < LLN–1.2 mg/dL; replete with 2 g IV weekly

- Grade 2: < 1.2 mg/dL–0.9 mg/dL; replete with 4 g IV weekly
- Grade 3: < 0.9 mg/dL–0.7 mg/dL; replete with 6–10 g IV daily to biweekly, and hold EGFRI until magnesium WNL; consider increase in subsequent intervals between treatment
- Grade 4: < 0.7 mg/dL; same as grade 3 repletion
- Grade 3 and 4: 6–10 g IV daily to biweekly, and hold EGFRI until magnesium WNL; consider increase in subsequent intervals between treatment
- If the magnesium level remains < 1.5 mg/dL at next visit, increase the dose of magnesium in 2-g increments or higher based on magnesium level correction and duration of EGFRI therapy, until the level is WNL.
- Consider initiating IV magnesium at higher doses for patients who are elderly (age ≥ 70 years), are at risk for dehydration, or have a history of cardiac arrhythmias or seizures.

Patients should have their serum magnesium assessed prior to each treatment, and the magnesium repletion should be begun early, as it is difficult to replete patients when their levels are low. Continue to monitor serum electrolytes including magnesium for 8 weeks after completing therapy.

Nursing assessment of patients with hypomagnesemia includes the neuromuscular system (e.g., muscular weakness, tremors, seizure, paresthesias, tetany, positive Chvostek and Trousseau signs, and vertical and horizontal nystagmus), ECG abnormalities (nonspecific T-wave changes, appearance of U wave, prolonged QT interval), and arrhythmias (premature ventricular contractions, torsades de pointes, ventricular tachycardia in crescendo and decrescendo pattern, and VF). Also, symptoms of accompanying hypocalcemia may be apparent before those of hypomagnesemia and hypokalemia.

When repleting magnesium, the following signs and symptoms indicate hypermagnesemia (magnesium > 4 g/dL): neurologic symptoms (muscular weakness, flaccid paralysis, ataxia, drowsiness, confusion, depressed reflexes); flushing, seating, and vasodilation; hypotension and depression of cardiac function; hypothermia; and respiratory depression.

Risk for severe dermatologic reactions, with risk for infection: See prior discussion on nursing management of skin rash and skin appendage assessment and management (see pp. 39–48, management of class effects). Median time to rash, nail toxicity, or ocular toxicity is 14 days after the first panitumumab dose; median time to most severe skin/ocular toxicity is 15 days after the first drug dose; and the median time to resolve after the last dose of panitumumab is 84 days. Severe dermatologic toxicities resulting in infection, abcesses requiring incision and drainage, sepsis, and death have been reported.

Risk for nausea and vomiting: Drug has low risk of causing nausea and/or vomiting. Administer oral antiemetic 60 minutes prior to drug dose if needed.

Reproductive risk: EGFR plays an important role in embryogenesis; thus, blocking this receptor in the fetus may result in altered fetal development. Teach patients of childbearing age to use effective contraception.

Small Molecule Oral Tyrosine Kinase EGFRIs

Oral agents obviate the need for IV access, avoid the risk of hypersensitivity reactions, and, in the case of EGFRIs, avoid the risk of hypomagnesemia. However, oral tyrosine kinase inhibitors bring with them their own challenges. Patient adherence to oral agents is difficult for some patients, and if the patient has a response, oral therapy becomes a life-long responsibility. Some tyrosine kinase inhibitors, such as erlotinib, cannot be given with food because it will increase the bioavailability of the drug. In addition, oral EGFRIs have a higher incidence of diarrhea, which can be dose-limiting. As the duration of therapy extends, patients have more problems with eye and facial hair issues. Lastly, oral tyrosine kinase inhibitors have more drug interactions, as many are metabolized by the P450 microenzyme system in the liver (see Chapter 5). Finally, as more patients have experiences with long durations of therapy, more is known about tyrosine kinase inhibitor interaction with signaling pathways in the heart.

Drug: Erlotinib (Tarceva)

Indication: Erlotinib is indicated for the treatment of patients with:
- Locally advanced or metastatic NSCLC after failure of at least one prior chemotherapy regimen
- First-line treatment of patients with locally advanced, unresectable or metastatic pancreatic cancer, in combination with gemcitabine

Class: Oral tyrosine kinase inhibitor of EGFR

Mechanism of Action: Mechanism of antitumor activity is not fully characterized, but drug inhibits the phosphorylation of the intracellular portion of the tyrosine kinase domain of the EGFR. This inhibits the activation of cell signaling that otherwise would tell the cell to divide, to avoid programmed cell death, and to release VEGF.

Pharmacokinetics: Drug bioavailability is about 60% after oral administration on an empty stomach, with peak plasma concentrations occurring 4 hours after ingestion. Food can increase drug bioavailability to 100% with increased toxicity. Drug is highly protein bound (90–95%). Median half-life of the drug is 36.2 hours. Drug is primarily metabolized by the cytochrome P450 microenzyme system (CYP3A4) and to a lesser degree by CYP1A2.

Dosage and Administration:
- Take dose on an empty stomach at least 1 hour before or 2 hours after food.
- NSCLC: 150 mg/day until disease progression or unacceptable toxicity.

- Pancreatic cancer with gemcitabine: 100 mg/day until disease progression or unacceptable toxicity.
- If needed, dose reduce in 50-mg increments.

Available as: 25-mg, 100-mg, and 150-mg tablets

Reconstitution and Preparation: None. Store in a tightly closed container out of reach of children and pets. Avoid touching the tablet directly. Wear gloves when handling tablets, and wash hands thoroughly afterward. Bring any tablets not used to the dispensing pharmacy for disposal.

Drug Interactions:
- **Inducers of CYP3A4** may increase the metabolism of erlotinib, thus decreasing the plasma drug concentration (e.g., aminoglutethamine, carbamazepine, dexamethasone, griseofulvin, modafinil, nafcillin, phenobarbital, phenytoin, primidone, rifabutin, rifampin, rifapentine, St. John's wort). Avoid coadministration if possible. If not, consider increasing erlotinib dose.
- **Inhibitors of CYP3A4** may decrease the metabolism of erlotinib resulting in increased plasma drug levels and increased toxicity (e.g., atazanavir, clarithromycin, diltiazem, erythromycin, GRAPEFRUIT or grapefruit juice, indinavir, isoniazid, itraconazole, ketoconazole, metronidazole, nefazodone, nelfinavir, ritonavir, saquinavir, telithromycin, verapamil, voriconazole). Avoid coadministration. If must coadminister, consider decreasing dose of erlotinib.
- **Inducers of CYP1A2** may decrease erlotinib serum levels (e.g., barbiturates, carbamazepine, cruciferous vegetables, grilled meat, primidone, rifampin, smoking). SMOKING decreases erlotinib serum levels, so patients SHOULD NOT SMOKE. If dose is increased while the patient is smoking, the dose must be reduced (to normal dose) once patient stops smoking.
- **Drugs that alter the pH** of the upper GI tract may alter erlotinib solubility and absorption, as drug solubility is pH dependent. For example, omeprazole decreases erlotinib AUC by 46%. Avoid concomitant use of erlotinib together with proton pump inhibitors, and consider replacement with antacids given a few hours prior to or after erlotinib dose.
- **CYP3A4 substrates:** Erlotinib increases the AUC of midazolam by 24% when coadministered; assess for excessive CNS depression.
- **Warfarin:** Coadministration of erlotinib with warfarin may increase international normalized ratio (INR) with or without bleeding; monitor patient's INR closely and dose accordingly; teach patient to report any signs or symptoms of bleeding immediately and to stop warfarin.

Contraindications: None

Warnings:

- ILD may rarely occur and may be fatal. Interrupt erlotinib if patient develops acute onset of new or progressive unexplained pulmonary symptoms (e.g., dyspnea, cough, fever). Discontinue erlotinib if ILD is diagnosed.
- Rarely, acute renal failure and renal insufficiency may occur; interrupt erlotinib if patient develops dehydration, and monitor renal function and electrolytes in patients at risk for dehydration; teach patient to stay well hydrated.
- Hepatic failure and hepatorenal syndrome may occur; monitor periodic LFTs, and interrupt or discontinue erlotinib if abnormal LFTs indicate severe changes.
- Monitor patients with hepatic impairment closely (total bilirubin > upper limit of normal [ULN]); use extreme caution in patients with bilirubin > 3 times ULN. Interrupt or discontinue erlotinib if severe hepatic dysfunction occurs.
- GI perforation has been reported; teach patient to come to emergency deparment/physician if he or she develops severe abdominal pain, constipation, and/or vomiting so that GI perforation can be ruled out; discontinue erlotinib if patient develops GI perforation. Patients at risk are those receiving antiangiogenic agents, corticosteroids, NSAIDs, or taxane-based chemotherapy, or those who have a history of peptic ulcer disease or diverticular disease.
- Bullous and exfoliative skin disorders, sometimes fatal, have been reported. Interrupt or discontinue erlotinib if they occur.
- Cerebrovascular accident (CVA) may occur and be fatal (i.e., in patients with pancreatic cancer).
- Microangiopathic hemolytic anemia with thrombocytopenia has been reported in patients with pancreatic cancer.
- Corneal perforation and ulceration have been reported; interrupt or discontinue erlotinib if they occur.
- EGFR activation is critical to the developing fetus. Women of childbearing potential should use effective contraception and should be advised to avoid pregnancy. Treatment should only be continued if potential benefit to mother is greater than risk to the fetus.
- INR can be increased with bleeding; monitor INR closely and adjust warfarin or other coumarin-derivative anticoagulant dose appropriately.
- Most common side effects occurring in > 50%:
  - NSCLC: Rash, diarrhea, anorexia, and fatigue
  - Pancreatic cancer: Fatigue, rash, nausea, anorexia
- The phase III SATURN trial shows that erlotinib (Tarceva) maintenance therapy significantly improves overall survival in NSCLC (N = 899).

Progression-free survival was 45% compared to 41% with placebo, and overall survival was 12 months vs 11 months with placebo. Overall survival did not depend on EGFR mutation status.[84]

Adverse Reactions (**bold** indicates most common, occurring > 25% of patients):

Cardiovascular: CVA (2.3%) in pancreatic patients, MI (2.3%) in pancreatic patients

Pulmonary: **Dyspnea (54%)**, **cough (33%)**, ILD (rare)

CNS/neurologic: **Fatigue (52%)**, conjunctivitis (12%), keratoconjunctivitis sicca (12%), abnormal eyelash growth, rare corneal perforation or ulcers

Dermatologic: **Rash (75%)**, pruritus (13%), dry skin (12%), rare bullous, blistering and exfoliative skin conditions (e.g., Stevens-Johnson syndrome/ toxic epidermal necrolysis)

GI: **Anorexia (52%)**, **nausea (33%)**, vomiting (23%), stomatitis (17%), abdominal pain (11%), abnormal LFTs (4%), rare GI perforation, hepatotoxicity

Hematologic: Infection (24%), rare microangiopathic hemolytic anemia with thrombocytopenia (0.8%)

Renal: rare acute renal failure, renal insufficiency

Teach patient to call provider if experiencing the following:
- New or worsening skin rash; signs/symptoms of infection of the rash (appearance of exudates); pain
- Diarrhea that persists > 24 hours; nausea and/or vomiting that is not relieved with antiemetic pills; serious or ongoing loss of appetite or stomach pain
- New or worsening shortness of breath or cough
- Fever
- Eye irritation

Nursing Discussion:
EGFR mutations affect the response to anti-EGFR therapy. Studies showed that patients with specific mutations tended to respond to erlotinib.[85] The mutations were specific activating mutations in exon 21 and deletions in exon 19. An exon is a part of the gene that codes for a protein or parts of the recipe for the protein, and it is numbered. The exons are copied by the mRNA, and enzymes then splice the different exons together so the mRNA contains the complete recipe before it takes it to the ribosomes to make the protein. The entrons are separated from each other by introns. In addition, the patients who responded had increased EGFR gene copy numbers (gene amplification) and also increased HER2 copy numbers (gene amplification).[85]

In NSCLC, frequent EGFR mutations involve either exon 19, characterized by in-frame deletions of specific amino acids, or exon 21 (a point mutation). Of the

EGFR mutations of responders, 90% had these two mutations, while the remaining 10% had mutations involving exons 18 or 20. The mutations in EGFR activate the kinase activity, and the tumor is dependent upon this mutation for survival (called oncogene addiction). Drugs such as erlotinib that block this activation of the tyrosine kinase (interfere with oncogene addiction) cause the tumor cells to undergo massive apoptosis.[86]

Response was associated with the following characteristics:

- Female
- No history of smoking
- Adenocarcinoma histology
- Asian ethnicity
- Development of rash

The patients who did not respond had primary resistance, which has been shown to occur as a result of having a mutation on exon 20 (specific activating insertion), *KRAS* mutations, absence of total EGFR protein expression, and absence of *PTEN* expression. *PTEN* (phosphatase and tensin homolog) is a tumor suppressor gene that makes a protein found in most cells. When it is absent, the message to the cell nucleus continues to be sent telling the cell to divide, invade, make VEGF, and metastasize.

For people who do respond, however, over time their tumors develop resistance mechanisms, or secondary resistance. This happens to tyrosine kinase inhibitors like erlotinib and gefitinib through secondary mutations in the EGFR tyrosine kinase domain and amplification (increased gene copy numbers) of the *MET* oncogene. *MET* proto-oncogene is mutated, forming an oncogene in many cancers. It makes the protein product c-Met, which is the receptor for the hepatocyte growth factor or scatter factor that helps cancer cells metastasize.[85]

Risk for severe dermatologic reactions, with risk for infection: See prior discussion on nursing management of skin rash and skin appendage assessment and management (see pp. 39–48, management of class effects). Median time to rash is 8 days after starting erlotinib. Rash is generally less severe than with the EGFRI MAbs.

Risk for diarrhea: Diarrhea is a dose-limiting toxicity. If there is an acute onset, make sure patient is taking erlotinib as directed on an empty stomach. Time of onset to diarrhea is 12 days. See class effect discussion for full nursing assessment and care planning.

Risk for nausea and vomiting: Drug has low to moderate risk of nausea and/or vomiting. Administer oral antiemetic 60 minutes prior to drug dose if needed.

Reproductive risk: EGFR plays an important role in embryogenesis; thus, blocking this receptor in the fetus may result in altered fetal development. Teach patients of childbearing age to use effective contraception.

Drug: Gefitinib (Iressa, ZD1839)

Indications: Gefitinib is indicated as monotherapy for the continued treatment of patients with locally advanced or metastatic NSCLC after failure of both platinum-based and docetaxel chemotherapies. In clinical trials, the response rate was 10%, and no survival advantage was seen; thus, gefitinib is restricted to patients who are or who have had a response to the drug.

Class: Oral tyrosine kinase inhibitor of EGFR

Mechanism of Action: Mechanism of antitumor activity is not fully characterized, but drug inhibits the phosphorylation of the intracellular portion of the tyrosine kinase domain of the EGFR. This inhibits the activation of cell signaling that otherwise would tell the cell to divide, to avoid programmed cell death, and to release VEGF. Drug resistance develops when the tumor uses alternative pathways to send the signal to the cell nucleus to divide, such as the *MET* oncogene signaling pathway via erbB3.[87]

Pharmacokinetics: Oral drug is slowly absorbed from the GI tract with peak plasma levels occurring 3–7 hours after dosing. Bioavailability is 60% and is unaffected by food intake. Drug is 90% protein bound to albumin. Drug is metabolized via the P450 microenzyme system, primarily the CYP3A4 enzyme system; it is excreted in the feces (86%). The elimination half-life is 48 hours with a steady state level achieved within 10 days.

Dosage and Administration:
- 250 mg PO daily, available through the IRESSA access program. May allow to dissolve in water and drink immediately.
- Briefly interrupt therapy (up to 2 weeks) for poorly tolerated diarrhea or skin reaction.
- Interrupt treatment immediately if ILD is suspected; if diagnosed, discontinue drug.
- Discontinue drug for hypersensitivity (e.g., angioedema, toxic epidermal necrolysis, erythema multiforme).
- Higher doses increase toxicity but not efficacy.

Available as: 250-mg tablets, in a bottle of 30 tablets

Reconstitution and Preparation: None. Store in a tightly closed container at room temperature, out of reach of children and pets. Avoid touching the tablet directly. Wear gloves when handling tablets, and wash hands thoroughly afterward. Bring any tablets not used to the dispensing pharmacy for disposal.

Drug Interactions:
- **Inducers of CYP3A4** may increase the metabolism of gefitinib, thus decreasing the plasma drug concentration (e.g., aminoglutethamine, carbamazepine, dexamethasone, griseofulvin, modafinil, nafcillin, phenobarbital,

phenytoin, primidone, rifabutin, rifampin, rifapentine, St. John's wort). Avoid coadministration if possible. If not, consider increasing gefitinib dose.

- **Inhibitors of CYP3A4** may decrease the metabolism of gefitinib, resulting in increased plasma drug levels and increased toxicity (e.g., atazanavir, clarithromycin, diltiazem, erythromycin, GRAPEFRUIT or grapefruit juice, indinavir, isoniazid, itraconazole, ketoconazole, metronidazole, nefazodone, nelfinavir, ritonavir, saquinavir, telithromycin, verapamil, voriconazole). Avoid coadministration. If must coadminister, consider decreasing dose of gefitinib.
- **Drugs that alter the pH** of the upper GI tract may alter gefitinib solubility and absorption, as drug solubility is pH dependent. For example, omeprazole decreases gefitinib AUC by 46%. Avoid concomitant use of gefitinib with proton pump inhibitors, and consider replacement with antacids given a few hours prior to or after gefitinib dose.
- **Warfarin:** Coadministration of gefitinib with warfarin may increase INR with or without bleeding. Monitor patient's INR closely and dose accordingly. Teach patient to report any signs or symptoms of bleeding immediately and to stop warfarin.
- **Vinorelbine:** Gefitinib may increase the neutropenic effect of vinorelbine.
- **Metaprolol:** Gefitinib may increase serum metaprolol levels by 30%; assess for metaprolol toxicity (e.g., bradycardia, hypotension), and lower metaprolol dose as needed.

Contraindications:
- Patients allergic to the drug or its components
- Women who are pregnant or breastfeeding

Warnings:
- **Pulmonary toxicity:** ILD may occur rarely (incidence of about 1%) but has been fatal in one-third of these patients. Mortality is increased in patients with concurrent idiopathic pulmonary fibrosis whose condition worsens while receiving gefitinib. Presentation is often acute, with onset of dyspnea, which may be associated with cough or low-grade fever, and quickly becomes severe, requiring hospitalization. If ILD is suspected, gefitinib should be immediately interrupted; if ILD is confirmed, the drug should be discontinued.
- **Fetotoxicity:** EGFR activation is critical to the developing fetus; thus, gefitinib may cause fetal harm. Women of childbearing potential should use effective contraception and be advised to avoid pregnancy. Treatment should be continued only if potential benefit to mother is greater than risk to the fetus.
- **Hepatotoxicity:** Transient increases in LFTs may occur, so baseline and periodic LFTs should be assessed. Consider drug discontinuance if changes are severe.

Adverse Reactions (**bold** indicates most common, occurring in > 25% of patients):

Cardiovascular: Peripheral edema (2%), QT prolongation

Pulmonary: Dyspnea (2%), ILD (1%)

CNS/neurologic: Asthenia (6%), amblyopia (2%), conjunctivitis (1%); eye pain, corneal erosion/ulcer, sometimes associated with abnormal eyelash growth

Dermatologic: **Rash (43%)**, **acne (25%)**, dry skin (13%), pruritus (8%), vesiculobullous rash (1%), rare toxic epidermal neurolysis

GI: **Diarrhea (48%)**, low-moderate risk of nausea (13%) and/or vomiting (12%), anorexia (7%), mouth ulcers (1%), transient increase in LFTs, rare pancreatitis

General: Angiogedema

Teach patient to call provider if experiencing the following:
- Severe or persistent diarrhea, nausea, anorexia, or vomiting, as these symptoms may lead to dehydration; design nursing assessment and teaching to prevent dehydration
- Onset or worsening of pulmonary symptoms (e.g., shortness of breath or cough)
- Eye irritation
- Any new symptom(s)

Nursing Discussion:
EGFR mutations affect the response to anti-EGFR therapy. Studies showed that patients with specific mutations tended to respond to gefitinib.[85] The mutations were specific activating mutations in exon 21 and deletions in exon 19. An exon is a part of the gene that codes for a protein or parts of the recipe for the protein, and it is numbered. The exons are copied by the mRNA, and enzymes then splice the different exons together so the mRNA contains the complete recipe before it takes it to the ribosomes to make the protein. The entrons are separated from each other by introns. In addition, the patients who responded had increased EGFR gene copy numbers (gene amplification) and also increased HER2 copy numbers (gene amplification).[85]

In NSCLC, frequent EGFR mutations involve either exon 19, characterized by in-frame deletions of specific amino acids, or exon 21 (a point mutation). Of EGFR mutations of responders, 90% had these two mutations, while the remaining 10% had mutations involving exons 18 or 20. The mutations in EGFR activate the kinase activity, and the tumor is dependent upon this mutation for survival (called oncogene addiction). Drugs such as gefitinib that block this activation of the tyrosine kinase (interfere with oncogene addiction) cause the tumor cells to undergo massive apoptosis.[86]

Response was associated with the following characteristics:

- Female
- No history of smoking
- Adenocarcinoma histology
- Asian ethnicity
- Development of rash

The patients who did not respond had primary resistance, which has been shown to occur as a result of having a mutation on exon 20 (specific activating insertion), *KRAS* mutations, absence of total EGFR protein expression, and absence of *PTEN* expression. *PTEN* is a tumor suppressor gene that makes a protein found in most cells. When it is absent, the message to the cell nucleus continues to be sent telling the cell to divide, invade, make VEGF, and metastasize.

For people who do respond, however, over time their tumors develop resistance mechanisms, or secondary resistance. This happens to tyrosine kinase inhibitors like erlotinib and gefitinib through secondary mutations in the EGFR tyrosine kinase domain and amplification (increased gene copy numbers) of the *MET* oncogene. *MET* proto-oncogene is mutated, forming an oncogene in many cancers. It makes the protein product c-Met, which is the receptor for the HGF or scatter factor that helps cancer cells metastasize.[85]

Risk for severe dermatologic reactions, with risk for infection: See prior discussion on nursing management of skin rash and skin appendage assessment and management (see pp. 39–48, management of class effects). Rash is generally less severe than with the EGFRI MAbs.

Risk for diarrhea: Diarrhea is a dose-limiting toxicity. If there is an acute onset, make sure patient is taking gefitinib as directed on an empty stomach. See class effect discussion for full nursing assessment and care planning.

Risk for nausea and vomiting: Drug has low to moderate risk of nausea and/or vomiting. Administer oral antiemetic 60 minutes prior to drug dose if needed.

Reproductive risk: EGFR plays an important role in embryogenesis; thus, blocking this receptor in the fetus may result in altered fetal development. Teach patients of childbearing age to use effective contraception.

Drug: Lapatinib (Tykerb, GW-572016)

Indications: Lapatinib is indicated in combination with capecitabine (Xeloda, a 5-FU prodrug) for the treatment of patients with advanced or metastatic breast cancer whose tumors overexpress HER2 and who have received prior therapy including an anthracycline, a taxane, and trastuzumab.

Class: Multitargeted EGFR tyrosine kinase inhibitor

Mechanism of Action: Lapatinib inhibits the intracellular tyrosine kinase domains of EGFR (erbB1) and HER2 (erbB2), thus stopping the cell proliferation messages sent from the cell surface when ligands bind to the receptors on the cell surface. This stops cell proliferation and invasion. HER2 overexpression occurs in approximately 20–25% of breast cancer patients and is associated with an aggressive type of breast cancer.

Pharmacokinetics: Drug has variable oral absorption with drug identifiable in the serum in 15 minutes. Peak concentrations occur in 4 hours with a steady state reached in 6–7 days with single daily dosing. Dividing the dose results in a twofold higher exposure at steady state. When given with food, systemic exposure is increased threefold with low-fat diet or fourfold with a high-fat diet. Drug is highly protein bound (> 99%). It is a substrate for transporter proteins (e.g., breast cancer resistance protein and P-glycoprotein); yet lapatinib is also able to inhibit these efflux transporters, which helps to keep the chemotherapy within the cancer cell. Drug is extensively metabolized by the CYP3A4 and CYP3A5 microenzyme systems. Terminal half-life of the drug is 14.2 hours, compared to 24 hours with daily dosing. Drug is eliminated by the liver (P450 system), with about 27% recoverable from the feces and < 2% from the urine.

Dosage and Administration:
- 1250 mg PO once daily for 21 days in combination with capecitabine 2000 mg/m^2 PO days 1–14; repeat cycle every 21 days. DO NOT divide lapatinib dose.
- Lapatinib should be given on an empty stomach, at least 1 hour before or 2 hours after a meal; capecitabine should be given twice daily within 30 minutes of a meal and 12 hours apart.
- Dose modify for liver or cardiac toxicity:
  - Cardiotoxicity: NCI-CTCAE version 3.0 grades 2–4: LVEF reflects heart's ability to work as a pump (normal is 55–70%). If LVEF falls to < 50% (grade 2–4) or below the institution's LLN, stop lapatinib for at least 2 weeks until symptoms resolve, with LVEF normal, then restart lapatinib at 1000 mg PO once daily.
  - Hepatic toxicity: Preexisting severe liver impairment (Child-Pugh class C): Reduce dose to 750 mg PO daily for patients with severe hepatic dysfunction. Systemic exposure of lapatinib (AUC) increased 14% in patients with moderate hepatic dysfunction but increased 63% in patients with severe hepatic dysfunction. Discontinue lapatinib if patient develops severe hepatotoxicity while receiving lapatinib.
  - Other NCI-CTCAE version 3.0 toxicities: Interrupt or discontinue lapatinib for grade 2 or greater toxicities, and reinstitute lapatinib when toxicity is grade 1 or less at a lower dose of 1000 mg daily.

Available as: 250-mg tablets in bottles of 250 tablets

Reconstitution and Preparation: None. Store in a tightly closed container at room temperature, out of reach of children and pets. Avoid touching the tablet directly. Wear gloves when handling tablets, and wash hands thoroughly afterward. Bring any tablets not used to the dispensing pharmacy for disposal.

Drug Interactions:

- **Inducers of CYP3A4** may increase the metabolism of lapatinib, thus decreasing the plasma drug concentration (e.g., aminoglutethamine, carbamazepine, dexamethasone, griseofulvin, modafinil, nafcillin, phenobarbital, phenytoin, primidone, rifabutin, rifampin, rifapentine, St. John's wort). Avoid coadministration if possible. If not, consider increasing lapatinib dose gradually to 4500 mg daily. If the interacting drug is stopped, reduce lapatinib dose to 1250 mg PO daily.
- **Inhibitors of CYP3A4** may decrease the metabolism of lapatinib resulting in increased plasma drug levels and increased toxicity (e.g., atazanavir, clarithromycin, diltiazem, erythromycin, GRAPEFRUIT or grapefruit juice, indinavir, isoniazid, itraconazole, ketoconazole, metronidazole, nefazodone, nelfinavir, ritonavir, saquinavir, telithromycin, verapamil, voriconazole). Avoid coadministration. If must coadminister, consider decreasing dose of lapatinib to 500 mg PO daily; if the interacting drug is discontinued, allow a 1-week washout period before increasing lapatinib dose to 1250 mg PO daily.
- Drugs metabolized by the CYP3A4 (e.g., atorvastatin, carbamazepine, cyclosporine, calcium channel blockers, diltiazem, fentanyl, verapamil, warfarin) and CYP2C8 (e.g., amiodarone, paclitaxel, pioglitazone) microenzyme systems: Lapatinib inhibits CYP3A4 and CYP2C8 pathways; assess for toxicity of drug coadministered with lapatinib.
- Lapatinib inhibits the P-glycoprotein (transport system), so if administered with drugs that are substrates of p-glycogen (e.g., cyclosporine, digoxin, loperamide, loratidine, ritonavir, sirolimus, tacrolimus), assess for toxicity of the drug resulting from increased substrate concentrations.
- Drugs that inhibit P-glycoprotein (e.g., amiodarone, cyclosporine, felodipine, nicaripine, propafenone, quinidine, tacrolimus, tamoxifen, testosterone) may increase lapatinib concentration with increased lapatinib toxicity; decrease lapatinib dose as needed.

Contraindications: None

Warnings:

- **Decreased LVEF** has been reported. Monitor baseline and periodic gated blood pool scans (multiple gated acquisition, or MUGA) or echocardiogram, and modify lapatinib dose as needed.

- **Hepatotoxicity:** May cause hepatotoxicity. Monitor LFTs baseline and every 4–6 weeks during treatment. Stop lapatinib and do not resume if patient develops severe changes in LFTs.
- **Severe diarrhea** may occur. Manage with antidiarrheal medications, and prevent dehydration and electrolyte imbalance by repleting fluids and electrolytes as needed.
- **ILD and pneumonitis** have occurred. Discontinue lapatinib if patient develops severe pulmonary symptoms.
- **QT prolongation:** Consider baseline assessment of QT interval on ECG and periodically during treatment. Avoid coadministration with other drugs that prolong the QT interval (e.g., atypical antipsychotics such as olanzapine; erythromycin, fluoroquinolone antibiotics; serotonin receptor blocker antiemetics; prochlorperazine), or monitor patient closely. Ensure electrolytes, such as magnesium, calcium, and potassium, remain normal.

Adverse Reactions (**bold** indicates most common, occurring in > 25% of patients):

Cardiovascular: QT prolongation, decreased LVEF

Pulmonary: Dyspnea (12%), rare ILD

CNS/neurologic: Insomnia (10%)

Dermatologic (with capecitabine): **Palmar–plantar erythrodysesthesia (hand–foot syndrome) (53%), rash (28%)**, dry skin (10%)

GI: **Diarrhea (65%), nausea (44%), vomiting (26%)**, stomatitis (14%), dyspepsia (11%); hepatotoxicity with increased LFTs (total bilirubin [45%], AST [49%], ALT [37%])

Hematologic: **Expected bone marrow depression with capecitabine anemia (56%)**, thrombocytopenia (18%), neutropenia (22%)

Musculoskeletal: Pain in extremity (12%), back (11%)

General: Mucosal irritation (15%)

Teach patient to call provider right away if experiencing the following:
- Severe or persistent diarrhea, nausea, or vomiting, as these symptoms may lead to dehydration; design nursing assessment and teaching to prevent dehydration
- Onset or worsening of pulmonary symptoms (e.g., shortness of breath or cough)
- Palpitations
- Any new symptom(s)

Nursing Discussion:

EGFRI rash: See discussion in class effects section (pp. 39–48) for assessment and management.

ILD: See discussion in class effects section (pp. 39–48) for assessment and management.

Diarrhea: Diarrhea is a significant toxicity of capecitabine, which is given together with lapatinib. Teach patient the importance of drinking 2–3 L/day in divided glasses every hour while awake to avoid dehydration. Antidiarrheal medications such as loperamide are effective. It is very important for the nurse to be proactive to prevent severe diarrhea by teaching the patient to take loperamide when diarrhea starts and to continue aggressive oral hydration. See section on class effects (pp. 39–48).

Hepatotoxicity: May be severe, so it is important to assess patient's baseline LFTs and monitor every 4–6 weeks. If the patient has severe hepatic impairment, the starting dose of lapatinib is 750 mg instead of 1250 mg PO daily. Hepatotoxicity occurs days to several months after starting treatment. If changes in the LFTs are severe, lapatinib therapy should be discontinued.

Decreased LVEF: LVEF reflects the percentage of blood pumped out of the left ventricle (LV) of the heart. It is calculated by the volume ejected from the LV divided by the volume of blood in the ventricle after it fills. Normal LVEF is 50% or 55–75%. Assess that a baseline MUGA or echocardiogram has been done and that the LVEF is normal. Test should be repeated periodically during therapy, and drug should be interrupted if LVEF falls to < 50% or is 20% less than baseline. Monitor patients with uncontrolled or symptomatic angina, arrhythmias, or CHF very closely. The mechanism of cardiotoxicity appears different from that of trastuzumab. Lapatinib appears to activate AMP-activated protein kinase,[*] which stimulates a metabolic stress response in human cardiomyocytes. This process protects the cardiac cells from TNFα, which is often elevated in patients with cancer as a result of high numbers of circulating proinflammatory cytokines.[88]

Prolonged QT interval: Assess patient's risk for prolonged QT interval (e.g., medication profile; baseline magnesium, calcium, and potassium values) and results of baseline ECG. If QT interval is prolonged, discuss plan with physician/nurse practitioner/physician's assistant. Ensure hypomagnesemia and hypokalemia are corrected before patient leaves the clinical area to start lapatinib therapy at home. If patient has risk, or if in doubt, repeat ECG (for QT interval) periodically during therapy. Torsades de pointes can occur when patients have hypomagnesemia, hypocalcemia, and hypokalemia with an increasing QT interval. Of note, the serotonin-receptor antagonist antiemetics have the potential to increase QT interval.

Lapatinib appears to cross the blood–brain barrier, so is being studied in combination with trastuzumab to see if the combination is superior to each drug used separately. Patients with HER2-positive breast cancer often develop brain metastasis on trastuzumab.

---

[*] AMP-activated protein kinase is an enzyme that is important for controlling cellular energy, including disposition of fatty acids and insulin secretion.

Drug self-administration: Drug regimen is complex in that lapatinib must be given as a single dose (five pills) 1 hour before or 2 hours after a meal, while capecitabine must be given within 30 minutes of a meal, and the doses 12 hours apart. An example of a regimen would be 8 a.m. capecitabine with breakfast, 10 a.m. lapatinib, and 8 p.m. capecitabine after dinner.

Lapatinib is available through a restrictive distribution program called *Tykerb* CARES. This program is intended to make it easier for patients to receive the drug if they need assistance with reimbursement issues and to help them adhere to the oral regimen. The physician should enroll the patient in the program to receive lapatinib as follows:

- Complete the *Tykerb* CARES enrollment form (obtained by phone, 1-866-4-TYKERB, or online at www.tykerb.com/hcp/resources-and-patient-support/tykerb-cares.html).
- Fax completed form back to GlaxoSmithKline at 1-866-272-9439, or call 1-866-4-TYKERB (1-866-489-5372) for instructions.

The program will teach patients about lapatinib and will verify the patient's insurance coverage or need for financial assistance. Once reimbursement is verified, specialty pharmacies that provide lapatinib will be identified (they are listed on the Web site). Prescriptions are filled by mail order and can be sent directly to the patient or to the provider.

Specific HER2-Inhibiting Drugs

Drug: Trastuzumab (Herceptin)

Indications: Trastuzumab is indicated for the treatment of patients with HER2-positive breast cancer:
- Adjuvant treatment of HER2-overexpressing node-positive or node-negative (ER/PR negative or with one high-risk feature) breast cancer, as part of a treatment regimen (doxorubicin, cyclophosphamide, paclitaxel, or docetaxel; OR docetaxel and carboplatin; OR as a single agent following multimodality anthracycline-based therapy)
- Treatment of HER2-overexpressing metastatic breast cancer in combination with paclitaxel for first-line treatment, OR as a single agent in patients who have received one or more chemotherapy regimens for metastatic disease

Class: HER2 receptor antagonist MAb, humanized

Mechanism of Action: Trastuzumab is an IgG_1 recombinant MAb that binds to the extracellular domain of the human EGF receptor-2 protein, HER2. HER2 is an oncogene. It blocks the HER2 (erbB2) receptors on cancer cells, which, because they have too many copies of the HER2 gene, have too many HER2 protein receptors on the outside of the cell. Of patients with breast cancer, 25–30% have

HER2 overexpression, connoting an aggressive type of breast cancer. These protein receptors turn on a signal telling the nucleus of the cell to make more cancer cells. By binding to the HER2 receptors on the outside of the cell, trastuzumab, a humanized MAb with a long half-life, continuously suppresses HER2 activity on the cell surface that may lead to tumor proliferation, thus preventing proliferation. In addition, it recruits immune cells and activates them. Because it is a strong stimulator of ADCC, it binds to the HER2 receptor, then calls in immune effector cells to destroy the breast cancer cell, leading to cell stasis and cell death.

Pharmacokinetics: Initial studies using a loading dose of 4 mg/kg followed by a weekly maintenance dose of 2 mg/kg produced a mean half-life of 5.8 days (range 1–32 days). When a loading dose of 8 mg/kg is given, followed by 6 mg/kg every 3 weeks, the mean half-life is 16 days (11–23 days). Drug reaches a steady state between weeks 16 and 32. Trastuzumab does not appear to alter the serum levels of coadministered chemotherapy agents.

Dosage and Administration:
- **Adjuvant breast cancer**, for a total of 52 weeks—dose and schedule options:
  - During and following paclitaxel, docetaxel, or docetaxel/carboplatin:
    - Initial dose of 4 mg/kg as an IV infusion over 90 minutes, then at 2 mg/kg as an IV infusion over 30 minutes weekly during chemotherapy for the first 12 weeks (paclitaxel or docetaxel) OR 18 weeks (docetaxel/carboplatin)
    - One week following the last weekly dose of trastuzumab, administer trastuzumab at 6 mg/kg as an IV infusion over 30–90 minutes every 3 weeks
  - As a single agent within 3 weeks following completion of multi-modality, anthracycline-based chemotherapy regimens:
    - Initial dose at 8 mg/kg as an IV infusion over 90 minutes
    - Subsequent doses at 6 mg/kg as an IV infusion over 30–90 minutes every 3 weeks
- **Metastatic breast cancer:**
  - Administer trastuzumab, alone or in combination with paclitaxel, at an initial dose of 4 mg/kg as a 90-minute IV infusion followed by subsequent once weekly doses of 2 mg/kg as a 30-minute IV infusion until disease progression.
- **Dose modifications:**
  - **Infusion reactions:**
    - Mild or moderate infusion reactions: Decrease infusion rate.
    - Clinically significant infusion reactions, dyspnea, or hypotension: Interrupt infusion.
    - Severe or life-threatening infusion reactions: Discontinue trastuzumab.

- **Cardiomyopathy:** Assess LVEF baseline and at regular intervals during treatment.
  - ◆ Hold trastuzumab for at least 4 weeks if (1) there is a ≥ 16% absolute decrease in LVEF from pretreatment values, or (2) LVEF is below institutional LLN and ≥ 10% absolute decrease in LVEF from pretreatment values.
  - ◆ Trastuzumab may be resumed if, within 4–8 weeks, the LVEF returns to normal and the absolute decrease from baseline is ≤ 15%.
  - ◆ Permanently discontinue trastuzumab for a persistent (> 8 weeks) LVEF decline or if trastuzumab dose had to be held more than three times for cardiomyopathy.

Available as: 440-mg lyophilized powder per multi-use vial. Requires refrigeration at 2–8°C (36–46°F). DO NOT FREEZE.

Reconstitution and Preparation:
- Reconstitute with 20-mL bacteriostatic water for injection USP containing 1.1% benzyl alcohol, which is supplied with each vial. DO NOT SHAKE.
- Reconstituted solution contains 21 mg/mL. Further dilute desired dose in 250 mL of 0.9% sodium chloride injection USP. DO NOT use dextrose (5%) solution.
- Vial is designed for multiple use and is stable for 28 days following reconstitution if kept at 2–8°C (36–46°F). If the patient is hypersensitive to benzyl alcohol, use 20-mL sterile water for injection without preservatives as a single-use solution (NOT multidose).

Drug Interactions: Paclitaxel in combination with trastuzumab increases trastuzumab serum levels 150%.

Contraindications: **None**

Warnings:
- **Cardiomyopathy** risk is greatest if given concomitantly with an anthracycline, so this is avoided. Incidence of CHF is 2% when trastuzumab is given with paclitaxel or docetaxel following AC (Adriamycin [doxorubicin], Cytoxan [cyclophosphamide]), and 2% when trastuzumab is given alone after chemotherapy. However, when docetaxel, carboplatin, and trastuzumab are given together, the incidence of CHF is only 0.4% (control is 0.3%). Follow LVEF assessment outlined under dose modifications. LVEF reflects the percentage of blood pumped out of the LV of the heart. It is calculated by the volume ejected from the LV divided by the volume of blood in the ventricle after it fills. Normal LVEF is 55–75%.
- **Infusion reactions** are characterized by fever and chills, and may also include nausea, vomiting, pain (sometimes at tumor site), headache, dizziness, dyspnea, hypotension, rash, and asthenia. However, serious and sometimes fatal infusion reactions can occur, often on the first infusion,

characterized by bronchospasm, anaphylaxis, angioedema, hypoxia, and severe hypotension. Death, when it occurred, happened within hours or days of the serious infusion reaction. Interrupt the infusion if the patient has dyspnea or clinically significant hypotension and begin medical intervention to reverse the reaction, including epinephrine, oxygen, corticosteroids, diphenhydramine, and bronchodilators.

- **Pulmonary toxicity and fusion reactions** occur and can be fatal, characterized by dyspnea, interstitial pneumonitis, pulmonary infiltrates, pleural effusions, noncardiogenic pulmonary edema, pulmonary insufficiency, hypoxia, ARDS, and pulmonary fibrosis. These conditions can occur after serious infusion reaction. Highest risk is in patients with extensive lung involvement by tumor, resulting in dyspnea at rest.
- **Exacerbation of chemotherapy-induced neutropenia:** Risk for febrile neutropenia is higher in patients receiving trastuzumab in combination with myelosuppressive chemotherapy. Fortunately, the risk of septic death is not increased.
- **HER2 testing should be performed by laboratories with demonstrated proficiency** to ensure accurate identification of HER2 overexpression and of HER2 gene amplification. HER2 overexpression can be tested by measuring HER2 protein using IHC or HercepTest. Gene amplification can be assessed by FISH tests. A negative FISH test does not rule out HER2 overexpression and potential benefit from trastuzumab. Overexpression means the gene product or protein is measured on the outside of the cell. Amplification means the actual extra numbers of the gene are counted to confirm gene amplification (inside the DNA).
- **Fetotoxicity:** May cause oligohydramnios during the 2nd and 3rd trimesters, and fetal harm when administered to a pregnant woman. Register pregnant patients at 1-800-690-6720.

Adverse Reactions (**bold** indicates most common, occurring in > 25% of patients):

- **Most common > 2% compared to control—adjuvant:** Fatigue, infection, neutropenia, anemia, myalgia, dyspnea, rash/desquamation, headache, diarrhea, nausea
- **Most common > 2% compared to control—metastatic:** Nausea, fever, infection, rash, increased cough, vomiting, diarrhea, headache, anemia

Cardiovascular: Peripheral edema (10%), tachycardia (5%), hypertension (4%), decreased LVEF (3.5%), palpitations (3%), cardiac arrhythmias (3%), CHF (2%), cardiac failure (0.5%), ventricular dysfunction (0.2%)

Pulmonary: Nasopharyngitis (8%), cough (5%), dyspnea (3%), rhinitis (2%), pharyngolaryngeal pain (2%), sinusitis (2%), pulmonary hypertension (0.2%), ILD (0.2%)

CNS/neurologic: Headache (10%), dizziness (4%), paresthesia (2%)

Dermatologic: Rash (4%), nail disorders (2%), pruritus (2%)

GI: Diarrhea (7%), nausea (6%), vomiting (3.5%), constipation (2%), upper abdominal pain (2%)

Hematologic: Increased febrile neutropenia when combined with myelosuppressive chemotherapy

Renal: Nephritic syndrome (rare) occurring 4–18 months after beginning therapy

Musculoskeletal: Arthralgia (8%), back pain (5%), myalgia (4%), bone pain (3%), muscle spasm (3%)

General: **Infusion reactions (40%) within 1–2 hours of starting the infusion (initial) with risk decreasing to 20% with subsequent infusions,** flu syndrome (10%; chills, fever, malaise), pyrexia (6%), allergic reactions (3%)

Teach patient to contact a healthcare professional immediately for any of the following: New onset or worsening shortness of breath, cough, swelling of the ankles/legs, swelling of the face, palpitations, weight gain of more than 5 pounds in 24 hours, dizziness, or loss of consciousness

Pregnancy:
- Teach women of reproductive potential to use effective contraception methods during treatment and for a minimum of 6 months following the end of treatment.
- Encourage pregnant women who are using trastuzumab to enroll in the Herceptin Pregnancy Registry.

Nursing Discussion:

Cardiac assessment: **The HER2 signaling pathway is a repair pathway.** Trastuzumab-induced injury to the heart is different from that induced by anthracycline chemotherapy, which results in death of the cardiomyocyte or heart cells, probably from free radical injury.[89,90] Trastuzumab-induced injury is not completely understood. It may be due to a drug–drug interaction, induction of immune-mediated destruction of cardiomyocytes, defects in HER2 signaling required for cardiac contractility, an indirect consequence of trastuzumab-related effects outside the heart, or a decrease in HER2-mediated survival of the cardiomyocytes.[91]

Trastuzumab-induced cardiotoxicity is not dose-related and may regress with stopping trastuzumab and/or effective cardiac management of CHF. In fact, some patients have a spontaneous 20% increase in LVEF to baseline when trastuzumab is continued at full dose and without cardiac medications.[91] Reversibility of trastuzumab heart failure has also been documented by others,[92] but does not occur in all patients.[93] However, Seidman et al. found that 80% of patients had symptomatic improvement with standard medical therapy.[94] Risk factors for development are previous anthracycline drug exposure (e.g., doxorubicin), prior chest wall radiation, and prior heart dysfunction (e.g., LVEF < 50% preexisting heart failure).

There is increasing discussion in the medical community about replacing anthracyclines in breast cancer management, as the combination of docetaxel (Taxotere), carboplatin, and trastuzumab (Herceptin), called the TCH regimen, has a very low incidence of cardiac dysfunction (0.4%, compared to 0.3% of the control and 1.9% in the doxorubicin arms) with equal efficacy.[95] The oral tyrosine kinase inhibitor lapatinib has less cardiotoxicity, with no patients withdrawing from treatment due to LVEF dysfunction, no cases of CHF, and a fall of only 1.9% in LVEF reduction, which was asymptomatic. Thus, lapatinib may be a good alternative and is being studied in the treatment of patients with HER2-positive breast cancer in the adjuvant, neoadjuvant, and metastatic settings.[90] LVEF was assessed baseline before the doxorubicin, after completion of a doxorubicin-containing regimen (e.g., AC), and before trastuzumab was started, and during trastuzumab, every 3 months. The patient's LVEF should be assessed every 6 months for 2 years after completing adjuvant trastuzumab therapy.

The following recommendations provide a framework to assess the patient's LVEF.[96] Cardiac monitoring of LVEF should be performed by echocardiogram or MUGA baseline and every 3 months with the same test. Patients who develop heart failure and LVEF < 40% should receive an angiotensin-converting enzyme inhibitor (ACEI) if they are asymptomatic patients; they should receive both an ACEI inhibitor and beta-blocker if they have a recent or remote history of MI regardless of heart failure to prevent progression and death.[97] Table 2-5 gives assessment and management guidelines that are generally accepted as the standard.

The nurse should do a focused cardiac assessment on patients who will be or are receiving trastuzumab.[99] The patient history should be reviewed for risk factors: family history, hypertension, diabetes, coronary artery disease, valvular heart disease, any prior MI or angina, and sleep apnea. In addition, the nurse should identify patient's smoking status and history; alcohol intake; and exposure to anthracyclines, trastuzumab, other HER2-targeted agents or tyrosine kinase inhibitors, or RT to the chest. Finally, the history should review if the patient has any symptoms of heart failure. The right side of the heart is thin and low pressure, so it fails first. Then, the blood backs into the lungs, and the left side of the heart fails. Symptoms of right-sided heart failure are related to fluid accumulation and include dyspnea, orthopnea (increased dyspnea when lying flat), paroxysmal nocturnal dyspnea, difficulty sleeping lying flat in bed (which can be approximated by asking how many pillows the person uses to sleep at night), increased abdominal girth, bloating, peripheral edema in lower extremities, decreased appetite, nausea, cough, weight gain. Because there is less blood returning to the heart and less blood being pumped out of the LV, the heart in-

Table 2-5   Assessment and Guidelines for Managing Asymptomatic Patients Receiving Trastuzumab

Relationship of LVEF to LLN* in asymptomatic patients	Absolute ↓ of < 10% from baseline	Absolute ↓ of 10–15% from baseline	Absolute ↓ of ≥ 16% from baseline
Within normal limits	Continue	Continue	Hold[†]
1–5% below LLN	Continue	Hold*	Hold[†]
≥ 6% below LLN	Continue	Hold*	Hold[†]

*LLN = 50–55%; †Repeat LVEF assessment after 4 weeks; if criteria are met, resume trastuzumab. If drug is held two consecutive times, or a total of three times, discontinue trastuzumab. Data from Mackey et al.[96]; Popat and Smith[90]; Goldberg and Jessup[97]; Hunt et al.[98]

creases its heart rate and breathing rate. Symptoms of left-sided heart failure are due to decreased cardiac output. They include chest pain, palpitations, fatigue, weakness, exercise intolerance, decreased alertness, confusion, lightheadedness, decreased urination, and urination at night (nocturia). Nocturia results when the person lies down and fluid that has seeped into the third space [extravascular spaces] comes back into the bloodstream, increasing venous return and blood flow to the kidneys.

The nurse then does a focused physical exam looking for signs of heart failure.[99] Signs include changes in skin appearance (color, moisture, texture), changes in BP, tachycardia, tachypnea (rapid breathing rate), decreased oxygen saturation, elevated jugular venous pressure, abnormal heart sounds (S_3 gallop, murmurs), adventitious lung sounds that should not be present in a normal exam (such as crackles, which reflect the air passing over airway secretions), edema, abdominal ascites, and enlarged liver in the RUQ of the abdomen.

Reassure patients that CHF is uncommon and that they are being closely followed with tests that show any changes in their heart's ability to pump. Teach patients that although uncommon, CHF may occur and that they should report new onset or worsening of shortness of breath, swelling of legs or ankles, swelling of the face, palpitations, weight gain of 5 or more pounds in 24 hours, dizziness, or loss of consciousness.

The nurse should review the baseline MUGA scan or echocardiogram. In general, the low limit of normal is 50–55%. It is important to know the baseline value so that decreases can be determined. In addition, review the results of patient's fasting lipid profile and any other tests for cardiac function/disease that the physician ordered based on the assessment. If the patient smokes, encourage smoking cessation strategies, including resources to help the person quit. During adjuvant trastuzumab, the LVEF should be repeated every 3 months routinely. If there is a decrease in the LVEF and the drug is held, then assessment is repeated after at least 4 weeks. If the patient has signs and symptoms of CHF, the nurse can discuss with the physician/nurse practitioner/physician's assistant assessing a B-type natriuretic peptide to determine if the patient is in failure and referral to a cardiologist.[100,101]

Risk for heart failure has been diagramed by the American Heart Association.[97] Stage A includes patients at risk for heart failure but without structural heart disease or symptoms of heart failure, such as patients with hypertension, atherosclerotic heart disease, diabetes, obesity, or metabolic syndrome; those using cardiotoxic anticancer agents; or those with a family history of cardiomyopathy. Therapy is aimed at controlling hypertension, abnormal lipid profile, and metabolic syndrome; assisting in smoking cessation; and encouraging regular exercise and reduction in alcohol intake and illicit drug use. At this stage, drugs that may be used are ACEIs, or angiotensin II receptor blockers (ARBs) for patients with vascular disease or diabetes.

Stage B patients have structural heart disease but no signs or symptoms of heart failure. This group includes patients with previous MI, left ventricular hypertrophy or remodeling, low ejection fraction, or asymptomatic valvular heart disease. Goals are the same as in stage A, and drugs include ACEIs, ARBs, and now beta-blockers. Implantable defibrillators can be implanted in patients at risks for arrhythmias.

Stage C includes patients with structural heart disease with prior or current symptoms of heart failure. Stage D includes patients who have refractory heart failure requiring specialized interventions, including palliative care.

HER2 overexpression has been demonstrated in 20% of patients with gastric cancer, and trastuzumab is being tested in this population.[102] In addition, certain patients with ovarian cancer or NSCLC may overexpress HER2, and they are being studied as well.

Investigational Agents

Drug: Trastuzumab-DM1

Indication: Investigational; being studied in breast cancer

Class: First in class HER2 antibody-drug conjugate (ADC)

Mechanism of Action: MAb trastuzumab is attached to a very toxic antimicrotubular poison DM1, via the linker molecule methylmethcathinone, which provides a stable bond between the two agents. Trastuzumab goes directly to and binds to the HER2 overexpressed antigen like a guided bullet. The trastuzumab-linker-DM1 is brought into the cell (internalized), and the linker then releases the DM1 cellular poison into the cell. The resulting intracellular damage kills the cell and spares normal cells. Trastuzumab in the conjugate drug has the same affinity to HER2 as trastuzumab alone. The drug binds to HER2 tightly, thus inhibiting cell signaling and cell proliferation. Trastuzumab alone is believed to act through three different mechanisms: (1) the antagonizing function of the growth-signaling properties of HER2, (2) signaling immune cells to attack and kill malignant cells with this receptor (ADCC), and (3) synergistic and/or additive effects seen with many chemotherapeutic agents. DM1 is a mitotic tubulin inhibitor 20 times more potent than vincristine. It is a maytansinoid derivative. Studies have shown the compound is active in HER2-positive, trastuzumab-refractory tumors. In addition, normal cell lines are unaffected.[103]

Pharmacokinetics: Trastuzumab alone has a mean half-life of 5.8 days when dosed weekly compared with a range of 1–32 days and a mean half-life of 16 days (range of 11–23 days) when given every 3 weeks. Steady state is reached between weeks 6 and 37. Metabolism of the conjugate molecule, including half-life and time to steady state, is currently being studied.

Dosage and Administration: Per protocol. One protocol studied 1.2–2.9 mg/kg. Maximum tolerated dose is 3.6 mg/kg when given every 3 weeks and 2.4 mg/kg when given weekly.[104–106] Activity and safety are similar between every 1-week and every three-week dosing.

Available as: Per protocol

Reconstitution and Preparation: Per protocol, as an IV infusion

Drug Interactions: Unknown

Adverse Reactions (**bold** indicates most common, occurring in > 25% of patients):

Cardiac: Decreased LVEF

Metabolic: Hypokalemia

Pulmonary: Dyspnea, pleural effusion

GI: **Elevated hepatic transaminases**, constipation

Hematological: **Anemia**, **thrombocytopenia**

Musculoskeletal: Chest pain, muscular weakness, arthralgias

General: Fatigue, headache

Nursing Issues: Drug has shown considerable activity in patients who have received extensive previous therapy with trastuzumab with tumor shrinkage. There appears to be some cardiac toxicity at maximum tolerated dose, but it did not require interruption of therapy and was not a dose-limiting toxicity.[106] Because normal cells are not targeted, there is infrequent and manageable toxicity.

Most common were thrombocytopenia grade 1, fatigue, constipation, arthalgias, headache, muscular weakness, musculoskeletal chest pain, dyspnea, and pleural effusion.

Drug: Pertuzumab (Omnitarg, rhuMab 2C4, investigational)

Indications: Investigational; being studied in breast, prostate, and ovarian cancers

Class: HER dimerization inhibitor; first drug of its class

Mechanism of Action: Pertuzumab is a recombinant, humanized MAb that blocks EGFR on the outside of the cell from partnering with a neighboring receptor (called dimerization), which is necessary to "turn on" the receptor or activate it to start sending a growth signal to the cell nucleus. Normally, a growth factor (ligand) attaches to the HER. The growth factor receptor then needs to dimerize or pair with another growth factor receptor to activate the receptor tyrosine kinase; for example, HER2 receptor needs to dimerize or pair with another HER, such as HER1. Pertuzumab is an IgG_1 MAb that binds to the dimerization domain of HER so the binding of the antibody directly inhibits the ability of HER2 to dimerize with other HER (EGFR) proteins. This disrupts the activation of downstream effectors, notably the AKT pathway (which is needed for cell survival), and the growth signal is not sent. The cell then undergoes programmed cell death. It appears to be active against tumors that do not overexpress HER2.

Pertuzumab appears to be synergistic with trastuzumab for the following reasons: (1) Trastuzumab alone continually suppresses HER2 activity and flags cancer cells for destruction by the immune system, but it does not inhibit HER2 dimerization, while (2) Pertuzumab inhibits HER2 dimerization, suppresses multiple HER2 signaling pathways, and also flags cancer cells for destruction by the immune system.[107]

Pharmacokinetics: Unknown. Drug may need to be administered with chemotherapy or trastuzumab to improve response.

Dosage and Administration: Per protocol. Studies have included doses 0.5–15 mg/kg every 3 weeks.

Available as: Per protocol

Reconstitution and Preparation: Per protocol, as an IV infusion

Drug Interactions: Unknown

Contraindications: Per protocol

Warnings: Per protocol

Adverse Reactions (**bold** indicates most common, occurring in > 25% of patients):

Cardiovascular: Rare drop in LVEF in patients with metastatic breast cancer who had previously received anthracycline drugs such as doxorubicin

Dermatologic: **Rash**

GI: **Diarrhea, nausea, vomiting**

General: **Fatigue**

Nursing Issues: Drug is being studied prospectively in the phase III CLEOPATRA trial comparing patients with trastuzumab with or without pertuzumab, as there appears to be synergy with the two agents. Side effects are mild and generally grade 1 or 2.[107]

HEPATOCYTE GROWTH FACTOR (HGF/C-MET) RECEPTOR PATHWAY TARGETS

HGF is a very powerful growth factor that can activate many different biologic events by turning on or activating the c-Met receptor on the cell surface (membrane). Multiple biologic processes that are critical in embryogenesis are started. HGF is the only known ligand for c-Met and is so named because it stimulates the growth of liver cells or hepatocytes. It is secreted by fibroblasts (mesenchymal cells). The proto-oncogene *MET* codes for the receptor tyrosine kinase c-Met on the cell membrane, also called hepatocyte growth factor receptor. The *MET* proto-oncogene can be turned on (transcribed) by HGF, hypoxia-inducible factor-1 (HIF1), and other growth factors.

As discussed in Chapter 1, *MET* stands for mesenchymal–epithelial transition factor, and it is critical in embryogenesis to make the germinal disc into a three-dimensional shape, allowing some cells to transform from epithelial-behaving cells to a mesenchymal cell shape and behavior so the cells can move to the correct anatomical parts prior to becoming specialized (a process called epithelial–mesenchymal transition); thus, angiogenesis, myoblast migration (muscle), bone remodeling, and nerve sprouting are ebabled.[108]

In the adult, *MET* is necessary for the liver to regenerate and for wound healing. Because it is potentially such a powerful receptor, the c-Met receptor is normally expressed only by stem cells and progenitor cells so it can move cells (invade) or regenerate injured tissue. C-Met membrane receptor, a protein receptor kinase, is expressed by epithelial and endothelial cells, neurons, hepatocytes, hematopoietic cells, and melanocyte cells, but HGF expression is found only in mesenchymal cells.[109] It regulates cell growth, cell motility, and cell shape once the ligand HGF binds to its receptor c-Met and activates a signaling cascade. It facilitates epithelial and endothelial cell function and has a role in tissue regeneration. In angiogenesis, it stimulates cell growth, motility, and invasion of the extracellular matrix. However, as discussed in Chapter 1, HGF is the ligand for the cell membrane protein kinase receptor c-Met and is very involved in cancer invasion and metastasis.

HGF is also called "scatter factor," as it helps cancer cells "scatter" or disseminate.[110] Thus, once again, embryological processes are reactivated by the cancer process, as the "software" is already programmed in the cells. It appears that cancer stem cells acquire the ability to express *MET* so that cancer cells can continue to proliferate, invade, and metastasize.[109] In this instance, it is the invasive growth pathway where cells can "scatter" or, with the help of MMPs, disassociate from their neighboring cells.[108,109] This is combined with the ability of HGF to activate c-Met to activate powerful pathways that drive cancer such as RAS, P13K, STST3, and beta-catenin, as well as angiogenesis. As one might imagine, if the *MET* proto-oncogene is mutated, amplified, or dysregulated, or if its ligand and/or receptor is overexpressed, or if it has abnormal autocrine loops or paracrine loops activating the receptor, cancer soon follows, as the activated c-Met receptor stimulates malignant cell growth, angiogenesis, invasion, and metastasis.[3] Each of these potential flaws is a target for anticancer therapy. The c-Met pathway elements are mutated or dysregulated in liver, gastric, breast, brain, and head and neck cancers. In addition, in hereditary papillary renal cancer, MET mutation and activation is the principal malignant flaw.

Specifically, signaling through the c-Met pathway involves connection (communication) with multiple other signaling systems, such as src, Grb2/SOS, P13 kinase, and Gab1, all of which result in changes that let the cell leave its secure anchorage in normal cells without dying, and to invade and metastasize. Changes in motility, shape, adhesion, and resistance to apoptosis enable the cell to achieve anchorage independence.[111,112] As c-Met helps transform cells into invasive malignant cells, it interacts with integrins to activate tissue invasion.[111] Integrin $\alpha6\beta4$ acts as a cofactor to c-Met signaling to help in cell growth and proliferation.[111] It interacts with *PTEN*, a tumor suppressor gene that codes for the protein PTEN, which, when normal, interferes with c-Met signaling.[113] Once HGF activates the c-Met receptor, the multiple signaling pathways can be summarized as follows[3,109]:

1. RAS pathway communicates the message to invade, scatter, and proliferate. HGF stimulation of the receptor is constant and sustained, so there is prolonged MAPK stimulation.

2. P13K pathway is activated by RAS, as it lies downstream from RAS, or by a separate docking site with resulting cell motility, reshaping or remodeling of the extracellular matrix, and survival via the AKT pathway.

3. STAT3 pathway, together with sustained MAPK signaling, results in HGF-stimulated branching of tissue. STAT3 is a protein that is phosphorylated by receptor-associated kinases, stimulating it to move from the cytoplasm of the cell into the nucleus, where it acts as transcription factor. It is critical for the renewal of embryonic stem cells.

4. Wnt signaling (specifically the beta-catenin pathway), once activated by

c-Met signaling, moves to the cell nucleus and turns on or off a number of genes.

5. Notch pathway is activated via the delta ligand (DLL3).

Drugs are being tested that target each of the potential targets. Two examples are:

- A neutralizing MAb targets the ligand HGF. AMG-102 is a IgG$_1$ human MAb that targets the ligand HGF.[114] In phase I clinical trials, a 20 mg/kg dose was shown to be safe and tolerable; dose limiting toxicities were dyspnea/hypoxia and GI bleed, while other toxicities were fatigue, constipation, anorexia, nausea, and vomiting.[3]

- Inhibit c-Met tyrosine kinase and other pathway biologic processes. XL880, now called GSK1363089, is an oral, small molecule inhibitor of multiple receptor tyrosine kinases c-Met and VEGFR, and it also inhibits PDGFR-β, c-KIT, FLT3, Tie-2, and RON (recepteur d'origine nantais, a receptor tyrosine kinase overexpressed or constitutively active in some epithelial cancers[115]). Drug has been studied in patients with gastric cancer who have MET amplification at 7q31 and who are sensitive to MET inhibition,[116] as well as in patients with hereditary papillary renal cell cancer.

INSULIN-LIKE GROWTH FACTOR RECEPTOR PATHWAY TARGETS

IGF-1 is very important in children's growth and is anabolic in the adult, affecting every cell in the human body. It is a ligand of and binds to the IGF-1R, where it is a powerful stimulator of AKT signaling, which, as previously discussed, leads to cell growth and proliferation, and avoidance of apoptosis. IGF-1 and insulin both bind to the IGF-1R but IGF-1 has a significantly stronger affinity than insulin. Once IGF-1 binds and activates IGF-1R, there is autophosphorylation and activation of the P13k/Akt/mTOR and MAPK pathways. As these pathways continue the signaling to the cell nucleus, the message tells the cell how to regulate cell growth, to protect the cell from apoptosis, to start differentiation of the cell, and to regulate angiogenesis via VEGF.[117]

Gunter et al. studied the rate of incident breast cancer among a case-cohort of nondiabetic women who were enrolled in the Women's Health Initiative Observational Study, a prospective cohort of 93,676 postmenopausal women.[118] They compared fasting serum samples of insulin, glucose, total IGF-1, free IGF-1, IGF binding protein-3, body mass index, and risk of breast cancer among 835 women who developed incident breast cancer and 816 randomly chosen women. They found that hyperinsulinemia is an independent risk factor for breast cancer and that this likely will help explain the obesity–breast cancer relationship related to insulin resistance. Kabat et al. also used a cohort of women from the Women's Health Initiative and used repeated measures to analyze breast cancer risk in postmenopausal women, finding that the link between elevated insulin level and breast cancer was strongest among lean women and weakest among obese women.[119] These findings suggest that insulin may be independent of obesity but that both hyperinsulinemia and high endogenous estradiol levels were independent risk factors, and as such could explain the association between obesity and the risk of breast cancer. However, the authors state that these results must be confirmed by additional studies.

Studies have shown that breast cancer cells are stimulated to proliferate at physiologic levels of insulin.[120] However, there are studies implicating the insulin receptor and the IGF-II receptor, which does not have any tyrosine kinase signaling ability.[3] Because of the potential toxicities (e.g., Type II diabetes, osteoporotic fractures, and ischemic heart disease), blockade of these potential targets has not been studied. No IGF-1R has been FDA approved yet, and all are still undergoing clinical testing. Agents being tested block the IGF-1R. Of interest, IGF-1R overexpression confers a poor prognosis in clear cell renal cell cancer, but expression can be inhibited by the von Hippel–Lindau (VHL) tumor suppressor gene. However, when the VHL tumor suppressor gene is inactivated, IGF-1R is upregulated (turned up).[121]

CP-721871 is being studied in a phase III study of patients with NSCLC, and a phase II study of patients with breast, colorectal, lung, or prostate cancer.[3] This agent is an IgG_2 MAb that blocks IGF-1 from binding to the IGF-1R receptor and thus prevents downstream signaling via the MAPK and P13K pathways. Other drugs that are being tested in phase II clinical trials that block IGF-1R are AMG-479 and IMC-A12.

INTRACELLULAR SIGNALING KINASES (E.G., SRC, P13K/AKT/MTOR; MAPK; SONIC HEDGEHOG PATHWAYS)

The first group of drugs were membrane RTK inhibitors that spanned the cell membrane, with a ligand-binding extracellular domain outside the cell, and inside the cell, an intracellular kinase domain.[122] MAbs are effective in blocking ligand binding, which prevents the message from being generated. If it is not blocked, ligand binding and receptor dimerization activate the message and it is sent across the cell membrane to the intracellular kinase, which can be blocked by small, oral tyrosine kinase inhibitors. These strategies to blocking the EGFR RTK either at the external domain of the receptor (e.g., via cetuximab) or the internal domain (tyrosine kinase, e.g., via erlotinib) have been discussed previously (see Figure 2-5).

Other strategies could be neutralization of the ligand, but if the ligand is critical for other human body functions, such as cellular repair, it cannot always be neutralized. We will see in Chapter 3 that neutralizing the ligand VEGF is an effective strategy. As we saw in the families of these receptors, there were multiple pathways within the cell that became activated as the message made its way like a bucket brigade downstream to the cell nucleus. Once the message reaches the nucleus, there are transcription factors in the nucleus that may also be abnormal from the malignant transformation, and the malignant process accelerates. This section will address the proteins involved in taking the message to the cell nucleus, the secondary messengers in the cytoplasm. There are other secondary messengers, such as calcium, but these will not be discussed. An example of a protein kinase that is a secondary messenger is that in Philadelphia chromosome-positive (Ph+) chronic myelocytic leukemia (CML), BCR-Abl, which is blocked by imatinib mesylate (Gleevec).[2] In addition, imatinib mesylate blocks c-kit and PDGFR.

PROTEIN KINASE SIGNALING PATHWAYS

Protein kinases attach a phosphate group to a side chain of a serine/threonine or tyrosine residue of proteins within the cell, called phosphorylation.[2] This action is how the message gets sent by a bucket brigade, from protein kinase to protein kinase. Each member of the bucket brigade gets phosphorylated to take the message the next step. It basically turns "on" the protein it attaches to, and then, once it passes it on, the protein is shut "off"—just like you turn on the light when you enter a dark room and turn the light back off when you leave the room. The actual process of phosphorylation changes the shape of the protein it attaches to. For example, the tumor suppressor protein p53 is the major police officer of the cell cycle, and it is heavily protected from becoming damaged. When it recognizes that a mistake in DNA in a dividing cell cannot be fixed, it sends the cell into programmed cell death, as it is important not to copy and reproduce DNA with mistakes in it, as happens in cancer. Once the protein is activated by phosphorylation, the cell undergoes apoptosis, but the p53 protein needs to be shut down so it does not cause other, perhaps normal cells to be killed. P53 protein gets a deactivation signal when it again is dephosphorylated or a phosphate group is removed.

Thus, the proteins involved in running the cell are tightly controlled in normal circumstances. Unfortunately, cancer subverts the activity of many proteins in the signaling cascade. Many of the tumor suppressor genes and oncogenes are protein tyrosine kinases (PTKs), representing about 0.3% of all genes, as they are critical for the complex signaling within a multicellular organism such as humans.[2] Most of these are transmembrane receptor kinases, like EGFR, VEGFR, PDGFR, and hepatic growth factor receptor (c-Met), while the others are cytoplasmic nonreceptor PTKs. As we have seen, in cancer, many of these PTKs are mutated, amplified, or dysfunctional, leading to uncontrolled cell proliferation, avoidance of apoptosis, invasion, angiogenesis, and metastasis.

The nonreceptor *tyrosine* kinases are in the cytoplasm (outside of the cell nucleus) where they take the signals that have come into the cell from outside and transduce or send them down to the other members of the bucket brigade to get the message to the cell nucleus. Some are attached to a transmembrane receptor, such as those for cytokines.[2] They are activated when the ligand binds to the outside of the receptor or by cellular events such as cell adhesion, influx of calcium, or the turning on of the cell cycle.[2] Examples are src, abl, and JAK. In contrast to the nonreceptor tyrosine kinase, there are also serine/threonine kinases, and they too live in the cytoplasm and have a large role in sending the message to the nucleus as members of the bucket brigade. Key players in cancer are raf, Akt/protein kinase B, and mitogen-activated protein extracellular regulated kinase (MEK).

Now it is time to look at each of these major, albeit selective, signaling pathways, and discuss individual drugs that block or disrupt signaling within the cell, again to prevent the message from ultimately getting to the nucleus of the cell where it operationalizes its malignant behavior. Many of these secondary messengers that carry the message in the bucket brigade are abnormal and overactive because of the influence by mutated, overexpressed, or amplified oncogenes. Our targets here are protein kinases, the enzymes that carry the message from one step to the next, always heading toward the cell nucleus (downstream). Other proteins that are excellent targets are the proteins involved in recycling the proteins in the cell, such as the proteasomes. The key pathways that will be discussed are the src, MAPK, P13K/Akt/mTOR, and SHH pathways.

The src Pathway

The src pathway is important in normal cells because it participates in control of the cell cycle, producing autocrine growth factors, deciding how the cell survives in light of threats to survival, and enabling cell motility for migration, all qualities that would allow a cell to transform into a malignant one.[123] Src was the first oncogene to be discovered, and the first protein kinase.[124] Src is involved in transforming normal cells into malignant ones, control of the cell cycle, reorganization of the cytoskeleton, and growth factor independent growth.[125] When the cell is stimulated to divide by a mitogen (mitosis), src is necessary for the cells to enter the cell cycle. When a mitogen such as platelet-derived growth factor (PDGF) stimulates the cell, src sends a signal starting a cascade of downstream messages that ultimately activate *myc*, a transcription factor. The myc gene (cMyc) is a proto-oncogene that codes for the transcription factor myc. However, the proto-oncogene is often mutated, making it an oncogene, and it is is often overexpressed in many cancers. When overexpressed, its transcription factor (*myc*) turns on the transcription of up to 15% of all the genes in the cell's DNA. It also recruits histone acetyltransferases (HATs) to help turn on some of the genes (see next section on epigenetic control).

Src family kinases appear to oppose the efforts of p53 to stop cell cycle progression when the cell should not pass through the control points, due to irreparable mutations, or other factors.[125] Thus, src may shut off p53, which normally keeps *myc* transcription in check, so that the cell cycle stays turned on and malignant cells continue to mutate and proliferate.[125] Src is implicated in cancers of the breast, colon and rectum, ovary, and lung, as well as some hematologic malignancies.[2]

Drug therapy is aimed at blocking src, which receives "go" signals from EGFR, c-Met, and IGF-1R activation, and also interacts with the downstream signaling cascades MAPK and P13k/Akt/mTOR.[3] If src is blocked, this would decrease or eliminate src control on cancer cell mitosis, adhesion, invasion, motility, and progression.[3] Drugs that inhibit the src pathway include dasatinib, which inhibits both src and abl protein kinases and is also effective against CML, which has become resistant to imatinib mesylate. Investigational src antagonists include the oral inhibitor bosutinib (SKI-606), which is being studied in phase I and II clinical trials of patients with breast and CML. Studies have shown that bosutinib inhibits breast cancer cell migration and invasion.[126]

Another key pathway that appears to play an important role in cancer is the STAT (signal transducers and activators of transcription) pathway. This pathway is made up of proteins in the cytoplasm of the cell that join together (dimerize) when activated by tyrosine phosphorylation.[127] This causes the activated STAT proteins to move into the cell nucleus then into the DNA, where they bind to gene promoters and regulate the expression of certain genes involved in malignancy. The STAT proteins that are activated by themselves (constitutively) without normal growth regulation, during malignant transformation, regulate pathways such as cell-cycle progression, apoptosis, angiogenesis, invasion, metastasis, and evasion of the immune system by tumor.[127] Many tumors have dysregulation of Stat 3 and Stat 4, and loss of Stat 1 function. Agents are being studied to target the flaws in the STAT signaling pathway.

The MAPK Pathway

The MAPK pathway is turned on in many cancers and helps cells to become anchorage independent (i.e., leave their home turf without being sent to programmed cell death) and to proliferate in other locations. The main targets in this pathway are Ras, Raf, and MEK.[2]

Ras is a gene family that makes some of the energy forms (e.g., GTPases, special hydrolase enzymes) used in taking the message from outside the cell into the cell and down to the cell nucleus. *Ras* genes are frequently mutated in cancer (e.g., colon and lung cancers, neuroblastoma), which makes them an important target because their jobs include regulation of cell differentiation (once differentiated, the cell no longer divides), cytoskeletal organization, and keeping proteins moving (like a traffic cop). The family contains over a hundred different proteins, and they are subdivided into eight main families, including Ras, Rho, and Arf. The Ras family's main job is cellular proliferation, Rho helps regulate the cell's actin cytoskeleton, and Arf helps in vesicle transport.[128] Normally, the ras gene, a proto-oncogene, codes for proteins that bring the message from the cell surface growth factor receptors to other protein messengers further down the signal cascade as part of the bucket brigade, activating downstream effectors such as the MAPK pathway, and the Rac/Rho pathway.[129] Once the message is sent to the nucleus, the ras protein is turned "off" and remains off until recruited again to the cell membrane to bring another message from the extracellular growth factor to inside the cell and down to the cell nucleus. If the ras proto-oncogene is mutated (e.g., H-ras, N-ras, K-ras) and activated, it becomes locked in an "on" position and keeps sending the message to divide even when there is no growth factor binding to the surface receptor and no message was actually generated. Ras mutations occur in 33% of human cancers and most often involve codons 12 and 61, on the short arm of chromosome 12.[2,128] K-ras mutations occur in patients with NSCLC (30%), CRC (50%), and pancreatic cancers (90%); H-ras mutations are found in bladder, kidney, and thyroid (50%) cancers; and N-ras mutations occur in melanoma, hepatocelllular cancer, and some hematologic malignancies (CML [65%] and in some acute leukemias [5–30%]).[2,3]

In order to become activated and to attach to the inner surface of the cell membrane, ras has a molecule added called farnesyl isoprenoid, in a process called prenylation; an enzyme called farnesyltransferase is needed to catalyze this addition. If the enzyme is inhibited, then the ras protein is blocked and, in many tumors, causes cells to undergo apoptosis. If farnesylation is not blocked and the ras protein goes to the cell membrane, then Raf-1 kinase is activated and phosphorylates two MAPK kinases (MEK1 and MEK2, which are also known as extracellular signal-regulated kinases-1 and -2). Once activated via phosphorylation, the MAPKs move to the nucleus, where they start a chain reaction leading to cell proliferation.[129] These oncogenes, or their products, are therapeutic targets being studied in clinical trials to block their function so that, for example, the abnormal ras proteins are not produced.

Ras has a place for src (src homology 2, SH2) to attach or an adaptor protein Grb2/SOS binds to ras, thus turning it "on." Just like a bucket brigade, ras then activates the next in line raf (a serine/threonine kinase). Raf activates the MAPK kinase, called MAPKK or MEK, which then turns on or activates MAPK, also called ERK (extracellular regulated kinase). Activated MAPK turns on (phosphorylates and activates) transcription factors c-jun, c-*myc*, and c-fos, which turn on cell proliferation genes in the cell's DNA, and which are mutated in over 50% of human cancers.[2]

Other members of the MAPK family that play a role in cancer are the JNK (Jun N-terminal kinase) and p38 MAPK pathways. JNK and p38MAPK help integrate signals that control cell proliferation, differentiation, survival, and migration.[130] These MAPK signaling pathways are also called stress-activated protein kinase pathways, and they are activated when the cell tries to respond and control environmental stresses, such as inflammation. They, like other normal pathways, are subverted by cancer, and are therefore used to stimulate tumor cell proliferation, survival, and migration of certain cells. Elements of either or both of these pathways are upregulated in some cancers, such as hepatocellular, brain, prostate, and head and neck cancers; thus, they are being studied closely to better undertstand their role in cancer and to develop agents that can target them.[130]

Drug strategies to block ras or its downstream signaling proteins include four approaches[2]:

- Inhibit Ras protein through antisense oligonucleotides
- Prevent membrane localization of Ras
- Locate viral vectors that will kill ras-transformed cells
- Inhibit ras function by inhibition of downstream ras effectors in the MAPK pathway

See Figure 2-5, which shows the Ras-MAPK signaling pathway in the context of other cellular signaling.

Sorafenib (Nexavar, BAY 43-9006) is a multitargeted protein kinase inhibitor that inhibits Raf-kinase, as well as two kinases involved in angiogenesis (VEGF-2, PDGF-β). It is approved for the treatment of metastatic renal cell and unresectable hepatocellular cancers. Drugs that are being studied in the blockade of the Ras-MAPK pathway include farnesyltransferase inhibitors (FTIs) and inhibitors of downstream proteins. Tipifarnib (Zarnestra, R115777) is an FTI. Other investigational agents being studied are lonafarnib (Sarasar, SCH-66336), another FTI, which is being studied in phase II clinical trials of patients with brain, breast, genitourinary, and head and neck cancers.[3] Blockade of downstream effectors are being studied as well, including Raf inhibitors such as RAF-265 (CHIR-265), similar to sorafinib, and the MEK inhibitor AZD-6244 (ARRY-142886).[3]

The Raf protein is a serine/threonine kinase, and there are three members of the Raf family (A-Raf, B-Raf, and C-Raf or Raf-1). Ras mutations can affect the MAPK pathway so that it is always "on," but Raf itself can also be mutated, such as in colon or rectal cancers and in melanoma (70%). In melanoma, B-raf mutation turns on ERK so that it keeps sending proliferation messages to the cell nucleus, which is required for melanoma cell proliferation.[3] In CRCs, because B-raf is the principal effector of K-ras, if it is mutated, the drugs panitumumab and cetuximab are ineffective.[40] There are two MEK proteins in the MEK family, MEK1 and MEK2. They are highly specific and phosphorylate or turn on Erk1 and Erk2.[3] MEK can become turned on by either upstream action (mutated Ras) or it can itself be turned on by malignancy. However, in many malignancies, it is constitutively activated.[3] The developed inhibitors do not compete or block the ATP-binding pocket, as do most kinase inhibitors, but they stabilize the inactive shape of the kinase by binding next to the ATP-binding pocket.[3]

The P13K/Akt/mTOR Pathway

The **P13K (phosphoinositide 3-kinase)** pathway is a very important signaling pathway that links oncogenes and many different receptors to carry out the critical functions of everyday cellular functioning. This pathway is the most commonly activated signaling pathway in cancer.[131] The family of P13Ks is divided into three classes. Class 1 is the one most implicated in cancer.[132] P13K receives messages from RTKs (e.g., EGFR, HER2, c-Met, other RTKs) and sends them downstream to the cell nucleus via its bucket brigade, which includes sending the message to AKT (a serine-threonine kinase also known as kinase B). AKT sends the message to mTOR, which controls many critical functions, including angiogenesis, and cell movement through the cell cycle. As can be seen in Figure 2-5, P13K receives messages about cell survival and also talks to other pathways that control cell proliferation, avoidance of apoptosis, and other critical functions. PTEN is a tumor suppressor protein that functions to keep P13K signaling in check by dephosphorylating P13K substrates and turning off the pathway. It tells cells to stop dividing and, if needed, to die (undergo apoptosis). However, PTEN is frequently mutated or, in cancer, has decreased expression (e.g., mutated in glioblastoma and endometrial and prostate cancers, and decreased expression in breast and lung cancers).[133,134] Nagata et al. found that in order for patients with HER2-positive breast cancer to respond to trastuzumab, an HER2-receptor antagonist, PTEN, had to be activated.[135] If PTEN activity was diminished or blocked, then response to trastuzumab was poor. P13K inhibitors rescued PTEN loss-induced trastuzumab resistance, suggesting a role for P13K inhibitors.[135]

AKT, a serine-threonine kinase (protein kinase B), plays a very active role in cancer. It is turned on directly by P13K. The protein is encoded by three genes, Akt1, Akt2, and Akt3. Akt1 stimulates protein synthesis, such as hypertrophy of muscles, cell growth, avoidance of apoptosis, and cell survival. Thus, Akt1 is most important in malignant transformation and metastasis. Akt2 function is unknown. However, it appears that the three different forms of the Akt protein have overlapping roles, and each may be involved in cancer.[132] When P13K activates Akt signaling, Akt sends the message to mTOR, leading to cell growth and survival. mTOR is a complex protein, and by blocking P13K signaling, a designed drug could also directly block mTOR as opposed to blocking only Akt.[132] Akt also plays a role in tumor resistance to therapy. Los et al. suggest that Akt may facilitate apoptosis under certain circumstances by increasing reactive oxygen species and suppressing antioxidant enzymes.[136] The authors suggest this may be an "Achilles' heel," which could be exploited to kill tumor cells expressing high levels of Akt activity by using oxidant therapy. Perhaps the best way to block Akt is to develop a multikinase inhibitor that blocks MEK as well.[132]

Investigational agents to block P13K are all in phase I testing. Akt inhibitors in phase II clinical trials include perifosine, in patients with brain, breast, gastrointestinal stromal tumor (GIST), head and neck, leukemia, NSCLC, melanoma, lymphoma, myeloma, and other cancers.[2]

For a discussion of mTOR, see Chapter 3.

Hedgehog (Sonic) Signaling Pathway

The SHH pathway is very important in the embryo. It is necessary to spatially orient the cells in embryo as they develop differently depending upon whether they are in the head or tail end, left or right positons.[137] For example, SHH signaling determines the number and placement of the digits on the hands and feet. In the adult, the SHH pathway appears to regulate adult stem cells that maintain and regenerate adult tissues.[138] SHH signaling plays an important role in controlling cell differentiation, growth, and proliferation.[139] See the Hedgehog receptors (Patched [Ptch1] and Smoothened [SMO]) on the right side membrane of the cell in Figure 2-5.

Hedgehog signaling regulates adult stem cells that are involved in maintenance and regeneration of adult tissues.[140] The signaling pathway is mediated by two receptors that oppose each other. See Figure 2-5 where the Ptch1 and SMO receptors are shown on the right border of the cell image. SMO is the only receptor that can initiate a signaling cascade, and it is opposed by Ptch1, which inhibits it and may act as a tumor suppressor. When the Hedgehog ligand binds to Ptch1, it is internalized, permitting SMO to move to the cell surface, where it becomes activated and starts the signaling cascade.[141] If Ptch1 is mutated, then SMO can continue to signal unopposed, leading to uncontrolled cell proliferation. Other ways SMO can be turned to the "on" position so it continues to signal indefinitely is if the Hedgehog ligand is overexpressed, if the SMO receptor is mutated, or if Ptch1 is inhibited.[139]

Cancer, as has been discussed, can reactivate primitive, embryologic signaling, as the programming or software for the pathway is already embedded in the cell's DNA. In cancer, the SHH pathway appears to reduce E-cadherin and the tight junctions so that cells can separate. It is also important in angiogenesis, where it increases angiopoietin-1 and -2, and metastasis.[142,143] In addition, it influences the cell cycle, specifically cyclins D1 and B1, decreases the expression of the genes responsible for apoptosis, and enhances the antiapoptotic genes so that tumor cells survive.[141] The authors suggest that the Hedgehog Ptch1 receptor functions as a "gatekeeper" tumor suppressor gene that inhibits cell cycle progression in the G_1–S phase as well as the G_2–M phase, and when it is mutated, there is rapid onset of tumor progression. SHH is implicated in the onset and progression of pancreatic cancer[143] and in basal cell carcinomas.[144] Hedgehog signaling likely plays an important role in tumor–stroma interactions, as Hedgehog signaling is activated in both epithelial and stromal compartments in pancreatic metastatic models.[145] The gatekeeper or tumor suppressor Ptch1 is the receptor for Hedgehog proteins, and in patients with sporadic basal cell carcinoma, it is mutated in 90% of at least one allele or gene copy of Ptch1, while another 10% have activating mutations in the SMO protein, both of which keep SMO in the activated or "on" state, as no longer can Ptch1 inhibit SMO.[144] In addition, SHH signaling is activated in other cancers, such as breast, brain, GI, prostate, and lung, and may be due to overexpression of the Hedgehog ligand.[145]

Tuveson et al. described the challenges of treating pancreatic ductal adenocarcinoma, and his team was able to show that using a Hedgehog inhibitor IPI-926 in combination with gemcitabine, in a genetically engineered mouse model of pancreatic cancer, the tumor could be treated.[146] The barrier was the stroma, and inhibition of the Hedgehog pathway decreased the tumor stroma and increased the number of blood vessels in the stroma, thereby improving drug delivery. However, ultimately, the tumor progressed with increase in the volume of the stroma and reduction in the number of blood vessels. Other investigators are studying the Hedgehog inhibitor GDC-0449, in combination with erlotinib, based on the premise that there is synergy by blocking both EGFR and Hedgehog, as both pathways interact.[133,147]

Thus, SHH pathway offers a number of attractive targets.[145] For example, cyclopamine binds directly with SMO to prevent Hedgehog signaling, and other SMO antagonists are being studied. It appears that vitamin D_3, together with Ptch1, can inhibit SMO, and these tests are ongoing.[148]

PROTEIN KINASE INHIBITORS

Drug: Imatinib Mesylate (Gleevec)

Indications: Imatinib mesylate is indicated for the treatment of patients with CML:
1. Initial treatment of newly diagnosed adult and pediatric patients with Ph+ chromosome CML in chronic phase
2. Ph+ CML in blast crisis, in accelerated phase, or in chronic phase after failure of interferon-α therapy
3. Pediatric patients with Ph+ chronic phase CML whose disease has recurred after SCT or who are resistant to interferon-α therapy

Imatinib is indicated for the treatment of:
1. Adult patients with relapsed or refractory Ph+ acute lymphoblastic leukemia (ALL)
2. Adult patients with myelodysplastic/myeloproliferative diseases (MDS/MPD) associated with PDGFR gene rearrangements
3. Patients with Kit (CD117)-positive unresectable and/or metastatic malignant GISTs
4. Adult patients following resection of Kit (CD117)-positive GIST (adjuvant)
5. Adult patients with aggressive systemic mastocytosis (ASM) without the

D816V c-Kit mutation or with unknown status
6. Adult patients with hypereosinophilic syndrome (HES) and/or chronic eosinophilic leukemia with or without FIP1L1-PDGFRα fusion kinase
7. Adult patients with unresectable, recurrent, and/or metastatic dermatofibrosarcoma protuberans

Class: Protein tyrosine kinase inhibitor

Mechanism of Action: Inhibits abnormal tyrosine kinase encoded by the Philadelphia chromosome (BCR-Abl) in CML, thus preventing cell proliferation. Drug also inhibits receptor tyrosine kinases for PDGF. Inhibits c-Kit receptor called stem cell factor receptor tyrosine kinases as well, which has resulted in marked responses in GIST. Of patients with GISTs, 15–85% have Kit mutations that result in constitutively active kinases; imatinib mesylate selectively inhibits this mutated tyrosine kinase.

Pharmacokinetics: Well absorbed after oral administration, with 98% bioavailability and maximum concentration 2–4 hours after dosing. Elimination half-life of imatinib is 18 hours and 40 hours for primary active metabolite N-desmethyl derivative. Drug is 95% protein bound. It is metabolized via CYP3A4 hepatic cytochrome P450 enzyme system, with 81% of the dose eliminated in 7 days, primarily via fecal route (68%) and, to a lesser degree, urinary (13%). Of drug dose, 25% is excreted unchanged in feces and urine.

Dosage and Administration:
- 400 mg/day orally (single dose) for patients in chronic phase of CML
- 600 mg/day orally (single dose) for patients in accelerated phase or blast crisis
- Treatment continued as long as patient derives benefit from drug
- In case of disease progression at any time, failure to achieve a satisfactory hematologic response after 3 months of treatment, failure to achieve a cytogenetic response after 6–12 months of treatment, or loss of a hematologic or cytogenetic response: Increase dose to 600 mg/day (chronic CML); increase to 800 mg/day, given as 400 mg twice daily (accelerated or blast crisis) if no severe adverse drug reactions occur.
- Adults with Ph+ ALL: 600 mg/day
- GIST dosing: 400 mg/day orally. Metastatic or unresectable GIST: may dose escalate to 800 mg/day (400 mg PO twice daily) if disease progression occurs and drug is well tolerated. Adjuvant therapy following complete resection: some studies continued dosing for 1 year; optimal time is unknown.
- MDS, MPD: 400 mg/day PO
- Pediatric dosing (newly diagnosed): 340 mg/m^2/day (not to exceed 600 mg/day)

- Pediatric dosing (recurrence after SCT or if intolerant of interferon-α therapy): 260 mg/m²/day
- Patients with mild to moderate hepatic impairment: 400 mg/day
- Patients with severe hepatic impairment: 25% dose reduction (e.g., 300 mg/day)
- Dose reduce for renal insufficiency: Moderate (creatinine clearance 20–39 mL/min) requires a 50% reduction in initial dose, which may be increased once it is established how the patient tolerates the drug, but doses > 400 mg/day are not recommended. Patients with creatinine clearance of 40–59 mL/min should not receive doses > 600 mg/day. Use drug cautiously (e.g., 100 mg/day if at all in patients with severe renal dysfunction).
- Dose reduce for severe neutropenia (ANC < 1.0 cells/mm³) and/or platelet count < 50,000/mm³ (see package insert).

Available as: 100-mg and 400-mg scored tablets in bottles of 120

Reconstitution and Preparation: None, as dose is oral. Administer dose orally, once daily (unless the total dose is 800 mg, which is given as 400 mg twice daily), with a meal and a large glass of water. Can dissolve tablet in water or apple juice if patient has dysphagia. If the dose is 800 mg and higher, 400-mg tablets should be used to reduce exposure to iron. Store at room temperature, 59–86°F (15–30°C), in a dry place, away from children and pets. Use gloves when handling the tablets, and return any unused drug in the bottle to the dispensing pharmacy for disposal.

Drug Interactions:
- CYP3A4 inhibitors (ketoconazole, itraconazole, erythromycin, clarithromycin, voriconazole, aprepitant) may increase imatinib plasma concentrations; do not coadminister, or monitor closely for imatinib adverse effects.
- CYP3A4 substrates (simvastatin): Imatinib decreases simvastatin metabolism with simvastatin serum levels increased 2–3.5 times. Use together cautiously, if at all, monitor BP, and dose reduce simvastatin if needed.
- CYP3A4 inducers (dexamethasone, phenytoin, carbamazepine, rifampicin, phenobarbital, St. John's wort) may increase metabolism of imatinib, so imatinib serum levels are reduced. Use together cautiously, if at all. When used with dexamethasone, phenytoin, carbamazepine, phenobarbital, rifabutin, or rifampin, increase imatinib dose by 50%. Do not take St. John's wort if taking imatinib.
- Other CYP3A4 substrates (cyclosporine, pimozide) increase plasma concentrations if coadministered with imatinib. Do not administer together because drug has a narrow therapeutic window.
- Other CYP3A4 substrates (triazolobenzadiazepines, dihydropyridine calcium channel blockers, HMG-CoA reductase inhibitors) may have increased serum levels when given together with imatinib. Use together cautiously, and monitor patient closely.

- Other CYP3A4 substrates: Eletriptan (Relpax) should not be administered within 72 hours of imatinib. Monitor vital signs closely.
- Warfarin: Do not give together with imatinib because imatinib inhibits warfarin metabolism by CYP2C9 enzymes. Use low molecular heparin or standard heparin instead.
- Acetaminophen: Systemic exposure of acetaminophen will be increased when coadministered with imatinib mesylate.

Contraindications: None

Warnings:
- **Edema and severe fluid retention:** Weigh patient regularly and manage unexpected, rapid weight gain with diuretics and dose interruption.
- **Cytopenias with risk for infection, bleeding, and fatigue:** Anemia, neutropenia, and thrombocytopenia have occurred. Manage with dose reduction or interruption, and rarely drug discontinuance. Monitor CBC weekly for first month, every other week for the second month, and periodically thereafter. Teach patient to self-assess and report temperature > 100.5°F, symptoms of infection or bleeding, or excessive fatigue. Teach patient to avoid contact with people who have colds and to wash hands frequently.
- **Severe CHF and left ventricular dysfunction** have been reported, especially in those with comorbidities, existing cardiac disease, or risk factors. Monitor patients closely and treat appropriately.
- **Severe hepatotoxicity** may occur. Assess LFTs baseline before starting the drug and monthly thereafter, or more frequently if clinically indicated. Monitor more closely when drug is combined with chemotherapy known to cause liver dysfunction. Dose modify depending upon laboratory findings, with a 25% dose reduction for patients with severe hepatic dysfunction.
- **Grade 3 or 4 hemorrhage** has been reported, especially in patients with newly diagnosed CML or GIST (GI lesions may be source).
- **GI perforations** have been reported.
- **Cardiogenic shock or left ventricular dysfunction** has been reported during drug initiation in patients with high eosinophil levels (HES, MDS/MPD, ASM). Monitor these patients very closely.
- **Bullous dermatologic reactions** such as erythema multiforme and Stevens-Johnson syndrome have been reported.
- **Hypothyroidism** in patients who have had a thyroidectomy and who are on levothyroxine replacement may occur. Monitor TSH levels closely in these patients.
- **Drug is fetotoxic**, so teach patients to use effective birth control measures and avoid pregnancy.

Adverse Reactions (**bold** indicates most common, occurring in > 25% of patients):

Cardiovascular: **Edema with increased weight**, **periorbital edema**, rare CHF, tachycardia, palpitations, angina

Pulmonary: Rare pleural effusions, ILD

CNS/neurologic: **Headache**, **nasopharyngitis**, dizziness, depression, blurred vision, nosebleeds, conjunctivitis, dry eye

Dermatologic: **Rash**, dry skin, alopecia, photosensitivity, rare hypersensitivity (e.g., bullous, erythema multiforme, Stevens-Johnson syndrome)

GI: **Nausea**, **vomiting**, **diarrhea**, **abdominal pain**, **elevated LFTs**, constipation, dyspepsia, anorexia, hypokalemia, stomatitis, rare increased serum amylase

Hematologic: **Hemorrhage**, **neutropenia**, **thrombocytopenia**, **anemia**

Musculoskeletal: **Muscle cramps**, **arthralgias**, myalgias, bone pain

General: **Fatigue**, pyrexia, night sweats

Nursing Discussion:
- Assess patient's laboratory parameters: CBC, platelets, LFTs (transaminases, bilirubin, alkaline phosphatase) baseline and then weekly × 4 CBC/differential, then every other week × 2, then monthly, along with monthly LFTs.
- Patients may develop resistance to the drug over time and require rescue with a second-generation agent.
- Review medication profile for interacting drugs, including OTC drugs such as aspirin and NSAIDs.
- Teach patient to use gloves when handling the tablet and to wash hands before and after wearing gloves. If pills remain in the bottle, return them to dispensing clinic or pharmacy for disposal.

Drug: Dasatinib (Sprycel)

Indications: Dasatinib is indicated for the treatment of adults with:
- Chronic, accelerated, or myeloid or lymphoid blast phase CML with resistance or intolerance to prior therapy including imatinib
- Ph+ ALL with resistance or intolerance to prior therapy

Class: Multitargeted kinase inhibitor

Mechanism of Action: Drug inhibits the following kinases: BCR-Abl, SRC-family (SRC, LCK, YES, FYN), c-KIT, EPHA2, and PDGFR-β. Drug forms a tighter bond with BCR-Abl kinase (300–1000 times more potently) than imatinib mesylate (Gleevec) and binds to both active and inactive forms (multiple forms of the ABL kinase).

Pharmacokinetics: Drug is rapidly absorbed after oral ingestion with peak serum levels in 0.5–6 hours and an overall mean half-life of 3–5 hours. If ingested with a high-fat meal, there is a 14% increase in the mean AUC exposure, but this is not considered clinically relevant. Drug and its active metabolite bind to plasma proteins 96% and 93%, respectively. Drug is extensively metabolized by the P450 microenzyme CYP3A4. Drug is excreted in the feces (85%) and to a lesser degree the urine (4%).

Dosage and Administration:
- Chronic-phase CML: 100 mg PO once daily
- Accelerated-phase CML, myeloid- or lymphoid blast-phase CML, or Ph+ ALL: 140 mg PO once daily
- Dose may be increased or decreased in 20-mg increments based on individual patient response or coadministration with drugs that either increase or decrease dasatinib serum levels (see drug interactions).
- Dose modifications for neutropenia: Monitor CBC weekly for the initial 2 months and then periodically.
- *Chronic phase CML* (starting dose 100 mg once daily): ANC $< 0.5 \times 10^9$/L or platelets $< 50 \times 10^9$/L: (1) Stop drug until ANC is $\geq 1 \times 10^9$/L or platelets $\geq 50 \times 10^9$/L; (2) resume treatment at initial starting dose if recovery occurs on or within 7 days; (3) if platelets $< 25 \times 10^9$/L or recurrence of ANC $< 0.5 \times 10^9$/L for > 7 days, stop drug as above, and resume drug at a reduced dose of 80 mg once daily (second episode) or discontinue drug (third episode).
- *Accelerated phase CML, Blast phase CML, and Ph+ALL* (starting dose 140 mg once daily): ANC $< 0.5 \times 10^9$/L or platelets $< 10 \times 10^9$/L: (1) Check to see if cytopenia is related to leukemia by assessing bone marrow aspirate or biopsy; (2) if cytopenia unrelated to leukemia, stop drug until ANC is $\geq 1.0 \times 10^9$/L or platelets $\geq 20 \times 10^9$/L and resume treatment at initial starting dose; (3) if recurrence of cytopenia, repeat step 1 and resume drug at reduced dose of 100 mg once daily (second episode) or 80 mg once daily (third episode); (4) if cytopenia is related to leukemia, consider dose escalation to 180 mg once daily.
- In clinical studies, adult patients with CML or Ph+ ALL who did not achieve a hematologic or cytogenic response at the recommended dosage were allowed to dose escalate to 140 mg once daily, or 180 mg once daily, respectively.

Available as: 20-mg, 50-mg, 70-mg, and 100-mg tablets, each in 60-tablet bottles, except the 100-mg tablets, which come in a 30-tablet bottle

Reconstitution, Preparation, Administration: Drug Administration: Oral, once in the morning and once in the evening, with or without food; do not crush or cut. Store at room temperature, 59–86°F (15–30°C), in a dry place, away from children and pets. Use gloves when handling the tablets, and return any unused drug in the bottle to the dispensing pharmacy for disposal.

Drug Interactions:
- CYP3A4 inhibitors (e.g., ketoconazole, itraconazole, erythromycin, clarithromycin, atazanavir, indinavir, nefazodone, nelfinavir, ritonavir, saquinavir, telithromycin): May decrease metabolism of dasatinib, thus increasing serum concentrations of dasatinib; avoid coadministration, and if they must be given together, decrease dose of dasatinib. Decrease dose by 20 mg in patients taking 100 mg daily, and decrease 40 mg in patients taking 140 mg daily. If reduced drug dosage is not tolerated, either the strong CYP3A4 inhibitor must be discontinued or dasatinib. After the strong inhibitor is discontinued, allow a washout period of approximately 1 week before dasatinib dose is increased.
- CYP3A4 inducers: Rifampin—decreases dasatinib serum concentrations by 81%; others (dexamethasone, phenytoin, carbamazepine, phenobarbital, St. John's wort)—avoid coadministration, and if they must be given together, increase dose of dasatinib. Patients receiving dasatinib should NOT take St. John's wort.
- Antacids (aluminum hydroxide/magnesium hydroxide): Decreases dasatinib AUC by 55%, as drug requires acid pH; avoid concurrent administration or administer 2 hours prior to or 2 hours after dasatinib dose.
- H_2 blockers/proton pump inhibitors (PPIs): Famotidine decreases dasatinib AUC 61%; avoid concurrent administration. Consider use of antacids rather than H_2 blockers or PPIs.
- Simvastatin, CYP3A4 substrates: Dasatinib is a time-dependent inhibitor of CYP3A4 and may decrease the metabolism of drugs primarily metabolized by CYP3A4, such as alfentanil, astemizole, terfenadine, cisapride, cyclosporine, fentanyl, pimozide, quinidine, sirolimus, tacrolimus, or ergot alkaloids; decreases simvastatin AUC 37%; avoid concurrent administration or administer cautiously.

Contraindications: None

Warnings:
- **Myelosuppression:** Severe thrombocytopenia, neutropenia, and anemia may occur, requiring dose interruption or dose reduction. Cytopenias are more common in patients with advanced-phase CML or Ph+ ALL than in chronic-phase CML. Monitor CBC, differential baseline, then weekly for the first 2 months, and monthly thereafter. Teach patients to self-assess for signs/symptoms of infection, bleeding, and excessive fatigue. Teach patients to report temperature > 100.5°F, bleeding, or excessive fatigue.
- **Bleeding-related events:** Most are associated with severe thrombocytopenia. Rarely severe bleeding, such as CNS hemorrhage (1%), GI bleeding/hemorrhage (4%), have occurred and have required treatment interruption and transfusions. Use drug cautiously in patients who are also receiving medications that inhibit platelet function or anticoagulants.

- **Fluid retention:** Fluid retention occurs commonly and may occasionally be severe; fluid retention (10%, e.g., edema, ascites) and pleural (7%) and pericardial (1%) effusions may occur. Severe pulmonary edema occurrs in 1% of patients. Assess patients closely and manage with appropriate medical care (e.g., assess patients for dyspnea and dry cough; signs/symptoms suggestive of pleural effusion should prompt a chest x-ray). Supportive care is usually effective and includes diuretics, short course of steroids, and rarely thoracentesis and oxygen therapy.
- **QT prolongaation:** Use drug cautiously in patients who have or are at risk for developing QT prolongation, such as those taking certain antiarrythmic drugs or those who have an electrolyte imbalance (e.g., hypokalemia, hypomagnesemia), congenital QT prolongation, or high cumulative antracycline doses. Assess baseline ECG with QTc measurement, and repeat periodically during treatment.
- **Drug is fetotoxic:** Teach patients to use effective contraception.
- **Although no drug modification is recommended, use cautiously in patients with hepatic impairment.**

Adverse Reactions (**bold** indicates most common, occurring in > 25% of patients):

Cardiovascular: **Fluid retention**, hypertension, arrhythmia

Pulmonary: **Dyspnea**, pleural effusion, pericardial effusion, CHF, cardiac dysfunction, pulmonary edema

CNS/neurologic: **Headache**, insomnia, depression, visual disturbance

Dermatologic: **Skin rash**, urticaria

Metabolic: Hypophosphatemia, hypokalemia, hypocalcemia, elevated LFTs

GI: **Diarrhea**, nausea, abdominal pain, vomiting, mucosal inflammation, anorexia

Hematologic: **Myelosuppression**, hemorrhage, febrile neutropenia

Musculoskeletal: Myalgias, arthralgias

General: **Fatigue**, fever

Nursing Discussion:
- Assess patient's laboratory parameters: CBC, platelets, LFTs (transaminases, bilirubin, alkaline phosphatase) baseline and then CBC/differential weekly × 8, then monthly. Assess baseline ECG for QTc interval and document in the chart. Assess if patient has risk factors (e.g., electrolyte imbalance), correct, if possible, and discuss with physician or midlevel practitioner.
- Patients may develop resistance to the drug over time and require rescue with a second-generation agent.

- Review medication profile for interacting drugs, including OTC drugs such as aspirin and NSAIDs.
- Teach patient to use gloves when handling the tablet and to wash hands before and after wearing gloves. If pills remain in the bottle, return them to dispensing clinic or pharmacy for disposal.

Drug: Nilotinib (Tasigna)

Indications: Nilotinib is FDA indicated for the treatment of chronic-phase and accelerated-phase Ph+ CML in adult patients resistant to or intolerant to prior therapy that included imatinib.

Class: Protein kinase inhibitor (specific for)

Mechanism of Action: Ph+ CML and ALL are caused by a reciprocal mutation involving two chromosomes in the bone marrow stem cells that causes genetic material to be exchanged between chromosomes 9 and 22, creating the Philadelphia chromosome. The result is a fusion gene formed when the breakpoint cluster region (BCR) from chromosome 22 is placed next to the *Abl* gene on chromosome 9, forming the BCR-Abl gene. The normal ABL gene is a proto-oncogene and makes a protein kinase messenger that is normally tightly controlled. In the fusion gene, which looks like a short and fat bowling ball, the protein kinase behaves like an oncogene and continues to send the message to the cell nucleus to divide, resulting in the formation of primitive leukemic cells. In fact, the BCR-Abl fusion gene causes cell proliferation, decreased adhesion/ increased migration, inhibition of apoptosis, degradation of regulatory proteins, and prevention of DNA repair. When the protein kinase is activated, it continues to send the message to the cell nucleus telling the cell to divide. However, the binding site is sometimes blocked (inactive) and sometimes active and able to bind to ATP, which turns it on. In addition, it can mutate, and a drug that was once able to block the ATP binding site may no longer fit into the ATP pocket. When a patient progresses on imatinib, it is because BCR-Abl is reactivated through a number of processes, such as amplification of BCR-Abl gene expression, or more than 30 point mutations in the BCR-Abl kinase domain that disable the drug from binding to the ATP binding site on the protein kinase. Nilotinib is a designer drug that is highly specific for and binds very tightly to the ATP binding site of ABL (more selective and 30 times more potent an inhibitor than imatinib mesylate). The drug is active against 32 of the 33 most common BCR-Abl mutations causing imatinib resistance. The drug also inhibits the KIT and PDGFR-A proteins found in patients with GIST.

Pharmacokinetics: The drug is metabolized via the cytochrome P450 microenzyme system in the liver (CYP3A4). A high-fat diet greatly increases drug bioavailability (82%), and thus, the drug must be given on an empty stomach.

Peak concentrations are reached 3 hours after drug administration. Serum protein binding is 98%. Elimination half-life with daily dosing is 17 hours, and steady state is reached by day 8. Metabolism occurs by oxidation and hydroxylation. Metabolites are not pharmacologically active. More than 90% of administered dose is eliminated within 7 days, primarily via the feces. Age, weight, gender, and ethnicity do not significantly affect pharmacokinetics.

Dosage and Administration: Oral.

- Nilotinib 400 mg orally twice daily, approximately 12 hours apart on an empty stomach (no food 2 hours before or 1 hour after the dose). Drink only water in the hour after the dose.
- Dose reduce for corrected QT (QTc) interval prolongation > 480 milliseconds. Stop the drug, assess serum potassium and magnesium, and replete if needed. Resume dose within 2 weeks if the QTc returns to < 450 milliseconds and to within 20 seconds of baseline. If the QTc is 450–480 milliseconds after 2 weeks, reduce the dose to 400 mg once daily. If following the dose reduction, the QTc returns to > 480 milliseconds, discontinue nilotinib. An ECG should be repeated approximately 7 days after any dose adjustment.
- Dose reduce for hematologic (ANC < 1.0×10^9/L and/or platelet count < 50×10^9/L). Stop nilotinib, and monitor blood counts. Resume within 2 weeks at prior dose if ANC > 1.0×10^9/L and platelets are > 50×10^9/L. If blood counts remain low for > 2 weeks, reduce dose to 400 mg once daily.
- Grade 3 or higher nonhematologic toxicities (serum lipase or amylase, elevated bilirubin, elevated hepatic transaminases): Hold nilotinib and monitor serum values; resume nilotinib at 400 mg once daily if serum levels return to ≤ grade 1.
- If patient requires a dose reduction, if appropriate, may gradually escalate base to 400 mg twice daily once condition has stabilized.
- Nilotinib can be given with hematopoietic growth factors such as erythropoietin or G-CSF if indicated.
- Nilotinib can be given with hydroxyurea or anagrelide if clinically indicated.

Available as: 200-mg hard gelatin capsules

Reconstitution and Preparation: Oral. Store at room temperature, 59–86°F (15–30°C), in a dry place, away from children and pets. Use gloves when handling the tablets, and return any unused drug in the bottle to the dispensing pharmacy for disposal.

Drug Interactions:

- CYP3A4 (strong) inhibitors (ketoconazole, itraconazole, clarithromycin, atazanavir, indinavir, nefazodone, nelfinavir, ritonavir, saquinavir, telithromycin, voriconazole, grapefruit juice) may increase imatinib plasma concentrations; do not coadminister. IF their administration is necessary, interrupt nilotinib therapy; if continued coadministration is necessary, adjust nilotinib dose to 400 mg daily (decrease by 50%), and monitor QTc interval closely for any prolongation. If the strong inhibitor is discontinued, a washout period should be allowed before increasing the dose of nilotinib back to 400 mg every 12 hours. Teach patient to avoid grapefruit and grapefruit juice.

- CYP3A4 substrates (simvastatin): Nilotinib decreases simvastatin metabolism with simvastatin serum levels increased 2–3.5 times. Use together cautiously, if at all, and monitor BP and dose reduce simvastatin if needed.
- CYP3A4 (strong) inducers (dexamethasone, phenytoin, carbamazepine, rifampicin, phenobarbital, St. John's wort) may increase metabolism of nilotinib so that nilotinib serum levels are reduced. Use together cautiously, if at all. When used with dexamethasone, phenytoin, carbamazepine, phenobarbital, rifabutin, or rifampin, increase nilotinib dose by 50%. If later the strong inducer is discontinued, the nilotinib dose should be decreased to the original dose. Teach patient to not take St. John's wort if taking nilotinib.
- Other CYP3A4 substrates (cyclosporine, pimozide) increase plasma concentrations if coadministered with nilotinib. Do not administer together because drug has a narrow therapeutic window.
- Other CYP3A4 substrates (triazolobenzodiazepines, dihydropyridine calcium channel blockers, HMG-CoA reductase inhibitors) may have increased serum levels when given together with nilotinib. Use together cautiously, and monitor patient closely.
- Other CYP3A4 substrates: Eletriptan (Relpax) should not be administered within 72 hours of nilotinib. Monitor vital signs closely.
- Warfarin: Nilotinib is a competitive substrate; thus, INR must be monitored closely and warfarin dose adjusted frequently.
- Drugs prolonging QTc (e.g., serotonin antagonists, other tyrosine kinase inhibitors): Do not use together, as will increase risk of prolonged QTc and sudden death.
- Nilotinib is an inhibitor of CYP3A4, CYP2C8, CYP2C9, and CYP2D6. It may be an inducer for CYP2B6, CYP2C8, and CYP2C9, thus affecting the serum levels of other drugs. See Chapter 5.

Contraindications:
- Patients with hypokalemia, hypomagnesemia, or long QT syndrome
- Drug is fetotoxic. Women of childbearing potential should use effective contraception and avoid pregnancy.
- Nilotinib should not be used by women who are breastfeeding.

Warnings:
- Myelosuppression: Associated with neutropenia, thrombocytopenia, and anemia. CBC should be assessed every 2 weeks for the first 2 months,

then monthly. Reversible by withholding dose, and dose reduction per manufacturer. Dose reduction may be required.

- QT prolongation: nilotinib prolongs the QT interval. Correct hypokalemia or hypomagnesemia prior to administration and monitor periodically. Avoid drugs known to prolong the QT interval and strong CYP3A4 inhibitors. Use caution in patients with hepatic impairment. Hypokalemia and hypomagnesemia can increase the QTc interval. When taking nilotinib, which also prolongs the QTc interval, the patient may develop torsades de pointes, a ventricular tachycardia that can result in sudden death. This can be prevented by ensuring that serum magnesium and potassium are WNL and by closely monitoring QTc by ECG.

- Obtain ECGs at baseline, 7 days after initiation, and periodically thereafter, as well as following any dose adjustments.

- Sudden deaths: There were sudden deaths reported in the safety population and the expanded access program. Ventricular repolarization abnormalities may have contributed to their occurrence.

- Nilotinib can cause elevated serum lipase: Use cautiously if at all in patients with a history of pancreatitis. Assess serum lipase and amylase regularly during treatment.

- Liver function abnormality may occur, with elevations in bilirubin, AST/ALT, and alkaline phosphatase. Monitor LFTs baseline and periodically during treatment.

- Nilotinib can cause electrolyte abnormalities, including hypophosphatemia, hypokalemia, hyperkalemia, hypocalcemia, and hyponatremia. Correct electrolyte abnormalities prior to initiating nilotinib and monitor periodically during therapy.

- Hepatic impairment: Nilotinib has not been studied in patients with hepatic dysfunction. Use nilotinib cautiously in this patient group, and monitor QTc interval on ECG closely.

- Drug interactions: Avoid concomitant use of strong inhibitors or inducers of CYP3A4. If patients must be coadministered a strong CYP3A4 inhibitor, dose reduction should be considered, and the QT interval should be monitored closely.

- Food effects: Food increases blood levels of nilotinib. Avoid food 2 hours before and 1 hour after a dose.

Adverse Reactions (**bold** indicates most common, occurring in > 25% of patients):

Cardiovascular: **QTc interval prolongation on ECG**, peripheral edema, palpitations, hypertension, flushing

Pulmonary: Pneumonia, cough dyspnea, nasopharyngitis

CNS/neurologic: **Headache**, intracranial hemorrhage, dizziness, paresthesia, vertigo

Dermatologic: **Rash**, **pruritus**, night sweats, eczema, urticaria, alopecia, erythema

Metabolic: Elevated lipase, amylase, hypokalemia, hyponatremia, hyperglycemia, hypophosphatemia, hyperkalemia, decreased albumin, hypocalcemia, hyperthyroidism

GI: **Nausea**, **diarrhea**, constipation, vomiting, decreased serum albumin, elevated LFTs (ALT, total bilirubin, AST, alkaline phosphatase), abdominal pain, dehydration, anorexia, dyspepsia, flatulence

Hematologic: **Neutropenia**, **thrombocytopenia**, anemia, febrile neutropenia, leucopenia

Musculoskeletal: Arthralgia, myalgias, pain in extremity, bone pain, muscle spasms, back pain

Genitourinary: Elevated serum creatinine

General: **Fatigue**, pyrexia, asthenia

Nursing Discussion:

QTc interval prolongation: Nilotinib can increase the QTc interval (the period of ventricular repolarization in the heart) on the ECG. Prolongation of the QTc can increase the risk of developing torsades de pointes (twisting about the points), an unusual variant of ventricular tachycardia that may result in sudden death, syncope, or seizures (Figure 2-9). Risk of developing this condition is also increased if the patient has hypomagnesemia and hypokalemia. Thus, the nurse should ensure that the patient's electrolytes are WNL and that any abnormalities are corrected before the patient begins nilotinib. In addition, a baseline ECG should be done and repeated 7 days after nilotinib initiation, and then periodically during therapy. Electrolytes should also be monitored closely and repleted as needed. Concomitant use of drugs that are strong inhibitors of the CYP3A4 will block metabolism of nilotinib, resulting in increased toxicity, including QTc prolongation. The nurse should carefully review the patient's medication profile along with the physician, midlevel practitioner, or pharmacist to ensure that there are no drug interactions.

Patient teaching takes on increased importance, as the patients must be able to take nilotinib safely—that is, 2 hours before or 1 hour after a meal. Only water should be taken in during the 1 hour after the dose. If patients take nilotinib with food, the bioavailability of the drug is greater, the serum drug levels higher, and the risk of toxicity higher.

Review medication profile for interacting drugs, including OTC drugs such as aspirin and NSAIDs. Teach patient to use gloves when handling the tablet and to wash hands before and after wearing the gloves. If pills remain in the bottle, return them to dispensing clinic or pharmacy for disposal.

Figure 2-9   Torsades de pointes.

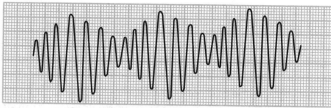

From *12-Lead ECG: The Art of Interpretation,* courtesy of Tomas B. Garcia, MD.

Lab monitoring: CBC/differential baseline, then every 2 weeks for the first 2 months, and then monthly; ECG to monitor QTc baseline, 7 days after first dose, then periodically as well as after any dose adjustments; monitor QTc closely in patients with liver impairment or receiving strong CYP3A4 inhibitors; monitor electrolytes baseline and correct prior to starting drug, especially magnesium and potassium; monitor magnesium, potassium, calcium, phosphorus, sodium; monitor serum lipase and glucose baseline in patients with a history of pancreatitis; monitor LFTs baseline and periodically.

Risk for neutropenia and thrombocytopenia: Grade 3 or 4 neutropenia occurred in 28% of patients in chronic-phase and 37% of patients with accelerated-phase; thrombocytopenia in 28–37% of patients; anemia in 8–23% of patients. Febrile neutropenia occurred in < 10% of patients with accelerated-phase CML. Assess baseline CBC, WBCs, differential, and platelet count baseline before initiating therapy, then every 2 weeks for the first 8 weeks, and then monthly. Assess for signs/symptoms of infection or bleeding. Teach patient the signs/symptoms of infection or bleeding and to report them immediately, and teach patient self-care measures to minimize risk of infection and bleeding. Measures include avoidance of crowds, proximity to people with infections, and OTC aspirin-containing medications. Discuss need for blood product support or growth factors with physician or nurse practitioner.

Potential alteration in nutrition related to GI symptoms: Nausea affects 31% of patients (1% grade 3 or 4), and vomiting affects 21% (< 1% grade 3 or 4). Diarrhea affects 22% (3% grade 3 or 4), whereas constipation affects 20%. Hepatotoxicity is characterized by transient and reversible increase in LFTs. Grade 3 or 4 lipase increased in 15–17% of patients and glucose in 11%. The largest increase in bilirubin was found in patients with (TA) 7 genotype (UGT1A1*28).**

** The enzyme UGT1A1*28 has a gene copy in some people (polymorphism) that has extra Thymidine-adenine (TA) repeats in the promoter region (7). This results in the liver's decreased ability to break down certain drugs, such as irinotecan, and causes an elevated level of unconjugated bilirubin in the blood. It is also found in people with Gilbert's syndrome and results in jaundice.

Teach patient to self-administer antiemetic 1 hour before each dose if needed and to call if nausea/vomiting develop. Discuss with physician more effective antiemetic regimen if nausea/vomiting develop despite antiemetics. Encourage small, frequent intake of cool, bland foods as tolerated if nausea develops. Refer to dietitian as needed for meal planning. Assess bowel elimination pattern baseline and at each visit. Teach patient to report diarrhea or constipation that does not respond to antidiarrheal or anticonstipation medications. Teach dietary modifications as appropriate. Monitor LFTs, serum, lipase, and glucose baseline and periodically during therapy. Discuss abnormalities with physician. Teach patient to report any abdominal pain with nausea or vomiting.

PROTEIN DYNAMICS: HEAT SHOCK PROTEINS AND UBIQUITIN–PROTEASOME INHIBITORS

The body is very careful to prevent uncontrolled cell proliferation, as well as the replication of damaged DNA, so it has many safeguards in place. One of them is the ubiquitin–proteasome system. It is clear that proteins are the key to all cellular processes. The genes that code for them are the instructions or recipe to make the protein. Some proteins are extremely important, such as the cyclins and cyclin-dependent kinases that regulate the cell cycle. The cell cycle is turned on when certain proteins are made and their level in the cell rises, but then the cell cycle needs to be turned off; thus, these proteins need to be destroyed so they cannot be used to turn the cell cycle back on for proliferation without the usual checkpoints. Proteins also have time-limited function in signal transduction (kinases), differentiation, and DNA repair, and these proteins need to be turned on and off.

There are two main ways the body breaks down damaged proteins or proteins that are no longer needed, such as those just described. The first way is with lysosomes, which degrade extracellular proteins. The second way, with proteasomes, does not use lysosomes and is used to remove endogenous proteins the cell has made inside the cell. How does the proteasome know which proteins to degrade so that the protein can stop working (i.e., stop turning the cell cycle), and the components of the protein (e.g., amino acids) can be recycled? Ubiquitin, which means found everywhere, is a small regulatory protein that attaches to the proteins that need to be destroyed and recycled. This process is found in all our cells, and in fact, in all plants and animals (eukaryotic cells). It is a highly conserved process that allows the tight regulation of the concentration of specific proteins so that critical processes can be turned off, such as the cell cycle, and signal transduction. In addition, it is important in destroying proteins that are damaged or misfolded, such as proteins that have been made by mutated genes. It is also important in regulating gene expression. Ubiquitin tags are attached to the short-lived protein, and there are actually three different enzymes that help to tag the protein (E1, E2, and E3). Once the tagging is complete and identified with its ubiquitin tag, the protein is escorted to the 26S proteasome, where it is degraded. The ubiquitin is released so it can go do the same job somewhere else in the cell.

There are many different proteasomes. The number of E3 molecules on the ubiquitin tag tells the protein which proteasome to go to. The 26S proteasome is one of the most important proteasomes. It is shaped like a barrel and is found both in the cell nucleus and in the cytoplasm. The barrel contains four stacked rings, called α or β subunits, which surround a core. The tagged protein is recognized by the ends of the barrel (called regulatory caps) and pulled in. One of the subunits helps the protein move into the center core, the protein is unfolded, and the subunit then begins to degrade the protein. The protein is cut into peptides, by destroying the peptide bonds, and then further divided into the component amino acids that were used to make the protein in the first place. ATP is the cell's energy source that is used to degrade the protein. These amino acids are then released and reused (recycled) to make new proteins.

Cells depend on effective ubiquinated proteasome degradation of key proteins used in running the cell. When it is inhibited by a proteasome inhibitor such as bortezomib (Velcade), the cell goes crazy and dies. On a molecular level, it appears to cause increased levels of IkB, an inhibitor of nuclear factor-kappaB (NF-kB).[149] Because it is not doing its job, misfolded proteins accumulate, ringing an alarm within the cell (unfolded protein response, which triggers endoplasmic reticulum stress). When the alarm is triggered, the cell interprets it as severe stress and initiates apoptosis. Interestingly, it was thought that green tea might enhance the effective cell killing started by bortezomib. However, the reverse was found, in that the green tea extract blocked proteasome inhibition by bortezomib; thus, patients taking bortezomib should not drink green tea or take green tea extracts.[149] Figure 2-10 shows the ubiquitin–protease pathway and the interaction with NF-κB. The protein-degradation pathway is very tightly regulated so that cells can quickly turn on or off proteins necessary to keep the cell functioning optimally. In some cancers that have mutations in tumor suppressor proteins, such as BRCA1, which is involved in DNA repair, there is a mutation disabling ubiquitin from linking to the mutated tumor suppressor protein; thus, it is not inactivated and continues to allow division of cells with damaged DNA. In addition, there are oncogenes (e.g., double minute 2 [MDM2] and S-phase kinase protein [SKP2]) that send messages for ubiquitin to tag proteins, such as p53 and p27, that regulate the cell cycle and would otherwise stop the cell from dividing.[150]

HSPs are also in this group of potential targets for anticancer therapy.[152] The body is very careful to have a rapid response team to help when the body is exposed to high temperatures or internal stress. Heat or stress causes the release of transcription factors that increase the expression of the HSPs (which is part of the heat shock response), mediated by heat shock factor (HSF). HSF is the

Figure 2-10 Ubiquitin-protease pathway and interaction with NF-κB.

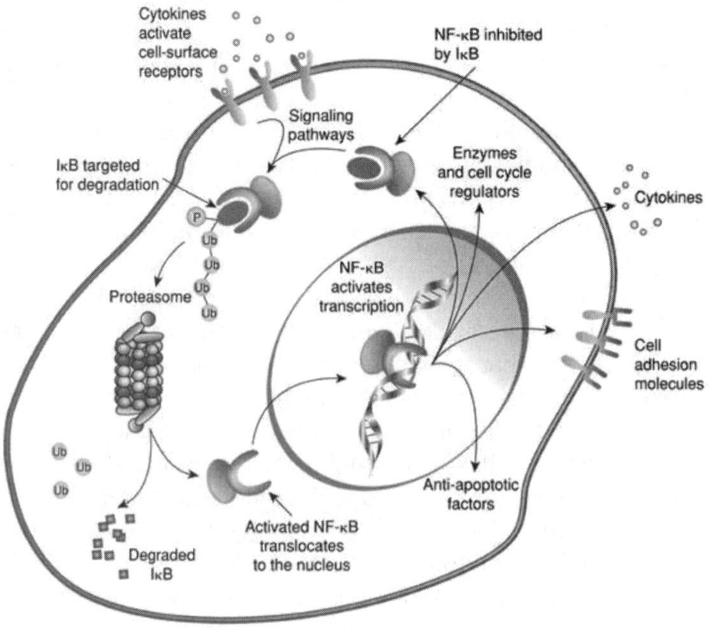

Lee Moffitt Cancer Center and Research Institute Inc.[151]

same molecule found in all living organisms, so it is a primitive protective mechanism for proteins. One has only to fry an egg to see the effects of heat on protein. HSPs play a role as molecular chaperones when they help fold proteins (they have to be folded correctly or they are unable to do their job), helping proteins cope with stress (e.g., inflammation, hypoxia), intracellular trafficking, and housekeeping (i.e., monitor protein health and help bring old proteins to the recycling bin or proteasome).[152]

Heat shock factor 1 (HSF1) is a transcription factor that upregulates (turns on the production) Hsp70 protein expression. Hsp70 and Hsp90 are HSPs that are highly expressed in cancer cells and are critical to the cancer cell's survival.[153] Interestingly, Hsp70 not only protects the proteins within the cell, but it also helps the cell survive. It does this by (1) helping keep proteins folded correctly as they are being synthesized, (2) helping to bring proteins through the cell membrane in a partially folded state, (3) protecting them from thermal and oxidative stress, (4) interacting with E3 ubiquitin ligase to bring old proteins to the proteasome, and lastly, and most importantly, (5) directly inhibiting apoptosis. It does this by blocking procaspase-9 to Apaf-1/dATP/chytochrome c in the second step of the cytochrome c pathway of apoptosis.[154] Hsp90 is also a molecular chaperone that is highly expressed in most normal as well as cancer cells and is necessary for cell survival. Similar to Hsp70, Hsp90 is able to clamp onto proteins to help in protein folding, cell signaling, protein degradation, and protein protection from stress (e.g., hypoxia, free radicals, radiation, chemotherapy). Some of the proteins that Hsp90 chaperones are EGFR, ErbB2 (HER2), c-Met, BCR-Abl, RET, CDK4, FLT3, androgen receptors, B-Raf, NF-kB, C-Raf, p53, and HIF-1α, which helps one appreciate how important this protein is as a target in cancer therapy.[3] On one hand, Hsp90 protects the integrity of proteins by making sure that damaged or mismade proteins are brought to S26 proteasome for degradation by the ubiquitin–proteasome pathway. However, on the other hand, Hsp90 appears to protect damaged proteins, as elevated levels of Hsp90 allow the cell to accumulate the protein products of mutated genes as well; this may be an evolutionary advantage. However, in the context of cancer, this function underscores how important Hsp90 is as an anticancer target.

Hsp90 is necessary to keep the 26S proteasome functioning effectively, as it is responsible for the ATPase activity of the proteasome.[155] However, even though it keeps the 26S proteasome in excellent functional shape, it is also able to help cancer protein kinases to survive in the cell cytoplasm (P13K-Akt). Not surprisingly then, Hsp is overexpressed in cancer cells. P13K and AKT are important proteins in cancer signal transduction, and if they are inhibited, the cell dies (undergoes apoptosis). Hsp90 stabilizes P13K and AKT proteins, so if Hsp90 can be blocked, it appears both P13K and AKT are also blocked, leading to cell death. Hsp90 is a good target for other reasons as well. Hsp90 protects or stabilizes mutated proteins such as the fusion oncogene BCR-Abl and p53, which is mutated in more than 50% of cancers.[156] In addition, Hsp90 plays an important role in angiogenesis. It is necessary for VEGF and the endothelial cell to make and release nitric oxide, both of which are necessary for angiogenesis.[157] Because of its wide-reaching effect on proteins, it influences tumor cell apoptosis (via Akt), TNF receptors, and NF-kB function, and through interaction with MMP2, it promotes invasiveness of the tumor so that it can metastasize.[158]

Clearly, Hsp70 and Hsp90 are attractive anticancer targets for three reasons.[3] First, targeting Hsp90 will leave most normal proteins alone, as tumor cells have increased expression of Hsp90 and drugs targeted to Hsp90 should accumulate in the tumor cells. Second, because Hsp90 chaperones so many important cellular proteins, many of which are signaling proteins in malignant pathways, multiple targets can be attacked by just targeting Hsp90. Third, as we have seen, there are multiple signaling pathways to accomplish the same goal. Thus, by targeting multiple pathways mediated by Hsp90, the likelihood of the tumor cells escaping, as they would with a single targeted pathway, lessens. Conceptually, targeting both Hsp90 and the ubiquitin–proteasome pathway also makes excellent sense. This results in a pile of unfolded proteins that become toxic to tumor cells.[159]

Despite a strong argument for targeting Hsp90, little success has been found so far. More work has been done studying Hsp90 and developing agents that target this protein. A geldanamycin analogue, 17-AAG, is a Hsp90 inhibitor that promotes the degradation of oncoproteins HER2, mutant p53, c-Raf, BCR-Abl.[3] The dose-limiting side effects are anemia, thrombocytopenia, dehydration, hyperglycemia, and GI effects. Other common toxicities are fatigue, anorexia, diarrhea, nausea, and vomiting.[3] Other agents being studied are tanespimycin (KOS-953), which is in phase III (for GIST, myeloma) and phase II (for pancreatic and renal cancer) testing, as well as retaspimycin (IPI-504), which is being studied in phase II trials (for GIST, NSCLC, prostate cancer). Alternatively, another strategy to attack the HSPs is via epigenetic routes, with HDAC inhibitors.[3]

Drug: Bortezomib (Velcade)

Indications: Bortezomib is FDA approved for the treatment of patients with:
- Multiple myeloma
- Mantle cell lymphoma who have received at least one prior therapy

Class: Proteasome inhibitor

Mechanism of Action: A reversible inhibitor of the 26S proteasome; inhibits the breakdown of ubiquinated intracellular proteins and disrupts the ubiquitin–proteasome pathway. This pathway normally regulates the intracellular concentration of specific proteins, thus controlling homeostasis. Cancer cells depend on the proteins that are available from this process to turn on the cell cycle and to make the apparatus of mitosis. When the ubiquitin–proteasome pathway is disrupted, the proteins are not available, and multiple signaling pathways within the cell are disrupted, encouraging the cell to undergo apoptosis. Cell cycle movement (cell division) stops. Cells are unable to migrate, and sensitivity to chemotherapy is increased. In addition, the drug appears to downregulate the NF-κB pathway, which is necessary for cell growth, avoidance of apoptosis, and adhesion. This downregulation may restore chemosensitivity. In multiple myeloma, it interferes with cellular adhesion molecules so that tumor cells cannot bind to the bone marrow.

Pharmacokinetics: After IV administration, the drug is rapidly cleared from the plasma, with a mean elimination half-life range of 40–193 hours after multiple dosing. Drug undergoes oxidative metabolism via cytochrome P450 enzymes 3A4, 2D6, 2C19, 2C9, and 1A2. Drug is deboronated into two metabolites that are then hydroxylated into several metabolites. The elimination path is unknown.

Dosage and Administration: 1.3 mg/m^2 administered as a 3- to 5-second bolus IV injection. Specific conditions as follows:

Multiple myeloma, previously untreated: Administered in combination with oral melphalan (9 mg/m^2) and prednisone (60 mg/m^2) given PO on days 1–4 of a 6-week cycle.

- Cycles 1–4, bortezomib is administered once weekly (days 1, 4, 8, 11, 22, 25, 29, and 32).
- Cycles 5–9, bortezomib is administered once weekly (days 1, 8, 22, and 29).
- At least 72 hours should elapse between consecutive doses of bortezomib.
- Dose modifications: For prolonged grade 4 neutropenia or thrombocytopenia with bleeding in the previous cycle, consider reduction of melphalan dose by 25% in next cycle.
- If platelet count is $\leq$ 30,000/mm^3 or ANC $\leq$ 750/mm^3 on a bortezomib dosing day other than day 1, bortezomib dose should be held.
- If bortezomib doses in consecutive cycles are held due to toxicity, bortezomib dose should be reduced by one dose level (from 1.3 mg/m^2 to 1 mg/m^2, or from 1 mg/m^2 to 0.7 mg/m^2).
- Grade 3–4 nonhematologic toxicities: Hold bortezomib until symptoms have resolved to grade 1 or baseline. Bortezomib may then be reinitiated with one dose level reduction (from 1.3 mg/m^2 to 1 mg/m^2, or from 1 mg/m^2 to 0.7 mg/m^2). For bortezomib-related neuropathic pain and/or peripheral neuropathy, hold or modify bortezomib.

Relapsed multiple myeloma or mantle cell lymphoma: Bortezomib is given twice weekly for 2 weeks (days 1, 4, 8, and 11) followed by a 10-day rest period (days 12–21).

- For extended treatment of more than 8 cycles, bortezomib may be given on the standard or maintenance schedule of once weekly for 4 weeks (days 1, 8, 15, and 22) followed by a 13-day rest period (days 24–35).
- At least 72 hours should elapse between consecutive doses of bortezomib.
- Dose modifications: Hold bortezomib for any grade 4 nonhematologic or grade 4 hematologic toxicity except for peripheral neuropathy, which is discussed separately. Once the toxicity symptoms have resolved, resume bortezomib at a 25% dose reduction (e.g., 1.3 mg/m^2 to 1.0 mg/m^2, or 1 mg/m^2 to 0.7 mg/m^2).

Peripheral neuropathy dose modifications:
- Grade 1 (paresthesias, weakness +/– loss of reflexes) without pain or loss of function: No action is taken.
- Grade 1 with pain or grade 2 (interfering with function but not with ADLs: Reduce bortezomib to 1 mg/m^2.
- Grade 2 with pain or grade 3 (interfering with ADLs): Hold bortezomib until toxicity resolves. When symptoms resolve, reinitiate with a reduced dose of bortezomib (0.7 mg/m^2), and change schedule to once a week.
- Grade 4 (sensory neuropathy that is disabling or motor neuropathy that is life-threatening or leads to paralysis): Discontinue bortezomib.

Available as: One single-use 10-mL vial contains 3.5 mg of bortezomib. Dose must be individualized to prevent overdose.

Reconstitution and Preparation: Store unopened vials at room temperature, 25°C (77°F), and protect from light. Reconstitute each vial with 3.5 mL 0.9% sodium chloride injection USP, forming a colorless and clear solution (stable for 8 hours at controlled room temperature). Final concentration is 1 mg/mL of bortezomib. Draw up prescribed amount (stable in syringe for 8 hours).

Drug Interactions:
- Potent CYP3A4 inhibitors (e.g., ketoconazole, ritonavir): Increase bortezomib exposure; monitor closely for toxicity or reduce dose of bortezomib.
- Patients receiving other drugs that are either inhibitors or inducers of CYP3A4 should be monitored closely for toxicity or reduced efficacy.
- In clinical trials, the addition of dexamethasone 20 mg PO given the day of and the day after bortezomib resulted in increased response rate in patients with stable disease or progressive disease on bortezomib alone.
- Green tea: Polyphenols in green tea may decrease the drug's ability to induce cancer cell death and can negate the drug's efficacy.

Contraindications: Patients with hypersensitivity to bortezomib, boron, or mannitol

Warnings:
- Women of childbearing age should use effective contraception to avoid becoming pregnant while being treated with bortezomib, as the drug decreases the chances of successful delivery of the fetus.
- Women should be advised against breastfeeding or becoming pregnant while being treated with bortezomib.
- Peripheral neuropathy is primarily sensory but may be severe. Patients should have a neurologic assessment prior to each drug dose, eliciting history (symptoms such as pain, burning, paresthesias, dysesthesias, weakness); patients should be asked to pick up a coin and squeeze the nurse's hand; and the nurse should observe patient walking into the exam room to see if there is any gait disturbance or if patient is holding onto the wall. If patient now wears sneakers, it may be an indication of numbness in the toes, but patient needs to validate this observation. Discuss your findings with physician or midlevel practitioner to determine dose modification or discontinuance depending upon severity. Patients report significant improvement in peripheral neuropathy grade after drug dose decrease or drug discontinuation, so peripheral neuropathy is largely reversible. Patients with preexisting severe neuropathy should be treated with bortezomib only after careful risk–benefit assessment.
- Hypotension can occur (incidence 13%). Caution should be used when treating patients receiving antihypertensives, those with a history of syncope, and those who are dehydrated. Teach patients to drink adequate fluid throughout the day (1–2 liters with one glass every hour while

awake). If the patient has nausea and vomiting, or diarrhea, teach patient self-administration of antiemetics or antidiarrheal medication and to call if these measures are ineffective in 24 hours.

- Patients with risk factors for or existing heart disease should be closely monitored. There are rare reports of decreased LVEF, CHF, and QTc prolongation.
- Acute diffuse infiltrative pulmonary disease has been reported, as has alveolitis, interstitial pneumonia, lung infiltration, and ARDS. Rare reports of pulmonary hypertension have been made. If the patient has worsening of any cardiac function, a prompt cardiovascular workup should occur.
- Nausea, diarrhea, constipation, and vomiting have occurred and may require use of antiemetic and antidiarrheal medications or fluid replacement.
- Thrombocytopenia or neutropenia can occur; CBC should be regularly monitored prior to each dose and throughout treatment.
- TLS, reversible posterior leukoencephalopathy syndrome (RPLS), and acute hepatic failure have been reported. For TLS, patients with high tumor burden who are beginning therapy should receive adequate TLS prophylaxis. For RPLS, ensure patients have well-controlled hypertension. If patient has change in mental status, confusion, lethargy, seizure, blindness, or other neurologic symptoms, stop bortezomib and evaluate the patient thoroughly. MRI will be diagnostic for RPLS. Manage with control of BP. See Chapter 3 for more on antiangiogenic agents. For acute hepatic failure, assess LFTs baseline and periodically during treatment. This condition appears to be reversible with drug discontinuance.
- Patients with diabetes may require close monitoring of blood glucose and adjustment of antidiabetic medication.

Adverse Reactions (**bold** indicates most common, occurring in > 25% of patients):

Cardiovascular: Hypotension, orthostatic hypotension, peripheral edema, hypertension

Pulmonary: Dyspnea, upper respiratory infection (URI), cough, pneumonia, bronchitis

CNS/neurologic: **Peripheral neuropathy**, **psychiatric disorders**, **neuralgia**, **headache**, **insomnia**, dizziness, blurred vision

Dermatologic: **Rash**, **pruritus**

Metabolic: **Increased hyperglycemia in patients with diabetes mellitus**

GI: **Diarrhea**, **moderate potential for nausea** and **vomiting**, **constipation**, **anorexia**, dysgeusia, dehydration, abdominal pain

Hematologic: **Thrombocytopenia with nadir day 11 and recovery by day 21; neutropenia, leucopenia, anemia**

Musculoskeletal: Back pain, pain in extremity, arthralgias, myalgias

General: **Pyrexia**, asthenia, rigors

Nursing Discussion:

Peripheral neuropathy: Of patients in clinical trials, 80% had a preexisting baseline peripheral neuropathy (PN); 37% of patients had new onset or aggravation of existing PN; and 14% developed grade 3 PN overall, with 5% occurring in patients without baseline PN symptoms. There were no patients with grade 4 PN. PN improved/resolved in 51% of patients who underwent a dose adjustment for grade 2 PN and in 73% of patients who discontinued the drug. Teach patient to report new onset or worsening of PN symptoms (paresthesias, dysesthesias), any changes in sensory function (temperature sensation, knowing where body parts are in relation to the whole, etc.), functional ability (especially senses of smell and taste), and ability to carry out ADLs. Assess severity of symptom(s) if they arise and potential for injury. If moderate, consult protocol and discuss medical intervention with physician. Teach patient measures to minimize symptoms and ensure safety. Discuss coadministered medication profile with physician, as concomitant administration of the following drugs increases risk of PN: amiodarone, antivirals, isoniazid, nitrofurantoin, or statins. Discuss adding agents that may decrease development or worsening of PN, such as glutamine. See Dosage and Administration.

Bone marrow depression with thrombocytopenia and neutropenia: Thrombocytopenia occurred in 43% of patients (27% grade 3 and 3% grade 4, with nadir day 11 and recovery by day 21) and neutropenia in 24% of patients (13% grade 3 and 3% grade 4; incidence higher in patients with multiple myeloma than mantle cell lymphoma). Febrile neutropenia occurred in < 1% of patients. Anemia incidence was 32%. Fever is common and higher in patients with multiple myeloma (37%) compared with mantle cell (19%). Assess baseline leukocyte, platelet, and Hgb/HCT, and monitor before each treatment, during therapy, and more often as needed. Hold drug for ANC < 1000/mm^3, and dose reduce 25% (see Dosage and Administration). Assess risk for infection and integrity of skin and mucous membranes, pulmonary status, and ability to clear secretions, as well as history of past infections, baseline and prior to each treatment. Teach patient to self-assess for signs/symptoms of infection and to call provider immediately or come to the emergency department if temperature > 100.5°F, shaking chills, rash, productive cough, burning on urination, or any signs/symptoms of infection or bleeding. Teach self-care strategies to minimize risk of infection and bleeding, including avoidance of OTC aspirin-containing medications.

Increased risk of herpes zoster: Risk of reactivation of herpes zoster in both newly diagnosed and relapsed multiple myeloma patients was 13%.[160] The incidence of herpes simplex was 2–8% in the patients receiving bortezomib compared to 1–5% in the control group. When patients received prophylactic antiviral therapy, previously untreated multiple myeloma patients had a decreased incidence (3%) compared to those who did not (17%). Rare cases of herpes meningoencephalitis and ophthalmic herpes have been reported postmarketing. Thus it is recommended that physicians consider prophylactic antiviral therapy.[160,161] For example, in some institutions, acyclovir 400 mg PO twice daily is used if the patient's renal function is normal.

Physicians should consider using antiviral prophylaxis in subjects being treated with Velcade. In the randomized studies in previously untreated and relapsed multiple myeloma, herpes zoster reactivation was more common in subjects treated with Velcade (13%) than in the control groups (4–5%). Herpes simplex was seen in 2–8% of subjects treated with Velcade and 1–5% in the control groups. In the previously untreated multiple myeloma study, herpes zoster virus reactivation in the Velcade, melphalan, and prednisone arm was less common in subjects receiving prophylactic antiviral therapy (3%) than in subjects who did not receive prophylactic antiviral therapy (17%). In the postmarketing experience, rare cases of herpes meningoencephalitis and ophthalmic herpes have been reported.

Nausea, vomiting, decreased appetite, diarrhea, constipation, and dehydration: Patients in clinical studies developed these symptoms with the following incidence: nausea (64%), diarrhea (51%), decreased appetite (43%), constipation (43%), vomiting (36%), dehydration (18%). Diarrhea, nausea, and vomiting occur 6–24 hours after infusion. Nausea is more common in patients with multiple myeloma. Diarrhea and constipation may occur during cycles 1 and 2, and then disappear. Patients with diabetes require close monitoring of their blood glucose and may require adjustments in their antidiabetic medication. Assess baseline weight and nutritional status, and monitor prior to each treatment. Assess glucose and electrolytes prior to each treatment to weekly, especially serum sodium and potassium; replete as necessary, and teach diet high in sodium and potassium. Teach patient that serum electrolytes may be decreased and to assess for signs/symptoms of hyponatremia (confusion, weakness, seizures), hypokalemia (muscle weakness, confusion, irregular heartbeats), hypercalcemia (constipation, thirst, confusion, muscle cramps, sleepiness), and hypomagnesemia (muscle cramps, headache, weakness). Teach patient that side effects may occur, self-care strategies, and to report them if symptoms do not resolve. Use aggressive antiemetics to prevent nausea and vomiting: serotonin antagonist IV prior to bortezomib dose and for 36 hours after each drug dose, if needed. If diarrhea develops after first treatment, teach patient to take loperamide prior to next dose of bortezomib and after every loose stool for 36 hours (not to exceed 8 tablets a day), as well as to use the bananas, rice, applesauce, toast diet. If patient develops constipation, teach preventive self-care (stool softener, flax-seed oil, Milk of Magnesia, prunes or prune juice every a.m. to ensure bowel movement at least every other day). Teach patient to drink 2 quarts of fluid daily, drinking 1 glass an hour while awake to prevent dehydration. Teach patient to report dizziness, lightheadedness, or fainting spells, and to avoid operating heavy machinery or driving a car if these occur. Develop symptom management plan with physician. Make referral to dietitian as appropriate. Teach diabetic patients to monitor their blood glucose closely, and discuss abnormalities and changes in their antidiabetic dose with their nurse practitioner, physician's assistant, or physician.

EPIGENETIC ABNORMALITIES (DNA METHYLTRANSFERASE AND HISTONE DEACETYLASE)

Epigenetics refers to the study of changes in gene expression that are inheritable but do not result in changes in DNA sequence.[162] It helps to explain how the environment, aging, and disease, together with an individual's genetic makeup determine the person's health. This subject was initially explored when it was observed that even though identical twins arise from a single fertilized egg and have identical DNA sequences, there are often differences in the phenotype (behavior) of each twin.[163] Although one's DNA does not change over time, the expression of certain genes does, as the result of interaction with the environment. Another definition of epigenetics is modifications of DNA or associated proteins but not DNA sequence that carries information during cell division.[164] Genes in DNA are turned on or off by transcription factors in the nucleus of the cell. However, epigenetics can influence what genes are turned on or off without changing the DNA, depending upon how tightly the DNA is coiled around histones (which give the three-dimensional shape to the DNA helix), or how methylated the DNA is. DNA is tightly wound around histones like thread around a spool; the DNA that can fit inside a cell, if unwound, would stretch 1.8 meters.[165] Histones are the principal protein in chromatin, which makes up the chromosome and which is composed of DNA, RNA, and proteins.

Normally, there is a epigenetic code that controls gene activity, as not all genes are turned on or expressed at the same time. The RNA polymerase, which is going to turn on the gene, identifies which genes to turn on by chemical tags that act like switches.[166] The more tightly DNA is wrapped around them, the less likely a gene is expressed, such as a tumor suppressor gene. When the switch is turned on at the epigenetic marked spots, the DNA unwinds, allowing that particular gene to be transcribed (Figure 2-11). Cancer processes can modify the epigenetic on and off switches so that tumor suppressor genes are turned off and/or oncogenes are turned on.

Epigenetic carcinogens refer to substances that increase the incidence of cancer but are not mutagenic, such as diethylstilbestrol (DES).[167] This risk of teratogenicity (birth defects) stays in the person who was exposed to DES during the person's lifetime. However, it appears now that the risk of fetal malformations persists and can be transmitted from fathers who were exposed during their mother's pregnancy, as well as to second and succeeding generations of chil-

Figure 2-11   The epigenetic code controls gene activity with chemical tags that mark DNA (diamonds) and the "tails" of histone proteins (triangles).

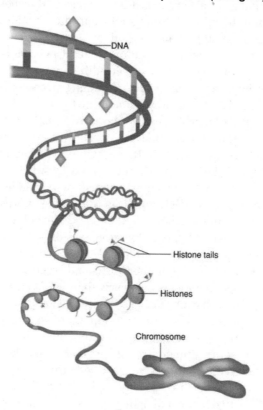

Image courtesy of the National Institutes of General Medical Sciences.[166] Public domain.

dren.[167] Interestingly, the package insert for Vidaza (5-azacitidine) cautions that men should be advised not to father a child while receiving the drug.[168]

Most mutations, as discussed in Chapter 1, involve changes in DNA that silence (tumor suppressor) or activate (oncogene) genes. However, epigenetics can help explain how the environment can influence gene expression. As discussed, epigenetics refers to the extra layer of instructions in the chromosome that influences which genes get turned off or silenced without altering DNA sequence. This silencing of genes without mutational changes in DNA (that occur during cell division or mitosis) is becoming more important and has been linked to the silencing of tumor suppressor genes in a number of malignancies. It can occur through DNA methylation and HDAC.[169] These two exciting areas offer new targets, and already, there are FDA-approved drugs to approach these molecular flaws.

Hypomethylating Agents

Whether the DNA is methylated or not influences gene transcription. DNA methylation means that a methyl group is added to part of the chemical structure (cytosine ring), and this methyl group sticks out into a major groove of the DNA helix so it inhibits or stops transcription of the gene located on that part of the DNA.[170] This occurs mostly in what are called CpG-rich islands located near promoter regions of genes. At least 50% of the human genes, including housekeeping genes, have these CpG island-containing promoter regions, but they are generally unmethylated.[171] Methylation of the CpG islands is brought about by DNMTs, and this occurs in or near promoter regions.[2]

Hypomethylation of areas that are normally methylated can lead to gene activation, such as the oncogene HRAS, while hypermethylation is linked to mutated mismatch DNA repair genes, such as MLH1.[164] In addition, hypomethylation is linked to chromosomal instability, and in the case of the mutidrug resistance gene MDR1, which is often overexpressed, leads to drug resistance in acute myelogenous leukemia.[164] Ehrlich describes the conundrum: Cancer-associated hypomethylation is as prevalent as cancer-linked hypermethylation, but they affect different DNA sequences.[172] Hypomethylation occurs in the genome, except in the CpG islands region, which is hypermethylated. Hypomethylation appears in areas with frequent and moderately repeated DNA sequences, and Ehrlich suggests that hypomethylation plays an independent role in tumorigenesis and progression, more so than does hypermethylation. This raises the question of whether anticancer hypomethylating agents may improve the short-term control of cancer, but may later speed tumor progression for those cells that survive DNA-demethylating–targeted therapy.[172]

Hypermethylation occurs in myelodysplastic syndrome and acute leukemia, and the activity of two hypomethylating agents, 5-azacitidine and decitabine, has led to their FDA approval for treating MDS. These agents get into the DNA and trap methyltransferases (enzymes that help put the methyl into the DNA) on the DNA strand so that there can be no further methylation when the cell goes to divide again. However, they do not remove methyl groups from existing genes. As expected, unlike chemotherapy, which kills or stops the growth of cancer cells right away, hypomethylating agents probably require prolonged therapy to achieve optimal efficacy. The major class of hypomethylating drugs is called DNA methyltransferase inhibitors (DNMTIs).[3] Another example of an FDA-approved agent is decitabine, which is FDA approved for MDS as well. Investigational agents being studied include zebularine, which is an oral agent, procainamide, procaine, and others.[3]

Histone Deacetylase Inhibitors

Another exciting group of agents being explored is the HDAC inhibitor class. The chromosomal DNA is wrapped around histones. The histones determine how tightly the chromatin or DNA is wrapped: If it is tightly wrapped, the gene is turned off or silenced; if it is loosely wrapped, the gene is turned on. Normally, HDACs complex with cell regulatory proteins to regulate gene transcription (i.e., copying the recipe for that gene's protein onto mRNA to be taken outside of the nucleus to the protein synthesis factory, or ribosome) and are key components of cell proliferation, angiogenesis, apoptosis, and cell differentiation. If genes need to be turned on, an acetyl group is added to the histones (acetylation), which loosens the DNA helix so it can be unwound, thus expressing the gene. In contrast, histone deacetylators remove the acetyl groups from proteins such as histones and transcription factors, causing the chromatin to be tightly wrapped and shutting off the genes. Addition of acetyl groups is controlled by HATs, and removal is controlled by HDACs.[3]

Some cancer cells have overexpression of HDACs, or they recruit extra HDACs to oncogene transcription factors, causing hypoacetylation, tightening of the chromatin structure, and gene silencing. HDAC inhibitors cause hyperacetylation, which decreases expression of oncogenes such as BCR-Abl and HER2, stops the cell cycle, induces apoptosis, and stops angiogenesis and cell motility.[173] HDAC inhibitors are intended to help malignant cells become normal again, as they target and accumulate in malignant cells. One example is vorinostat (Zolinza), recently FDA approved for the treatment of progressive or recurrent symptoms of cutaneous T-cell lymphoma (CTCL). Investigational HDAC inhibitors include phenylbutyrate (Buphenyl), which is being studied in phase II trials of patients with cancers of the brain, colon, rectum, and leukemia, as well as valproic acid (Depakote) and belinostat (PXD101), which are being studied in similar phase II trials.[3]

Drug: 5-azacitidine (Vidaza)

Indications: 5-azacitidine is indicated for the treatment of patients with MDS of the following subtypes:
- Refractory anemia
- Refractory anemia with ringed sideroblasts (if accompanied by neutropenia or thrombocytopenia or requiring transfusions)
- Refractory anemia with excess blasts
- Refractory anemia with excess blasts in transformation
- Chronic myelomonocytic leukemia (CMMoL)

Class: Pyrimidine nucleoside analog of cytidine. Classified as a nucleoside metabolic inhibitor. Demethylating or hypomethylating agent, with pyrimidine antimetabolic activity.

Mechanism of Action: Azacitidine causes hypomethylation of DNA, which may restore normal gene function to genes responsible for cell division and differentiation of the bone marrow. It also causes direct cytotoxicity on abnormal hematopoietic cells in the bone marrow. Cells that divide frequently are killed, while nonproliferating cells are relatively unharmed, as they are insensitive to azacitidine. Its cytotoxic effect is mediated by interference with nucleic acid metabolism by acting as a false metabolite when incorporated into DNA and RNA; cell cycle phase specific for S phase.

Pharmacokinetics: Rapidly absorbed following SQ administration, with peak plasma level in 30 minutes. Bioavailability of SQ administered drug is 89% of IV dose. Of the total administered dose, 85% is excreted in the urine and < 1% in feces. Mean elimination half-life is about 4 hours in both SQ- and IV-administered drug.

Dosage and Administration:
- Premedicate with antiemetic.
- 75 mg/m^2 SQ injection (or IV) daily for 7 days, repeated every 4 weeks for at least 4–6 cycles. Complete or partial responses may take longer to achieve.
- Dose may be increased to 100 mg/m^2 after 2 cycles if initial dose ineffective and toxicity manageable (i.e., no toxicity except nausea and vomiting).
- Decrease or hold dose if significant bone marrow depression.
- If baseline WBCs > 3000/mm^3, ANC > 1500/mm^3, and platelets > 75,000/mm^3, modify dose based on nadir counts.
  - ANC < 500/mm^3, platelets < 25,000/mm^3, give 50% dose next course.
  - ANC 500–1500/mm^3, platelets 25,000–50,000/mm^3, give 67% of dose next course.
  - ANC > 1500/mm^3, platelets > 50,000/mm^3, give 100% dose.
- If baseline WBC < 3000/mm^3, ANC < 1500/mm^3, or platelets < 75,000/mm^3, dose modifications and bone marrow biopsy cellularity at time of nadir used, unless there is clear improvement in differentiation (% mature granulocytes is higher with ANC higher than at onset of treatment); see package insert.
- Dose modification based on renal function and serum electrolytes:
  - If unexplained decreases in serum bicarbonate < 20 mEq/L, dose reduce 50% in next cycle.
  - If elevations of BUN or serum creatinine occur, delay next dose until values return to normal or baseline, and reduce dose by 50% in next cycle.

Available as: Lyophilized powder in 100-mg single-use vials

Reconstitution and Preparation:
- Drug is a lyophilized powder in 100-mg single-use vials.
- For SQ administration: Reconstitute aseptically with 4 mL sterile water for injection, adding diluent slowly into the vial.
  - Invert vial 2–3 times and gently rotate, yielding a cloudy suspension containing 25 mg/mL.

- ▪ For SQ administration, divide doses greater than 4 mL into two syringes and administer within 1 hour of reconstitution at room temperature.
- ▪ Reconstituted solution may be kept in the vial or drawn in a syringe(s) and refrigerated at 2–8°C (36–46°F) immediately for later use for up to 8 hours. After removal from the refrigerator, the suspension may be allowed to equilibrate to room temperature for up to 30 minutes prior to administration.
- ▪ For SQ administration: Resuspend contents of syringe by vigorously rolling syringe between palms until a uniform, cloudy suspension appears. Rotate sites for each injection if two syringes are needed (doses greater than 4 mL). Give injection at least 1 inch from an old site and never into areas that are bruised, tender, red, or hard.
- For IV administration: Reconstitute required vials to deliver ordered dose using 10 mL sterile water for injection; vigorously shake or roll vial until dissolved and solution is clear. The resulting concentration is 10 mg/mL. Withdraw ordered amount and inject into a 50–100 mL infusion bag of either 0.9% sodium chloride or lactated Ringer injection. Drug is incompatible with 5% dextrose solutions, Hespan, and solutions containing bicarbonate.
- Administer IV over 10–40 minutes but within 1 hour of reconstitution of the vial.
- Use PPE when handling drug.

Drug Interactions: Incompatible with 5% dextrose-containing solutions, Hespan, bicarbonate-containing solutions

Contraindications:
- Patients with advanced malignant hepatic tumors
- Patients with hypersensitivity to azacitidine or mannitol

Warnings:
- Anemia, neutropenia, and thrombocytopenia can occur. Perform CBCs prior to each treatment cycle and as needed to monitor response and toxicity.
- Hepatotoxicity: Use cautiously in patients with severe preexisting liver impairment, as patients with extensive liver metastases have experienced coma and death, especially in patients with serum albumin < 30g/L.
- Renal abnormalities may occur; monitor patients with renal impairment for toxicity, as azacitidine and its metabolites are primarily excreted by the kidneys.
- Monitor liver chemistries and serum creatinine prior to starting therapy and before each cycle. In patients receiving drug in combination with chemotherapy, renal tubular acidosis (serum bicarbonate < 20 mEq/L) together with an alkaline urine and hypokalemia (K < 3 mEq/L) occurred

in patients receiving drug and etoposide for CML. If unexplained serum bicarbonate < 20 mEq/L or elevated BUN or serum creatinine occur, dose should be reduced or held. Monitor patients with renal impairment closely, as drug is excreted by the kidneys.

• Women of childbearing potential should avoid pregnancy and use effective contraception, as drug is fetotoxic.

• Men should not reproduce while receiving the drug.

• Mothers should not nurse while receiving the drug.

• Monitor renal function closely in elderly patients, as they are more likely to have decreased renal function.

• Baseline and prior to each treatment: Monitor CBC with platelets and differential; BUN, creatinine, LFTs. Monitor nadir counts following cycle 1 to dose cycle 2. Monitor counts weekly if blood counts do not recover by day 28 of the cycle.

Adverse Reactions (**bold** indicates most common, occurring in > 25% of patients):

Cardiovascular: Hypotension, hypertension, peripheral edema

Pulmonary: Nasopharyngitis, pneumonia, URI, dyspnea, rhinitis

CNS/neurologic: Dizziness, headache, anxiety, insomnia, confusion, depression

Dermatologic: **Ecchymosis**, petechiae, dry skin, rash, urticaria, skin nodule

Metabolic: Hypokalemia

GI: **Nausea**, **vomiting**, **diarrhea**, **constipation**, abdominal tenderness, mouth hemorrhage, stomatitis, anorexia

Hematologic: **Anemia**, **neutropenia**, **thrombocytopenia**, **leucopenia**, febrile neutropenia

Musculoskeletal: Arthralgia, chest wall pain, myalgia

Renal: Hematuria, urinary tract infection, rare renal failure

General: **Pyrexia**, **injection site erythema**, rigors, weakness, injection site reactions (bruising, granuloma, pain, pigmentation changes, itching, swelling), lethargy, malaise, rare anaphylaxis

Nursing Discussion:

Bone marrow suppression and risk of infection: Leukopenia is dose-limiting, with nadir occurring days 14–17 after drug administration; it lasts 2 weeks, with recovery 14 days later. Thrombocytopenia and anemia also occur. Bone marrow depression lessens once patient has a response to therapy. Monitor CBC, neutrophil, and platelet count prior to drug administration and at nadir; assess for signs/symptoms of infection, bleeding, and anemia. Teach patient/family signs/symptoms of infection, bleeding, and anemia, and instruct to report them to nurse or physician immediately. Teach patient to avoid aspirin-containing OTC medications.

Potential alteration in nutrition, as nausea, vomiting, diarrhea, and constipation may occur: Nausea and vomiting are dose-related and occur in about 70.5% and 54.1% of patients, respectively, beginning 1–3 hours postchemotherapy. Symptoms tend to be worse in the first 1–2 cycles and increase in incidence with increasing doses. Diarrhea develops in 36.4% of patients, with incidence increasing as dose increases. Constipation occurs in about 33% of patients and is worse during the first 2 cycles of therapy. Anorexia affects 20% of patients, and stomatitis occurs in 7% of patients. Assess nutritional status baseline and periodically at visits. Premedicate with antiemetics before injection, and teach patient self-administration of antiemetics at home; encourage small, frequent feedings as tolerated; if severe vomiting occurs, treat with alternative antiemetics and assess for signs/symptoms of fluid and electrolyte imbalance. Monitor serum potassium, as hypokalemia may be a side effect of treatment. Assess baseline bowel elimination status. Instruct patient to report onset of diarrhea and administer antidiarrheals as ordered. If diarrhea is protracted, ensure adequate hydration, monitor total body fluid balance, and teach/reinforce perineal hygiene. Instruct patient to monitor for constipation and to use measures to prevent constipation if that is a problem. If patient has anorexia, teach patient to identify nutrient-dense foods and to eat small frequent meals, including a bedtime snack. Teach patient strategies to increase appetite, depending upon an individualized assessment. Teach patient to self-assess oral mucosa and to use a systematic cleansing of teeth/mouth after meals and at bedtime. Monitor LFTs periodically during therapy, and discuss abnormalities with physician.

Potential alteration in comfort related to skin (injection site) reaction, fever, fatigue, arthralgias, and myalgias: Fever occurs in 54% of patients, with rigors affecting about 25%; other reactions include fatigue (36%), arthralgias (22%), injection site erythema (35%), injection site pain (23%), injection site bruising (14%), and injection site reaction (14%). Injection site discomfort was more pronounced during the first and second cycles of therapy. If patient prefers, change to IV administration. Monitor temperature and teach patient to self-assess temperature. Teach patient that pyrexia may occur and how to self-administer antipyretics. Teach patient to notify nurse/physician if rigors occur and are severe. Teach measures to reduce discomfort related to myalgias if they occur, such as application of heat and NSAIDs. Teach patient strategies to conserve energy, such as alternating activity with rest. Teach patient to rotate sites used for injection and local measures to increase comfort.

Drug: Decitabine (Dacogen)

Indications: Decitabine is indicated for the treatment of patients with MDS, including previously treated, untreated, as well as secondary MDS or all French-American-British subtypes, and CMMoL.

Class: Pyrimidine antimetabolite, hypomethylating agent

Mechanism of Action: Drug is a pyrimidine analogue and prevents DNA synthesis in the S phase, leading to cell death. Drug is incorporated into DNA and inhibits DNMT, causing hypomethylation and cellular differentiation or apoptosis. Methyltransferase is an enzyme necessary for the expression of cellular genes. The cells in tumors that have progressed or that are resistant to therapy characteristically have DNA hypermethylation. Decitabine "traps" DNMT, thus greatly reducing its activity, which results in the synthesis of DNA that is hypomethylated. DNA hypomethylation activates genes that have been silent, causing the cell to differentiate and then to die (i.e., cell death through disorganized gene expression or extinction of clones of cells that were terminally differentiated). Research has shown that the drug modulates tumor suppressor genes, the expression of tumor antigens, other genes, and overall cell differentiation.

Pharmacokinetics: Biphasic distribution, with mean terminal phase elimination half-life of 0.5 ± 0.31 hours. Drug is not plasma-bound to serum proteins. Metabolism is not fully characterized but appears to involve deamination in the liver, granulocytes, intestinal epithelium, and whole blood. Metabolism does not appear to involve the P450 microenzyme system.

Dosage and Administration:
- First treatment cycle: 15 mg/m^2 IV continuous infusion over 3 hours, repeated every 8 hours for 3 days. Premedicate with antiemetic therapy.
- Subsequent treatment cycles: Repeat initial cycle every 6 weeks for a minimum of 4 cycles (a complete or partial remission may take more than 4 cycles).
- Dose modifications: Delay next cycle until ANC ≥ 1000/µL and platelets ≥ 50,000/µL, and dose reduce as follows:
  - Recovery requiring more than 6 but fewer than 8 weeks, delay drug up to 2 weeks and then temporarily reduce dose to 11 mg/m^2 every 8 hours (33/m^2 per day, 99 mg/m^2 per cycle) upon restarting therapy.
  - Recovery requiring more than 8 but fewer than 10 weeks, assess bone marrow aspirate for disease progression; if no progression, delay dose up to 2 more weeks and reduce dose to 11 mg/m^2 every 8 hours (33 mg/m^2 per day, 99 mg/m^2 per cycle) upon restarting therapy; maintain or dose increase in subsequent cycles as clinically indicated.
  - If any of the nonhematologic toxicities are present, do not restart until toxicity has resolved: serum creatinine ≥ 2 mg/dL, serum glu-

tamic pyruvic transaminase ≥ 2 times ULN; total bilirubin > 2 times ULN; active or uncontrolled infection

Available as: Sterile lyophilized white to almost white powder in a single-dose vial containing 50 mg of decitabine. Store vials at 25°C (77°F) with excursions up to 15–30°C (59–86°F) permitted.

Reconstitution and Preparation: Aseptically add 10 mL sterile water for injection (USP); upon reconstitution, each mL contains approximately 5.0 mg of decitabine at pH 6.7–7.3. Immediately after reconstitution, further dilute with 0.9% sodium chloride injection, 5% dextrose injection, or lactated Ringer injection to a final drug concentration of 0.1–1.0 mg/mL. Use within 15 minutes of reconstitution, or must use cold infusion fluids (2–8°C) to further dilute the drug, then store at 2–8°C (36–46°F) for up to a maximum of 7 hours until administration.

Drug Interactions: None known, but not formally studied

Contraindications: Patients hypersensitive to decitabine

Warnings:
- Drug is potentially fetotoxic, so women of childbearing age should avoid pregnancy by using effective contraception.
- Men should not reproduce while receiving decitabine and for 2 months following drug discontinuation.
- Decitabine causes neutropenia and thrombocytopenia. CBCs, differential, and platelets should be monitored baseline and before each cycle. Early institution of growth factors and/or antimicrobial agents may be needed to prevent infection in patients with MDS.
- Drug was not studied in patients with renal dysfunction (serum creatinine > 2.0 mg/dL), liver transaminases more than double normal, or serum bilirubin > 1.5 mg/dL.
- Baseline CBC, differential, platelets, serum creatinine, electrolytes, and LFTs should be performed, and at a minimum, CBC/differential and platelets should be assessed prior to each cycle; because hyperglycemia, hypomagnesemia, hypokalemia or hyperkalemia, and hyponatremia can occur, serum glucose and electrolytes should be monitored.

Adverse Reactions (**bold** indicates most common, occurring in > 25% of patients):

Cardiovascular: **Peripheral edema**, chest discomfort, chest pain, pulmonary edema, hypotension, rare MI, CHF

Pulmonary: **Cough**, pneumonia, pharyngitis, hypoxia, postnasal drip, sinusitis

CNS/neurologic: **Headache**, **insomnia**, dizziness, confusion, lethargy, hypoesthesia, anxiety, malaise, blurred vision, rare intracranial hemorrhage

Dermatologic: Pallor, rash, erythema, cellulitis, itching, alopecia, urticaria, facial swelling, injection site reactions, swelling

Metabolic: **Hyperglycemia**, hypoalbuminemia, hypomagnesemia, hypokalemia, hyponatremia, hyperkalemia, dehydration

GI: **Nausea, vomiting, constipation, diarrhea**, abdominal pain, stomatitis, dyspepsia, ascites, gingival bleeding, hemorrhoids, tongue or lip ulceration, dysphagia, abdominal distention, gastroesophageal reflux disease, glossodynia, anorexia

Hematologic: **Neutropenia, thrombocytopenia, anemia, febrile neutropenia, leukopenia**, lymphadenopathy, thrombocythemia, candidiasis infection, catheter infection, bacteremia, petechiae

Musculoskeletal: Arthralgias, limb pain, back pain, tenderness, pain, myalgia

Renal: Increased BUN, urinary tract infection, rare renal failure

General: Rare anaphylaxis, rigors

Nursing Discussion:

Bone marrow suppression and risk of infection: Dose-limiting factor is bone marrow suppression. In MDS studies, the incidence of neutropenia was 90%, with 29% of patients developing febrile neutropenia. Thrombocytopenia occurred in 89% of patients. Drug is extensively metabolized in the liver and partially excreted by the kidneys. Anemia occurs in 82% of patients. Assess baseline CBC and differential; assess platelet count and renal and hepatic function tests prior to initial and subsequent cycles of chemotherapy. Drug should be held if ANC < 1000/µL, platelets < 50,000/µL, BR > 2.0 times ULN, AST > 2 times ULN, creatinine > 2.0 mg/dL (see Dosage and Administration). Assess for signs/symptoms of infection, bleeding, and fatigue. Teach patient signs/symptoms of infection or bleeding, to report these immediately, and to come to the emergency department or clinic if febrile or bleeding. Teach patient self-care measures to minimize risk of infection and bleeding. Measures include avoidance of crowds and proximity to people with infections, and avoidance of OTC aspirin-containing medications.

Potential alteration in nutrition, as nausea, vomiting, diarrhea, and constipation may occur: Nausea and vomiting may occur, are mild to moderate, and are preventable by antiemetic medicines. Nausea occurs in 42% of patients and vomiting in 25%. Stomatitis occurs in 12% of patients. Premedicate patient with antiemetic. If patient develops nausea and/or vomiting, encourage small, frequent intake of cool, bland foods. Instruct patient to report nausea, and teach self-administration of antiemetic medications. If nausea and vomiting occur and are severe, assess for signs/symptoms of fluid/electrolyte imbalance. Teach patient to self-administer antidiarrheal medications if needed. Assess baseline oral mucous membranes. Teach patient oral assessment, hygiene measures, and to report any alterations.

Potential alteration in comfort related to skin (injection site) reaction, fever, fatigue, arthralgias, and myalgias: Pyrexia affects 53% of patients, with rigors in 22% of patients. Peripheral edema affects 25%, arthralgias 20%, and pain 13%. Catheter site pain, erythema, and injection site swelling occur in 5% of patients. Assess comfort level and symptoms experienced at baseline and prior to each dose, then prior to each cycle. Teach patient to alternate rest and activity periods. Teach patient to report fevers > 100.5°F and rigors right away, and to come to the clinic or emergency department. Teach patient symptomatic management of pain. Assess catheter and injection sites to rule out infection and to manage comfort.

Drug: Vorinostat (Zolinza)

Indications: Treatment of patients with cutaneous manifestations of CTCL who have progressive, persistent, or recurrent disease on or following two systemic therapies.

Class: HDAC inhibitor

Mechanism of Action: Histones are proteins that give structure and support to the DNA helix and DNA coils around the histones. Some tumors have excess HDAC, which causes the DNA to stay tightly packed. Because the DNA cannot be transcribed, genes are not expressed and are thus silenced, including important tumor suppressor genes. Vorinostat inhibits the enzymatic activity of HDAC1, HDAC2, and HDAC3 (class I) and HDAC6 (class II). This results in increased histone acetylation and uncoiling of DNA so that the DNA is open; genes are expressed and can be transcribed for protein synthesis. These proteins are critical in normal cell-cycle regulation. The drug induces cell cycle arrest and apoptosis in some transformed cells; the mechanism of action of antineoplastic effect has not been fully characterized.

Pharmacokinetics: After oral ingestion, the drug becomes 71% protein bound. It is metabolized via glucuronidation and hydrolysis followed by beta-oxidation, resulting in two inactive metabolites. Drug is eliminated primarily through metabolism, with < 1% of drug recoverable in the urine. Food slightly increases the extent of absorption but slows the rate; in clinical trials, the drug was taken with food.

Dosage and Administration:
- 400 mg orally once daily with food
- Dose modify for thrombocytopenia and anemia
- If the patient is intolerant of therapy, dose may be reduced to 300 mg PO once daily with food. If needed, the dose can be further reduced to 300 mg PO with food for 5 consecutive days each week.
- Teach patient to swallow capsules whole, not to crush or open them.

Available as: 100-mg capsules. Drug is available from a restricted distribution program called ACT (Accessing Coverage Today). Application for the ACT program is available by calling 1-866-363-6379 or online at www.zolinza.com/vorinostat/zolinza/consumer/about/act-program.jsp. Once completed, the form must be faxed back to ACT at 1-866-363-6389 for approval. The drug prescription is filled through specialty pharmacies and delivered directly to the patient's preferred pharmacy. ACT will teach patients about the drug, verify prescription coverage, send refill reminders, and assist with obtaining financial assistance if needed. Drug is available free to patients who have an annual gross income at or below 500% of the federal poverty level.

Reconstitution and Preparation: None, drug is oral

- Teach patient not to open or crush capsules and to take as a single dose once daily with food.
- Teach patient to keep the medication out of reach of children or pets and to use gloves when handling the drug. Teach patient to wash hands before putting on gloves and after removing gloves.
- Teach patient to return any unused drug in the original container to the pharmacy or clinic where care is received.

Drug Interactions:
- Coumarin-derivative anticoagulants may cause prolongation of prothrombin time (PT) and INR; monitor PT and INR closely, and adjust dose accordingly.
- Drugs that prolong the QTc interval (e.g., atypical antipsychotics such as risperidone, fluoroquinolone antibiotics such as levofloxacin, procainamide) may increase risk of QT prolongation because drug increases risk; avoid concomitant administration.
- Insulin and hypoglycemic agents may require increased doses of glucose-lowering agents because drug can cause hyperglycemia.
- Diuretics that cause potassium wasting may potentiate drug-induced hypokalemia; avoid concomitant administration.
- Valproic acid and other HDAC inhibitors may increase thrombocytopenia, with risk of GI bleeding; avoid concomitant use, or monitor platelet count closely if coadministered.

Contraindications: None

Warnings:
- Pulmonary embolism and deep vein thrombosis (DVT) have been reported. Monitor patient for pertinent signs and symptoms, especially if patient has a history of DVT. Teach patient to report right away any pain in the calf, difficulty breathing, or chest pain.

- Dose-related thrombocytopenia and anemia have occurred and may require dose modification or discontinuation.
- GI disturbances (e.g., nausea, vomiting, and diarrhea) may occur. Patients may require antiemetics, antidiarrheals, and fluid and electrolyte replacement (to prevent dehydration). Control preexisting nausea, vomiting, and diarrhea before beginning therapy with vorinostat.
- Hyperglycemia may occur. Adjustment of diet and/or therapy for increased glucose may be necessary. Monitor serum glucose closely in diabetic or prediabetic patients. Adjust diet and/or antidiabetic therapy based on increased glucose results.
- Qtc prolongation has been observed. Monitor electrolytes and ECGs at baseline and periodically during treatment. Normal QTc is 0.30–0.44 second (0.45 second for women). Grade 1 QTc prolongation is defined as > 0.45 second (450–470 msec), grade 2 > 0.47 second (470–500 milliseconds) or an increase of > 60 milliseconds above baseline, grade 3 is > 0.50 second (500 milliseconds). Use extreme caution when administering the drug to patients with a congenital long QT syndrome or patients taking antiarrhythmic medications that prolong the QTc interval. Correct hypokalemia and hypomagnesemia, as these may increase the risk of torsades de pointes, a crescendo ventricular tachycardia associated with sudden death (see dasatinib and nilotinib discussion). Assess patients who have diarrhea, nausea, or vomiting closely, and replete fluid and electrolytes as needed.
- Monitor blood cell counts and chemistry tests, including electrolytes (including potassium, magnesium, calcium), glucose, and serum creatinine, every 2 weeks during the first 2 months of therapy and monthly thereafter.
- Severe thrombocytopenia and GI bleeding have been reported with concomitant use of Zolinza and other HDAC inhibitors (e.g., valproic acid). Monitor platelet count.
- Drug has not been studied in patients with hepatic dysfunction. Because the drug is extensively metabolized in the liver, use caution in administering it to patients with hepatic dysfunction, and monitor closely. Similarly, although the drug is not excreted in the urine, the drug should be used cautiously in patients with renal dysfunction.
- Fetal harm can occur when drug is administered to a pregnant woman. Teach women of childbearing age to use effective contraception and avoid pregnancy.
- Monitor CBC and chemistry tests (electrolytes, glucose, serum creatinine, magnesium) every 2 weeks during first 2 months and monthly thereafter; assess ECG with QTc measurement baseline and periodically during treatment.

Adverse Reactions (bold indicates most common, occurring in > 25% of patients):

Cardiovascular: Peripheral edema, prolongation of QTc interval, pulmonary embolism, DVT; rare MI, ischemic stroke, syncope

Pulmonary: Cough, URI

CNS/neurologic: Dizziness, headache

Dermatologic: Alopecia, itching, rare exfoliative dermatitis

Metabolic: **Hyperglycemia**, hypokalemia

GI: **Diarrhea, nausea, dysgeusia**, anorexia, decreased weight, dry mouth, vomiting, constipation, GI hemorrhage

Hematologic: **Thrombocytopenia**, anemia, leucopenia, neutropenia, bacteremia

Musculoskeletal: Muscle spasms

Renal: Increased serum creatinine, proteinuria

General: **Fatigue**, chills, fever, rare secondary malignancy (squamous cell carcinoma, T-cell lymphoma)

Nursing Discussion:

Bone marrow suppression with thrombocytopenia: Thrombocytopenia occurs in 25.6% (grade 3 or 4 in 5.8%) of patients, and anemia in 14% (grade 3 or 4 in 2.3%). Monitor CBC and platelet count baseline and periodically during therapy. Assess for signs and symptoms of bleeding, fatigue, and anemia. Teach patient to self-assess for signs and symptoms of bleeding and anemia and to call if they occur. Assess patient medication profile and any OTC medications such as those containing aspirin or NSAIDs that would increase the risk of bleeding. Instruct patient to avoid these drugs and not to begin any OTC medications without first discussing with nurse or physician. Teach patient to alternate rest and activity periods if feeling fatigued and to organize shopping and chores in a way to minimize energy expenditures.

Potential alteration in nutrition, related to nausea, diarrhea, anorexia, dehydration, and hyperglycemia: In clinical trials, these side effects occurred with the following frequency: diarrhea 52%, nausea 41%, dysgeusia 28%, anorexia 24%, dry mouth 16%, vomiting 15%, and constipation 15%. Hyperglycemia occurred in 69% of patients who received the 400 mg daily dose. Transient decreases in serum creatinine occurred in 46.5% of patients, and proteinuria in 51% of patients. Assess weight, bowel elimination status, baseline nutritional status, renal status, and glucose level, and monitor during therapy. Teach patient that symptoms can occur and ways to minimize this effect, such as self-administration of antinausea and antidiarrheal medications, and to report symptoms that do not resolve with established plan. Teach patient to identify nutritionally dense (high calories and protein in the smallest amount) foods and to keep them handy in the refrigerator. Teach patient to eat small, frequent meals and to have a bedtime snack. Teach patient that goal is to take in at least 2 quarts of fluid a day and to try to drink a glass of fluid every hour while awake. Monitor patients at risk, such as the elderly, for dehydration closely. Teach patient signs and symptoms of hyperglycemia (i.e., excessive thirst, frequent urination) and to report these. Discuss any abnormalities with a physician.

Risk of QTc prolongation: The QTc interval is the period of ventricular repolarization in the heart. Prolongation of the QTc can increase the risk of developing torsades de pointes, an unusual variant of ventricular tachycardia that may result in sudden death, syncope, or seizures. Risk of developing this condition is also increased if the patient has hypomagnesemia and hypokalemia. Thus, the nurse should ensure that the patient's electrolytes are WNL and that any abnormalities are corrected before the patient begins vorinostat. In addition, a baseline ECG should be done and repeated periodically during therapy. If it is prolonged, it should be reassessed more frequently. Electrolytes should also be monitored closely and repleted as needed. Concomitant use of drugs that prolong the QTc should be avoided. The nurse should carefully review the patient's medication profile along with the physician, midlevel practitioner, or pharmacist to ensure that there are no other drugs that may prolong the QTc.

TUMOR VASCULATURE AND MICROENVIRONMENT

The tumor vasculature and microenvironment (e.g., angiogenesis with VEGF and VEGFR inhibitors; hypoxia-inducible factor; endothelium, and vascular-disrupting agents) are discussed in Chapter 3.

REFERENCES

1. Astra Zeneca. Arimidex challenges tamoxifen as gold standard treatment in women with advanced post-menopausal breast cancer. Available at http://www.astrazeneca.com/search/? itemId=3892537. Accessed October 4, 2009.

2. Adjei AA, Hidalgo M. Treating cancer by blocking cell signals. *J Clin Oncol.* 2005;23(23):5279-5280.

3. Ma WW, Adjei AA. Novel agents on the horizon for cancer therapy. *CA Cancer J Clin.* 2009;59(2):111-136.

4. Brambilla E, Gazdar A. Pathogenesis of lung cancer signaling pathways: roadmap for therapies. *Eur Respir J.* 2009;33:1485-1497.

5. Weiner GJ. Monoclonal antibody mechanisms of action in cancer. *Immunol Res.* 2007;39:271-278.

6. Types of monoclonal antibodies. Genmab Web site. http://www.genmab.com/ScienceAnd Research/IntroductionToAntibodies.aspx. Accessed September 17, 2009.

7. Adams GP, Weiner M. Monoclonal antibody therapy of cancer. *Nat Biotech.* 2005;23:1147-1153.

8. Iannello A, Ahmad A. Role of antibody-dependent cell-mediated cytotoxicity in the efficacy of therapeutic anti-cancer monoclonal antibodies. *Cancer Metastases Rev.* 2005;24:487-499.

9. National Cancer Institute. Common Terminology Criteria for Adverse Events v3.0 (CTCAE). http://ctep.cancer.gov/protocolDevelopment/electronic_applications/docs/ctcaev3.pdf. Published August 9, 2006. Accessed September 17, 2009.

10. Lieberman P, Kemp SF, Oppenheimer J, et al. The diagnosis and management of anaphylaxis: an updated practice parameter. *J Allergy Clin Immunol.* 2005;115:S483-S523.

11. Sampson HA, Munoz-Furlong A, Campbell RL, et al. Second symposium on the definition and management of anaphylaxis: summary report—second National Institute of Allergy and Infectious Disease/Food Allergy and Anaphylaxis Network symposium. *J Allergy Clin Immunol.* 2006;117:391-397.

12. Scarlet C. Anaphylaxis. *J Infus Nurs.* 2006;29:39-44.

13. Lenz HJ. Management and preparedness for infusion and hypersensitivity reactions. *Oncologist.* 2007;12(5):601-609.

14. Kang SP, Saif MW. Infusion-related and hypersensitivity reactions of monoclonal antibodies used to treat colorectal cancer—identification, prevention and management. *Supportive Oncol.* 2007;5(9):451-457.

15. Lundin J, Kimby E, Bjorkholm M. Phase II trial of subcutaneous anti-CD52 monoclonal antibody alemtuzumab (Campath-1H) as first-line treatment for patients with B-cell chronic lymphocytic leukemia (B-CLL). *Blood.* 2002;100(3):768-773.

16. Sehn LH, Donaldson J, Filewich A, et al. Rapid infusion rituximab in combination with corticosteroid containing chemotherapy or as maintenance therapy is well tolerated and can safely be delivered in the community setting. *Blood.* 2007;109(10):4171-4173.

17. Salar A, Casao D, Cervera M, et al. Rapid infusion of rituximab with or without steroid-containing chemotherapy: 1-year experience in a single infusion. *Eur J Haematol.* 2006;77(4):338-340.

18. Spectrum Pharmaceuticals, Inc. *Zevalin package insert.* Irvine, CA, 2009.

19. Murray J, Witzig T, Wiseman G, et al. Zevalin therapy can convert peripheral Blood BCL-2 status from positive to negative in patients with low-grade follicular or transformed non-Hodgkins's lymphoma (NHL). *Am Soc Clin Oncol.* 2000;77[Abstract].

20. Weber J. Review: anti-CTLA-4 antibody ipilimumab: case studies of clinical response and immune-related adverse events. *Oncologist.* 2007;12:864-872.

21. Beck KE, Blansfield JA, Tran KQ, et al. Enterocolitis in patients with cancer after antibody blockade of cytotoxic T-lymphocyte-associated antigen 4. *J Clin Oncol.* 2006; 24(15):2283-2289.

22. Blansfield JA, Beck KE, Tran K, et al. Cytotoxic T-lymphocyte–associated antigen-4 blockage can induce autoimmune hypophysitis in patients with metastatic melanoma and renal cancer. *J Immunotherapy.* 2005;28:593-598.

23. Marmor MD, Skaria KB, Yarden Y. Signal transduction and oncogenesis by ErbB/HER receptors. *Int J Radiat Oncol Biol Phys.* 2004;58(3):903-913.

24. Sliwkowski MX. In: Harris JR, Lippman ME, Morrow M, Osborne CK, eds. *Diseases of the Breast.* 3rd ed. Philadelphia, PA: Lippincott Williams & Wilkins; 2004:415-426.

25. Ritter CA, Arteaga CL. The epidermal growth factor receptor-tyrosine kinase: a promising therapeutic target in solid tumors. *Semin Oncol.* 2003;30:3-11.

26. Ejskjaer K, Serensen BS, Poulsen SS, et al. Expression of the human epidermal growth factor system in human endometrium during the menstrual cycle. *Gynecol Oncol.* 2007;104:158-167.

27. Britten CD. Targeting ErbB receptor signaling: a pan-ErbB approach to cancer. *Mol Cancer Ther.* 2004:1335-1342.

28. Linggi B, Carpenter G. ErbB receptors: new insights on mechanisms and biology. *Trends Cell Biol.* 2006;16:649-656.

29. Wong R, Cunningham D. Using predictive biomarkers to select patients with advanced colorectal cancer for treatment with epidermal growth factor receptor antibodies. *J Clin Oncol.* 2008;26(35):5668-5670.

30. Amado RG, Wolf M, Peeters M, et al. Wild-type KRAS is required for panitumumab efficacy in patients with metastatic colorectal cancer. *J Clin Oncol.* 2008;26:1626-1634.

31. Van Cutsem E, Lang I, D'haens G, et al. KRAS status and efficacy in the first-line treatment of patients with metastatic colorectal cancer treated with FOLFIRI with or without cetuximab: the CRYSTAL experience. *J Clin Oncol.* 2008;26(May 20 suppl):5S. Abstract 2.

32. Jimeno A, Messersmith WA, Hirsch FR, Franklin WA, Eckhardt SG. KRAS mutations and sensitivity to epidermal growth factor receptor inhibitors in colorectal cancer: practical application of patient selection. *J Clin Oncol.* 2009;27:1130-1136.

33. Epidermal growth factors and cancer. abcam Web site. http://www.abcam.com/index.html?pageconfig=resource&rid=10723&pid=10628. Accessed September 17, 2009.

34. Stern HM. EGFR family heterodimers in cancer: Pathophysiology and treatment. In: Haley JD, Gullick WJ, eds. *Cancer Drug Discovery and Development: EGFR Signaling Networks in Cancer Therapy.* New York, NY: Humana Press; 2008:15-31.

35. Hsieh AC, Moasser MM. Targeting HER proteins in cancer therapy and the role of the non-target HER3. *Br J Cancer.* 2007;97:453-457.

36. Sergina NV, Rausch M, Wang D, et al. Escape from HER-family tyrosine kinase inhibitor therapy by the kinase-inactive HER3. *Nature.* 2007;445(7126):437-441.

37. Feng SM, Sartor CI, Hunter D, et al. The HER4 cytoplasmic domain, but not its C terminus, inhibits mammary cell proliferation. *Mol Endocrinol.* 2007;21(8):1861-1876.

38. Allegra CJ, Jessup JM, Somerfield MR, et al. American Society of Clinical Oncology provisional clinical opinion: testing for KRAS gene mutations in patients with metastatic colorectal carcinoma to predict response to anti-epidermal growth factor receptor monoclonal antibody therapy. *J Clin Oncol.* 2009;27:2091-2096.

39. National Comprehensive Cancer Network. *NCCN Clinical Practice Guidelines in Cancer: Breast Cancer* v1.2009. Available at http://www.nccn.org/professionals/physician_gls/PDF/colon.pdf. Accessed October 4, 2009.

40. Di Nicolantonio F, Martini M, Molinari F, et al. Wild-type *BRAF* is required for response to panitumumab or cetuximab in metastatic colorectal cancer. *J Clin Oncol.* 2008;26(35):5705-5712.

41. Romond EH, Perez EZ, Bryant J, et al. Trastuzumab plus adjuvant chemotherapy for operable HER2 breast cancer. *N Engl J Med.* 2005;353:1673-1684.

42. Herbst RS. Review of epidermal growth factor receptor biology. *Int J Radiat Oncol Biol Phys.* 2004;59(suppl 2):21-26.

43. Imclone, Inc. *Erbitux package insert.* Branchburg, NJ, July 2009. Available at http://package inserts.bms.com/pi/pi_erbitux.pdf. Accessed October 4, 2009.

44. Lacouture M. Mechanisms of cutaneous toxicities to EGFR inhibitors. *Nat Rev Cancer.* 2006;6:803-812.

45. National Institutes of Health. NIH image bank. http://media.nih.gov/imagebank/display.aspx?ID=639. Accessed September 17, 2009.

46. Lynch TJ, Kim ES, Eaby B, et al. Epidermal growth factor receptor inhibitor-associated cutaneous toxicities: an evolving paradigm in clinical management. *Oncologist.* 2007;12:610-621.

47. Perez-Soler R. Can rash associated with HER1/EGFR inhibition be used as a marker of treatment outcome? *Oncologist.* 2003;17(11):1-5.

48. Cunningham D, Humblet Y, Siena S, et al. Cetuximab monotherapy and cetuximab plus irinotecan in irinotecan-refractory metastatic colorectal cancer. *N Engl J Med.* 2004;351:337-345.

49. Amgen, Inc. Vectibix prescribing information. Thousand Oaks, CA: Amgen, Inc; Feb 2009.

50. Melosky B, Burkes R, Rayson D, et al. Management of skin rash during EGFR-targeted monoclonal antibody treatment for gastrointestinal malignancy: Canadian recommendations. *Curr Oncol.* 2009;16(1):16-26.

51. Bender A, Zapolanski T, Watkins S, et al. (2008). Tetracycline suppresses ATP gamma S-induced CXCL8 and CXCL1 production by the human dermal microvascular endothelial cell-1 (HMEC-1) cell line and primary human dermal microvascular endothelial cells. *Exp Dermatol.* 2008;17(9): 752-760.

52. Segaert S, Van Cutsem E. Clinical signs, pathophysiology and management of skin toxicity during therapy with epidermal growth factor receptor inhibitors. *Ann Oncol.* 2005;16(9):1425-1433.

53. Lacouture ME, Basti S, Patel J, Benson A. The SERIES Clinic: an interdisciplinary approach to the management of toxicities to EGFR inhibitors. *J Support Oncol.* 2006;4(236):236-238.

54. Scope A, Agero AL, Dusza SW, et al. Randomized, double-blind trial of prophylactic oral minocycline and topical tazarotene for cetuximab-associated acne-like eruptions. *J Clin Oncol.* 2007;25: 5390-5396.

55. Jatoi A, Rowland K, Sloan JA, et al. Tetracycline to prevent epidermal growth factor receptor inhibitor-induced skin rashes: results of a placebo controlled trial from the North Central Cancer Treatment Group (N03CB). *Cancer.* 2008;113:847-853.

56. Wong S, Osann K, Lindgren A, Byun T, Mummaneni M. Pilot cross-over study to evaluate Regenecare topical gel in patients with epidermal growth factor receptor (HER1/EGFR) inhibitors-induced skin toxicity: the final analysis. *J Clin Oncol.* 26:2008(May 20 suppl; abstr 20507).

57. Ocvirk J, Rebersek M. Managing cutaneous side effects with K_1 vitamine crème reduces cutaneous toxicities induced by cetuximab. *J Clin Oncol.* 26:2008(May 20 suppl; abstr 20750).

58. Lacouture ME, Mitchell EP, Shearer H, et al. Impact of pre-emptive skin toxicity (ST) treatment (tx) on panitumumab (Pmab)-related skin toxicities and quality of life (QOL) in patients with metastatic colorectal cancer (mCRC): results from STEPP *Proceedings of the 2009 Gastrointestinal Cancers Symposium.* American Society Of Clinical Oncologists, abstract 291. http://www.asco.org/ASCOv2/Meetings/Abstracts?&vmview=abst_detail_view&confID=63& abstractID=10549. Accessed September 18, 2009.

59. Eaby B, Culkin A, Lacouture ME. An interdisciplinary consensus on managing skin reactions associated with human epidermal growth factor inhibitors. *J Clin Oncol.* 2008;12(2):283-290.

60. Dick SE, Crawford GH. Managing cutaneous side effect of epidermal growth factor receptor (HER1/EGFR) inhibitors. *Comm Oncol.* 2005;2:492-496.

61. O'Keefe P, Parrilli M, Lacouture ME. Toxicity of targeted therapy: focus on rash and other dermatologic side effects. *Oncol Nurse Edition.* 2006;20(13):1-6.

62. Segaert S. Management of skin toxicity of epidermal growth factor receptor inhibitors. *Targeted Oncol.* 2008;3(4):1776-2596.

63. Bernier J, Bonner J, Vermorken JB, et al. Consensus guidelines for the management of radiation dermatitis and coexisting acne-like rash in patients receiving radiotherapy plus EGFR inhibitors for the treatment of squamous cell carcinoma of the head and neck. *Ann Oncol.* 2008;19(1):142-149.

64. Basti S. Ocular toxicities of epidermal growth factor receptor inhibitors and their management. *Cancer Nurs.* 2007;30(4S):S10-S16.

65. Nair RR, Warner BB, Warner BW. Role of epidermal growth factor and other growth factors in the prevention of necrotizing enterocolitis. *Semin Perinatol.* 2008;32(2):107-113.

66. Hallquist-Viale P, Sommers R. Nursing care of patients receiving chemotherapy for metastatic colorectal cancer: implications of the treatment continuum concept. *Semin Oncol Nurs.* 2007;23:22-35.

67. Benson AB 3rd, Ajani JA, Catalano RB, et al. Recommended guidelines for the treatment of cancer treatment-induced diarrhea. *J Clin Oncol.* 2004;22(14):2918-2926.

68. Oncology Nursing Society. Systematic Review/Meta-analysis Diarrhea. In: *Putting Evidence Into Practice.* Pittsburgh, PA: ONS; 2007.

69. National Cancer Institute. Cancer therapy evaluation program, common terminology for adverse events, version 3.0. Available at http://ctep.cancer.gov/protocolDevelopment/electronic_applications/docs/ctcaev3.pdf. Accessed October 4, 2009.

70. Ando M, Okamoto I, Yamamoto N, et al. Predictive factors for interstitial lung disease, antitumor response, and survival in non–small-cell lung cancer patients treated with gefitinib. *J Clin Oncol.* 2006;24:2549-2556.

71. Sandler AB. Nondermatologic adverse events associated with anti-EGFR therapy. *Oncology.* 2006;20(suppl 2):35-40.

72. Higenbottam T, Kuwano K, Nemery B, Fujita Y. Understanding the mechanisms of drug-associated interstitial lung disease. *Br J Cancer.* 2004;91(suppl 2):S31-S37.

73. Tammaro KA, Baldwin PD, Lundberg AS. Interstitial lung disease following erlotinib (Tarceva) in a patient who previously tolerated gefitinib (Iressa). *J Oncol Pharm Pract.* 2005;11:127-130.

74. Ando M, Okamoto I, Yamamoto N, et al. Predictive factors for interstitial lung disease, antitumor response, and survival in non-small-cell lung cancer patients treated with gefitinib. *J Clin Oncol.* 2006;24(16):2549-2556.

75. Shah NT, Kris MG, Pao W, et al. Practical management of patients with non–small-cell lung cancer treated with gefitinib. *J Clin Oncol.* 2005;23:165-174.

76. Tabernero J, Cervantes A, Martinelli E, et al. Optimal dose of cetuximab (C) given every 2 weeks (q2w): a phase I pharmacokinetic (PK) and pharmacodynamic (PD) study of weekly (q1w) and q2w schedules in patients (pts) with metastatic colorectal cancer (mCRC). 2006 ASCO Annual Meeting Proceedings Part I. *J Clin Oncol.* 2006;24(June 20 suppl).

77. Pirker R, Szczesnna A, von Pawel J, et al. FLEX: A randomized, multicenter, phase III study of cetuximab in combination with cisplatin/vinorelbine (CV) versus CV alone in the first-line treatment of patients with advanced non-small cell lung cancer (NSCLC). *J Clin Oncol.* 2008;26 (May 20 suppl, abstr 3).

78. Lieberman P. Anaphylaxis. *Med Clin North Am.* 2006;90:77-95.

79. Chung CC, Mirakhur B, Chan E, et al. Cetuximab-induced anaphylaxis and IgE specific for galactose-α-1,3-galactose. *N Engl J Med.* 2008;358(11):1109-1117.

80. McEvoy GK (ed). AHFS drug information 2009 (online). Bethesda, MD: American Society of Health-Sustem Pharmacists. http://online.statref.com/document.aspx?fxid=1&dpcod=596/. Accessed April 23, 2009.

81. Saif MW. Management of hypomagnesemia in cancer patients receiving chemotherapy. *J Support Oncol.* 2008;6:243-248.

82. Fakih M. Management of anti-EGFR targeting monoclonal antibody-induced hypomagnesemia. *Oncology.* 2008;22:74-76.

83. Hecht JR, Mitchell E, Childiac T, et al. A randomized phase IIIB trial of chemotherapy, bevacizumab, and panitumumab compared with chemotherapy and bevacizumab alone for metastatic colorectal cancer. *J Clin Oncol.* 2009;27(5):672-680.

84. 13th World Conference on Lung Cancer; July 31–August 4, 2009; San Francisco, CA.

85. Gadzar AF. Activating and resistance mutations of EGFR in non-small-cell lung cancer: role in clinical response to EGFR tyrosine kinase inhibitors. *Oncogene.* 2009;28(suppl 1):S24-S31.

86. Gridelli C, Bareschino MA, Schettino C, et al. Erlotinib in non-small cell lung cancer treatment: current status and future development. *Oncologist.* 2007;12:840-849.

87. Engleman JA, Zejnullaha K, Mitsudomi T. MET amplification leads to gefitinib resistance in lung cancer by activating ERBB3 signaling. *Science.* 2007;316:1039-1043.

88. Force T, Kerkela R. Cardiotoxicity of the new cancer therapeutics: mechanisms of, and approaches to, the problem. *Drug Discov Today.* 2008;13(17-18):778-784.

89. Force T, Krause DS, Van Etten RA. Molecular mechanisms of cardiotoxicity of tyrosine kinase inhibition. *Nat Rev Cancer.* 2007;7:332-344.

90. Popat S, Smith IE. Therapy insight: anthracycline and trastuzumab—the optimal management of cardiotoxic side effects. *Nat Clin Pract Oncol.* 2008;5(6):324-335.

91. Floyd JD, Perry MC. Cardiotoxicity of cancer therapy. In: Perry MC, ed. *The Chemotherapy Source Book.* 4th ed. Philadelphia, PA: Lippincott Williams & Wilkins; 2008:179-190.

92. Ewer MS, Vooletich MT, Durand J-B, et al. Reversibility of trastuzumab-related cardiotoxicity: new insights based on clinical course and response to medical treatment. *J Clin Oncol.* 2005;23(31):7820-7826.

93. Telli ML, Hunt SA, Carlson RW, Guardino AE. Trastuzumab-related cardiotoxicity: calling into question the concept of reversibility. *J Clin Oncol.* 2007;25(23):3525-3533.

94. Seidman A, Hudis C, Pierri MK, et al. Cardiac dysfunction in the trastuzumab clinical trials experience. *J Clin Oncol.* 2002;20;1215-1221.

95. Slamon D, Eiermann W, Robert N, et al. Phase III trial comparing AC-T with AC-TH and with TCH in the adjuvant treatment of HER2 positive early breast cancer patients: second interim efficacy analysis. *San Antonio Breast Cancer Symposium 2006*; abstract 52.

96. Mackey JR, Clemons M, Cote MA, et al. Cardiac management during adjuvant trastuzumab therapy: recommendations of the Canadian Trastuzumab Working Group. *Curr Oncol.* 2008;15(1):24-35.

97. Goldberg LR, Jessup M. Stage B heart failure: management of asymptomatic left ventricular systolic dysfunction. *Circulation.* 2006;113:2851-2860.

98. Hunt SA, Abraham WT, Chin MH, et al. ACC/AHA2005 guideline update for the diagnosis and management of chronic heart failure in the adult: a report of the American College of Cardiology/American heart Association task force on practice guidelines: developed in collaboration with the American College of Chest Phsyicians and the International Society for Heart and Lung Transplantation: endorsed by the Heart Rhythm Society. *Circulation.* 2005;112;e154-e235.

99. Loerzel VW, Dow KH. Cardiac toxicity related to cancer treatment. *Clin J Oncol Nurs.* 2003; 7:557-562.

100. Lenihan DJ, Esteva FJ. Multidisciplinary strategy for managing cardiovascular risks when treating patients with early breast cancer. *Oncologist.* 2008;13:1224-1234.

101. Martin M, Esteva FJ, Alba E, et al. Minimizing cardiotoxicity while optimizing treatment efficacy with trastuzumab: review and expert recommendations. *Oncologist.* 2009;14:1-11.

102. Kim MA, Jung EJ, Lee HS, et al. Evaluation of *HER-2* gene status in gastric carcinoma using immunohistochemistry, fluorescence in situ hybridization, and real-time quantitative polymerase chain reaction. *Hum Pathol.* 2007;38(9):1386-1393.

103. Phillips GDL, Li G, Dugger DL, et al. Targeting HER2 positive breast cancer with trastuzumab-DM1, an antibody-cytotoxic drug conjugate. *Cancer Res.* 2008;68(22):9280-9290.

104. Krop IE, Mita M, Burris HA, et al. A phase I study of weekly dosing of trastuzumab-DM1 (T-DM1) in patients with advanced HER2+ breast cancer. *San Antonio Breast Cancer Symposium* 2008; abstract 3136.

105. Modi S, Beeram M, Krop IE, et al. A phase I study of trastuzumab-DM1 (T-DM1), a first-in-class HER2 antibody drug conjugate (ADC), in patients (pts) with HER2+ metastatic breast cancer (BC). *ASCO Breast Symposium* 2007; abstract 168.

106. Vogel CL, Burris HA, Limentani S, et al. Trastuzumab-DM1 (T-DM1) in HER2-positive metastatic breast cancer. *J Clin Oncol.* 2009;27(suppl; abstr 1017):15s.

107. Cortes J, Baselga T, Petrella K, et al. Pertuzumab monotherapy following trastuzumab-based treatment: activity and tolerability in patients with advanced HER2-positive breast cancer. *J Clin Oncol.* 2009;27(suppl; abstr 1022):15s.

108. Boccaccio C, Comoglio PM. Invasive growth: a MET-driven genetic programme for cancer and stem cells. *Nat Rev Cancer.* 2006;6(8):637-645.

109. Gentile A, Trusolino L, Comoglio PM. The Met tyrosine kinase receptor in development and cancer. *Cancer Metastases Rev.* 2008;27(1):85-94.

110. Walter KA, Hossain MA, Luddy C, et al. Scatter factor/hepatocyte growth factor stimulation of glioblastoma cell cycle progression through G(1) is c-Myc dependent and independent of p27 suppression, Cdk2 activation, or E2F1 dependent transcription. *Mol Cell Biol.* 2002;22(8):2703-2715.

111. Recio JA, Merlino G. Hepatocyte growth factor/scatter factor activates proliferation in melanoma cells through p38 MAPK, ATF-2 and cyclin D1. *Oncogene.* 2002;21(7):1000-1008.

112. Weinberg RA. *The Biology of Cancer.* New York: Garland Science; 2008:147-188.

113. Abounader R, Reznik T, Colantuoni C, et al. Regulation of c-Met dependent gene expression by PTEN. *Oncogene.* 2004;23(57):9173-9182.

114. Gordon MS, Mendelson D, Sweeney C, et al. Interim results from a first-in-human study with AMG-102, a fully human monoclonal antibody that neutralizes hepatocyte growth factor (HGF), the ligand to c-Met receptor in patients (pts) with advanced solid tumors. *J Clin Oncol.* 2007;18S(suppl):abstract 3551.

115. Thomas RM, Toney K, Fenoglio-Preiser C, et al. The RON receptor tyrosine kinase mediates oncogenic phenotypes in pancreatic cancer cells and is increasingly expressed during pancreatic cancer progression. *Cancer Res.* 2007;67:6075-6079.

116. Jhawer MP, Kindler HL, Wainberg ZA, et al. Preliminary activity of XL880, a dual MET/VEGFR2 inhibitor, in MET amplified poorly differentiated gastric cancer (PDGC): interim results of a multicentered phase II study. *J Clin Oncol.* 2008;26(May 20 suppl; abstr 4572).

117. Martins AS, Mackintosh C, Martin DH, et al. Insulin-like growth factor 1 receptor pathway inhibition by ADW742 alone or in combination with imatinib, doxorubicin, or vincristine, is a novel therapeutic approach in Ewing Tumor. *Clin Cancer Res.* 2006;12(11):3532-3538.

118. Gunter MJ, Hoover DR, Yu H, et al. Insulin, insulin-like growth factor-I, and risk of breast cancer in postmenopausal women. *J Natl Cancer Inst.* 2009;101(1):48-60.

119. Kabat GC, Kim M, Caan BJ, et al. Repeated measures of serum glucose and insulin in relation to postmenopausal breast cancer. *Int J Cancer.* June 2, 2009. doi:10.1002/ijc.24609.

120. Yee D. Targeting insulin-like growth factor pathways. *Br J Cancer.* 2006;94:465-468.

121. Yuen JSP, Akkaya E, Wang Y, et al. Validation of the type 1 insulin-like growth factor receptor as a therapeutic target in renal cancer. *Mol Cancer Ther.* 2009;8(6):1448-1459.

122. Krause DS, Van Etten RA. Turosine kinases as targets for cancer therapy. *N Engl J Med.* 2005;353(2):172-187.

123. Belsches-Jablonski AP, Demory ML, Parsons JT, Parsons SJ. The Src pathway as a therapeutic strategy. *Drug Discov Today Ther Strateg.* 2005;2(4):313-321.

124. Martin GS. The hunting of the Src. *Nature Rev Mol Cell Biol.* 2001;2:467-475.

125. Courtneidge SA. Role of Src in signal transduction pathways. *Biochem Soc Trans.* 2002;30(2): 11-17.

126. Vultur A, Buettner R, Kowolik C, et al. SKI-606 (bosutinib) a novel Src kinase inhibitor, suppresses migration and invasion of human breast cancer cells. *Mol Cancer Ther.* 2008;7(5):1185-1194.

127. Haura EB, Turkson J, Jove R. Mechanisms of disease: insights into the emerging role of signal transducers and activators of transcription in cancer. *Nat Clin Pract Oncol.* 2005;2(6):315-324.

128. Wennerberg K, Rossman KL, Der CJ. The Ras superfamily at a glance. *J Cell Sci.* 2005;118:843-846.

129. Rowinsky EK, Windle JJ, Von Hoff DD. Ras protein farnesyltransferase: a strategic target for anticancer therapeutic development. *J Clin Oncol.* 1999;17(11):3631-3652.

130. Wagner EF, Nebreda AR. Signal integration by JNK and p38 MAPK pathways in cancer. *Nat Rev Cancer.* 2009;9:537-549.

131. Liu P, Cheng H, Roberts TM, Zhao JJ. Targeting the phosphoinositide 3-kinase pathway in cancer. *Nat Rev Drug Discov.* 2009;8:627-644.

132. Engelman JA. Targeting PI3K signaling in cancer: opportunities, challenges and limitations. *Nat Rev Cancer.* 2009;9:550-562.

133. Mahalingam D, Kelly KR, Swords RT, et al. Emerging drugs in the treatment of pancreatic cancer. *Expert Opin Emerg Drugs.* 2009;14(2):311-328.

134. Waite KA, Eng C. Protean PTEN: form and function. *Am J Hum Genet.* 2002;70(4):829-844.

135. Nagata Y, Lan KH, Zhou X, et al. PTEN activation contributes to tumor inhibition by trastuzumab, and loss of PTEN predicts trastuzumab resistance in patients. *Cancer Cell.* 2004;6:117-127.

136. Los M, Maddika S, Erb B, Schulze-Osthoff. Switching Akt: form survival signaling to deadly response. *BioEssays.* 2009;31(5):492-495.

137. Lum L, Beachy PA. The Hedgehog response network: sensors, switches and routers. *Science.* 2004;304:1755-1759.

138. Liu S, Dontu G, Mantle ID, et al. Hedgehog signaling and Bmi-1 regulate self-renewal of normal and malignant human mammary stem cells. *Cancer Res.* 2006;66(12):6063-6071.

139. Rubin LL, de Sauvage FJ. Targeting the hedgehog pathway in cancer. *Nat Rev Drug Discov.* 2006;5:1026-1033.

140. Beachy PA, Karhadkar SS, Berman DM. Tissue repair and stem cell renewal in carcinogenesis. *Nature.* 2004;432:324-331.

141. Adolphe C, Hetherington R, Ellis T, Wainwright B. Patched 1 functions as a gatekeeper by promoting cell cycle progression. *Cancer Res.* 2006;66:2081-2088.

142. Lee SW, Moskowitz MA, Sims JR. Sonic hedgehog inversely regulates the expression of angiopoietin-1 and angiopoietin-2 in fibroblasts. *Int J Mol Med.* 2007;19(3):445-451.

143. Bailey JM, Mohr AM, Hollinsworth MA. Sonic hedgehog paracrine signaling regulates metastases and lymphangiogenesis in pancreatic cancer. *Oncogene.* July 27, 2009; doi:10.1038 /onc.2009.220.

144. Epstein EH. Basal cell carcinomas: attack of the hedgehog. *Nat Rev Cancer.* 2008;8:743-754.

145. Xie J. Activation of Hedgehog singaling in human cancer: basic mechanisms and clinical implications. In: *AACR Educational Book.* AACR 100th Annual Meeting 2009; April 18-22, 2009. http://educationbook.aacrjournals.org. Accessed August 15, 2009.

146. Olive KP, Jacobetz MA, Davidson CJ, et al. Inhibition of Hedgehog signaling enhances delivery of chemotherapy in a mouse model of pancreatic cancer. *Science.* 2009;324(5933):1457-1461.

147. Kasper M, Jaks V, Fiaschi M, Toftgard R. Hedgehog signaling in breast cancer. *Carcinogenesis.* February 23, 2009. doi:10.1093/carcin/bgp048

148. Bijlsma MF, Spek CA, Zivkovic D, et al. Repression of smoothened by patched-dependent (pro) vitamin D_3 secretion. *PLoS Biol.* 2006;4(8):e232.

149. Golden EB, Lam PY, Kardosh A, et al. Green tea polyphenols block the anticancer effects of bortezomib and other boronic acid-based proteasome inhibitors. *Blood.* 2009;113(23):5927-5937.

150. Nalepa G, Rolfe M, Harper JW. Drug discovery in the ubiquitin-proteasome system. *Nat Rev Drug Discov.* 2006;5:596-613.

151. Cancer Control. Lee Moffitt Cancer Center and Research Institute. Medscape. http://img .medscape.com/fullsize/migrated/463/787/cc463787.fig2.jpg. Published 2003. Accessed September 18, 2009.

152. Dai C, Whitesell L, Rogers AB, Lindquist S. Heat shock factor 1 is a powerful multifaceted modifier of arcinogenesis. *Cell.* 2007;130(6):1005-1018.

153. Didelot C, Lanneau D, Brunet M, et al. Anti-cancer therapeutic approaches based on intracellular and extracelllar heat shock proteins. *Curr Med Chem.* 2007;14(27):2839-2847.

154. Beere HM, Wolf BB, Cain K, et al. Heat shock protein 70 inhibits apoptosis by preventing recruitment of procaspase-9 to the Apaf-1 apoptosome. *Nat Cell Biol.* 2000;2(8):469-475.

155. Imai J, Maruya M, Yashiroda H, et al. The molecular chaperone Hsp90 plays a role in the assembly and maintenance of the 26S proteasome. *Embo J.* 2003;22(14):3557-3567.

156. Calderwood SK, Khaleque MA, Sawyer DB, Ciocca DR. Heat shock proteins in cancer: chaperones of tumorigenesis. *Trends Biochem Sci.* 2006;31(3):164-172.

157. Fontana J, Fulton D, Chen Y, et al. Domain mapping studies reveal that the M domain of hsp90 serves as a molecular scaffold to regulate Akt-dependent phosphorylation of endothelial nitric oxide synthase and NO release. *Circ Res.* 2002;90(8):866-873.

158. Whitesell L, Lindquist SL. Hsp90 and the chaperoning of cancer. *Nat Rev Cancer.* 2005;5(10):761-772.

159. Neckers L. Heat shock protein 90: the cancer chaperone. *J Biosci.* 2007;32:517-530.

160. Velcade [package insert]. Cambridge, MA: Millenium Pharmaceuticals; June 2008.

161. Chanan-Khan A, Sonneveld P, Schuster MW, et al. Analysis of herpes zoster events among the bortezomib-treated patients in the phase III APEX study. *J Clin Oncol.* 2008;26(29):4784-4790.

162. Feinberg AP. Epigenetics at the epicenter of modern medicine. *JAMA.* 2008;299(11):1345-1350.

163. Kaminsky ZA. DNA methylation profiles in monozygotic and dizygotic twins. *Nat Genetics.* 2009;41:240-245.

164. Feinberg AP, Tycko B. The history of cancer epigenetics. *Nat Rev Cancer.* 2004;4(2):143-153.

165. Ward R, Bowman A, El-Mkami H, et al. Long distance PELDOR measurements on the histone core particle. *J Am Chem Soc.* 2009;131(4):1348-1349.

166. National Institute of General Medical Sciences. RNA and DNA revealed: new roles, new rules. In: *The New Genetics.* http://publications.nigms.nih.gov/thenewgenetics/chapter2.html. Accessed September 18, 2009.

167. Newbold RR, Padilla-Banks E, Jefferson WN. Adverse effects of the model environmental estrogen diethylstilbestrol are transmitted to subsequent generations. *Endocrinology.* 2006; 147(suppl 6):S11-S17.

168. Vidaza [package insert]. Summit, NJ: Celgene Corp; August 2008.

169. Claus R, Lubbert M. Epigenetic targets in hematopoietic malignancies. *Oncogene.* 2003;22:6489-6496.

170. Herman JG, Baylin SB. Gene silencing in cancer in association with promoter hypermethylation. *N Engl J Med.* 2003;349:2042-2054.

171. Jones P. DNA methylation and cancer. Presented at: Breakthroughs in Therapeutic Epigenetics: An Emerging Clinical Approach, symposium held in conjunction with the 41st Annual Meeting of the American Society of Clinical Oncology; May 2005; Orlando, FL.

172. Ehrlich M. DNA methylation in cancer: too much, but also too little. *Oncogene.* 2002;21(35): 5400-5413.

173. George P, Bali P, Annavarapu S, et al.Combination of the histone deacetylase inhibitor LBH589 and the hsp90 inhibitor 17-AAG is highly active against human CML-BC cells and AML cells with activating mutation of FLT-3. *Blood.* 2005;105:1768-1776.

CHAPTER 3

Tumor Vasculature

TARGETING ANGIOGENESIS

Folkman, nearly four decades ago, demonstrated that tumors could not grow beyond 1–2 mm, the diffusion distance of oxygen, without the formation of new blood vessels, a process called angiogenesis.[1] Angiogenesis is a critical process during embryogenesis and also during wound healing, rebuilding the endometrial lining in women after menstruation, making the placenta during pregnancy, and enabling bone and muscle growth. Angiogenesis can also be activated during pathologic conditions, such as inflammation, atherosclerosis, and age-related macular degeneration.

Process of Angiogenesis

The body very carefully regulates angiogenesis via the "angiogenic switch." The switch is turned on when proangiogenic factors (the most important being hypoxia) are greater than antiangiogenic factors, which oppose angiogenesis.[2] When proangiogenic factors are stronger than opposing factors, the angiogenic switch is turned to the "on" position, driving angiogenesis. In the normal human, the angiogenesis switch is most often in the "off" position. For example, when cells do not get enough oxygen, they become hypoxic and release a substance called hypoxia-inducible factor (HIF), which is a transcription factor that leads to the production of vascular endothelial growth factor (VEGF). VEGF then goes to the endothelial cell, binds to the VEGF receptor (VEGFR), and starts sending a message to the cell nucleus to make more endothelial cells (proliferation) and for these new cells to migrate, forming blood vessels that will bring oxygen to the hypoxic cells. Figure 3-1 shows the process of angiogenesis. Table 3-1 presents pro- and antiangiogenic factors.

Angiogenesis is normally a very orderly, systematic process. Tissues requiring new blood vessels, such as injured tissue (e.g., wound), release angiogenic growth factors, such as VEGF, that diffuse into neighboring tissues, where they seek capillaries, and more specifically, receptors on the endothelial cells that line the nearby capillary or blood vessel. Once VEGF binds to the VEGFR on the endothelial cells, it tells the cells to proliferate and migrate. It does this by activating a signaling cascade by which this message is sent from outside the cell through the membrane of the cell (kinase domain) and then, as if by a bucket brigade, to the cell nucleus. The message tells the nucleus which genes need to be copied

Figure 3-1   Process of angiogenesis.

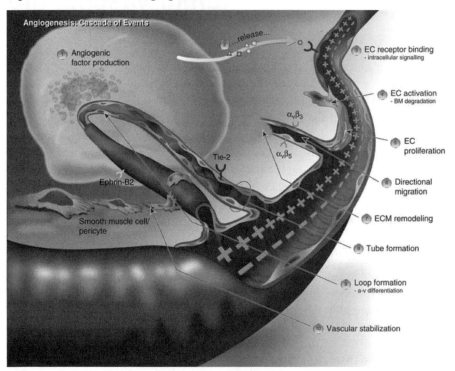

Reproduced with permission from the Angiogenesis Foundation.[3]

to give the protein recipes needed for cell proliferation and migration. In addition, recipes for proteins like matrix metalloproteinases (MMPs) are also copied so that the enzymes can be made. MMPs, when released, will dissolve the extracellular matrix (ECM) so that a path is made for the new and fragile blood vessel to travel to the injured tissue.

Once the recipes are copied and taken to the ribosomes to make the correct proteins, cells begin to proliferate and move through dissolved holes in the basement membrane in existing capillaries toward the injured tissue. The new cells start to sprout, and the endothelial tip cell leads the new vessel as it moves out of the existing blood vessel. The formation of the tip cell is initiated by VEGF, but differentiation is maintained by fibroblast growth factor receptor (FGFR) and VEGF signaling.[4] The tip cell needs to communicate with the endothelial cells behind it, so Notch ligands delta-like 4 (DLL4) and Jagged1 become expressed on the cell, and it is via the Notch signaling pathway that the message is sent to the cells in the rear to follow the tip cell as the vessel moves toward the tumor.

Table 3-1   Proangiogenic and Antiangiogenic Factors

Proangiogenic factors	Antiangiogenic factors
Fibroblast growth factor (FGF), FGF-1 (acidic), and FGF-2 (basic): promote proliferation and differentiation of endothelial cells, muscle cells, and fibroblasts	Angiostatin (plasminogen fragment)
Vascular endothelial growth factor (VEGF): increases permeability	Fibronectin fragment
VEGF receptor (VEGFR) and neuropilin-1 (NRP-1, co-receptor for VEGF): promote endothelial cell survival	Heparinases Heparin hexasaccharide fragment
Angiopoietin 1 and its receptor Tie2: stabilize vessels	Endostatin
Platelet-derived growth factor (PDGF) and its receptor PDGFR: increase ECM production	Alpha, beta, and gamma interferons (IFs)
Integrins $\alpha_v\beta_3$, $\alpha_v\beta_5$, $\alpha_5\beta_3$: bind matrix macromolecules and proteinases	Plasminogen activator inhibitor
Ephrin: determines whether it is an artery or a vein	Retinoids
Hepatocyte growth factor (HGF)/ scatter factor (SF)	Metalloproteinase inhibitors (TIMPs)
Transforming growth factors α and β (TGFα, TGFβ)	Transforming growth factor β (TGFβ)
Tumor necrosis factor alpha (TNFα)	Thrombospondin-1 (TSP-1)
Plasminogen activators: remodel ECM, release and activate growth factors	
Hypoxia	

Data from Kerbel RS. Molecular origins of cancer: Tumor angiogenesis. *N Engl J Med.* 2008;358:2039-2049; Ramanujan S, Koenig GC, Padera TP, Stoll BR, Jain RK. Local imbalance of proangiogenic and antiangiogenic factors: A potential mechanism of focal necrosis and dormancy in tumors. *Cancer Res.* 2000;60:1442-1448.

The tip cell has filopodia (membrane ruffles that move the cell along), and it strategizes with $\alpha_v\beta_3$ integrin, which will pull the tip cell and its followers (stalk cells) along in the path made by membrane type 1 matrix metalloproteinase (MT1MMP or MMP14), which dissolves (remodels) the ECM in the blood vessel path, making a highway to the tumor. Under electron microscopy, the ECM looks like a jungle with many obstructions to the advancing fragile, newly forming blood vessel; thus, a discrete path needs to be created. The following stalk cells and their covering pericytes make a basement membrane and contacts between the stalk cells.

It appears that VEGF-A, which is necessary for endothial cell proliferation, migration, and survival, is also responsible for controlling the tubular sprouting of the new vessel[5] (see Figure 3-1). The sprouting endothelial cells roll up to form a blood vessel tube. Integrins, specialized adhesion molecules $a_v\beta_3$ and $a_v\beta_5$, act like grappling hooks to pull the sprouting new blood vessel toward the injured tissue. The MMPs continue to dissolve the ECM in front of the advancing blood vessel so it can easily grow toward the injured tissue. Angiopoietin-1 and -2 play roles in helping the new blood vessels survive and communicate via the Tie2 receptors. They are also essential for blood vessel maturation. Blood vessel tubes connect to form blood vessel loops as shown in Figure 3-1, allowing blood from the existing blood vessel to circulate to the injured tissue.

EphrinB2 (EphB2) induces the migration of endothelial cells through the P13K pathway and helps to make adult blood vessels. EphB2 and EphB4 receptors are thought to help the endothelial cells move and form into a cord-line blood vessel; they also communicate with stromal-derived factor (SDF-1) in coordinating endothelial cell movement. SDF-1 is a chemokine that also regulates the movement of primitive stem cells. It binds to its cell surface receptor CXCR4.[6] It has been implicated in breast cancer metastasis, as breast cancer cells highly express CXCR4 receptors, and common metastatic sites express their ligand CXCL12/SDF-1 alpha, such as the axillary lymph nodes and lung.[7]

Once formed, smooth muscle cells and pericytes give the new vessel structural support. Endothelial cells release platelet-derived growth factor (PDGF), which binds to the PDGF receptor (PDGFR) located on the cell membrane of the pericyte. Pericytes attach to the exterior of the new blood vessel, protecting the new blood vessel like the shingles of a house. Because they are located in the basement membrane of the capillaries, they serve to stabilize the walls of the blood vessel so that blood will flow smoothly. Pericytes also express receptors for PDGF-β (PDGFR-β) and, together with the endothelial cells that express PDGF-β, help the blood vessels mature.[8] The principal driver of angiogenesis in tumors is hypoxia, which causes tumors to release VEGF. The VEGF family is a subfamily of the PDGF family and has the following members: VEGF-A, VEGF-B, VEGF-C, VEGF-D (also known as FIGF), and placental growth factor. VEGF-A was discovered first and called VEGF. It is responsible for proliferation and migration of endothelial cells, activates integrin $a_v\beta_3$, stimulates vasodilation, induces microvessel permeability, helps create blood vessel lumen, and creates the fenestrations in the blood vessel.[9] VEGF-C is important in lymphangiogenesis.

Within the VEGF-A group, there are three receptors, that are called transmembrane receptor tyrosine kinases (RTKs). They include VEGFR-1 (Flt-1), VEGFR-2 (KDR/Flk-1), and VEGFR-3 (Flt-4). The different forms of VEGF all have specific receptors to which they bind. VEGF is the principal ligand for VEGFR-1 and VEGFR-2, but not VEGFR-3. VEGF-3 has VEGF-C as its ligand, and it regulates the endothelial cells in the lymphatic vessels during lymphangiogenesis.

The neuropilins (NP1 and NP2, called NRP1 and NRP2) are coreceptors for the VEGFRs, and they increase the attraction (binding affinity) of VEGF to their receptor VEGFR. Their role in cancer, however, is not clear.[10] NRP1 helps integrate endothelial cell survival, together with VEGFR; it is also implicated in cell migration and invasion. NRP2 may play a role in tumorigenesis.[11] VEGFR-1 is found on endothelial cells and monocytes and may modulate VEGF-2 signaling. Interestingly, VEGF has a stronger affinity to VEGFR-1 than VEGFR-2, so VEGFR-1 may act as a negative regulator of angiogenesis by preventing VEGF from binding to VEGFR-2.[10] VEGFR-2 is the most well known, as it appears to mediate all the known VEGF effects.[12]

Within the endothelial cell, intracellular signal transduction involves similar pathways as other cancer cells. VEGF-A binds to its receptor VEGFR-1,2 on the endothelial cell. The receptors dimerize (come together), causing autophosphorylation, which activates signal transduction. Thus the receptor is turned on and a message is sent down the receptor into the cell to its internal domain tyrosine kinase. The message then travels as if by a bucket brigade (downstream) via three separate pathways to the cell nucleus[13]:

- The RAS → Raf → MEK → ERK pathway results in endothelial proliferation.
- The P13K → AKT pathway results in endothelial cell survival and vascular permeability.
- The p38MAPK → HSP27 pathway results in endothelial cell migration.

Like other embryological processes that are subverted by malignant transformation, angiogenesis is also a key process in tumor formation and metastasis. Both the tumor and the stroma regulate the pathways, driving angiogenesis in cancer. VEGF is commonly overexpressed in many solid tumors.[10]

As illustrated by Figure 3-1, angiogenesis is an orderly series of events:

1. Diseased or injured tissues produce and release angiogenic growth factors (proteins) that diffuse into the nearby tissues.
2. The angiogenic growth factors bind to specific receptors located on the endothelial cells of nearby preexisting blood vessels.

3. Once growth factors bind to their receptors, the endothelial cells become activated. Signals are sent from the cell's surface to the nucleus.
4. The endothelial cell's machinery begins to produce new molecules, including enzymes. These enzymes dissolve tiny holes in the sheathlike covering (basement membrane) surrounding all existing blood vessels.
5. The endothelial cells begin to divide (proliferate) and migrate out through the dissolved holes of the existing vessel toward the diseased tissue (tumor).
6. Specialized molecules called adhesion molecules (integrins $a_v\beta_3$, $a_v\beta_5$) serve as grappling hooks to help pull the sprouting new blood vessel forward.
7. Additional enzymes (MMPs) are produced to dissolve the tissue in front of the sprouting vessel tip in order to accommodate it. As the vessel extends, the tissue is remolded around the vessel.
8. Sprouting endothelial cells roll up to form a blood vessel tube.
9. Individual blood vessel tubes connect to form blood vessel loops that can circulate blood.
10. Finally, newly formed blood vessel tubes are stabilized by specialized muscle cells (smooth muscle cells, pericytes) that provide structural support. Blood flow then begins.

Tumor cells as they proliferate need new blood vessels to bring in oxygen and glucose (food) and remove waste products.[14] Hypoxia is a very strong proangiogenic factor and significantly drives new blood vessel formation. In cancer, the process of angiogenesis is very similar to that depicted in Figure 3-1 and is driven by hypoxia and local oncogenes. However, the blood vessels that are formed are very different. Key targets include VEGF, VEGFR-1 and -2, angiopoietin-1 and -2, Tie2, the integrins that pull the new blood vessel sprout toward the tumor, MMPs, and the pericytes. The hypoxic tumor cells release factors, such as VEGF-A, thus activating the endothelial cell via the VEGF receptor (VEGFR-1 and -2) and starting a process called "sprouting angiogenesis." As we have seen in normal angiogenesis, the activated endothelial cell starts proliferating and then releases proteases (enzymes) that dissolve the basement membrane of the blood vessel so the new endothelial cells can migrate from the vessel and make a new blood vessel tube. These new endothelial cells migrate out of the holes in the basement membrane into the surrounding extracellular matrix and make solid sprouts that link to the existing blood vessel and pull the sprout toward the tumor (source of growth factors). As the endothelial cells migrate to form the blood vessel tube, they are pulled along by integrins (adhesion molecules) that pull the tube along like grappling hooks. The sprouts are linked to make loops, the loops pull together to form a complete tube, and blood begins to flow to the tumor.

However, the formed blood vessels are very different. Tumor blood vessels are poorly made. They are characterized by highly branched and tortuous vessels, with some vessels being very narrow while others are dilated. Some branches lead to dead ends; others are so narrow that blood cannot reach parts of the tumor and it necroses. This poor vessel construction may be due to the antagonistic relationship between angiopoietin-1 and angiopoietin-2. Together, these molecules stimulate the endothelial cells to recruit pericytes and smooth muscle to the newly forming blood vessel, as this is necessary for the blood vessel to mature and survive. If there is an imbalance in the angiopoietin-1 and -2, together with a high level of VEGF, poor construction of the tumor blood vessels may result. The vessels are highly permeable, with fenestrations (or windows) in them. This permeability is caused by VEGF (which when first discovered, was called "permeability factor"), and it allows fluid to leak into the interstitial spaces of the tumor and raise interstitial pressure. Often, chemotherapy does not reach the tumor due to high interstitial pressure in the tumor, as well as the blinded, tortuous, and narrow blood vessels. Hypoxic tumor cells become resistant to the administered chemotherapy. Microvessel density (MVD) is a surrogate for the extent of tumor angiogenesis.[15] Tumors with high MVD are usually aggressive, and predictive of early recurrence, high potential for metastasis, and poor survival.[16] Antiangiogenic drugs work by preventing new blood vessel formation and normalization of existing vasculature so that the interstitial pressures in the tumor no longer prevent the entry of chemotherapy.

In the stroma, tumor-associated macrophages (TAMs) and proinflammatory molecules help to drive angiogenesis. In fact, it appears that angiogenesis begins in the stroma long *before* the basement membrane has been broken down.[17] Cross-talk between tumor cells, endothelial cells, and stromal cells is mediated by the Notch pathway, stimulating tumor angiogenesis.[18] Notch signaling is activated when the bordering endothelial, tumor, and stromal cells touch each other (cell-to-cell contact) between the Notch receptor, which is on the endothelial cell, and its ligand. Its ligand, either Jagged1 (which is strongly proangiogenic), or delta-like 1 (DLL1) or delta-like 4 (DDL4) (which are negative regulators of angiogenesis), is present on the tumor cell. If Jagged1 binds to Notch, this activates the Notch pathway and starts the proliferation and differentiation of the endothelial cells, in concert with VEGF. For example, Jagged1 is found expressed in squamous cell head and neck cancer cells and is induced via the mitogen-activated protein kinase pathway by hepatocyte growth factor (HGF, scatter factor), EGF, and TGFα, which not only drive angiogenesis but also tumor cell proliferation and progression.[19] DLL4 controls the degree of sprouting by turning down the activity (downregulation) of VEGFR-2. The endothelial cells of tumor blood vessels highly express the Notch ligand DLL4, and it is controlled by VEGF. High levels of VEGF cause increased expression of DDL4 found in the endothelial tip cell or the endothelial cells growing in the hypoxic tumor center.[20]

The Notch signaling pathway is very complex. Research continues to try to refine our understanding of the many roles, relationships, and interactions with other signaling pathways so effective targeted agents can be developed.[21] Not only can tumor and tumor endothelial cells activate Notch signaling, but so too can inflammatory cells.

In addition, tumors can make their blood vessels by having the myofibroblasts in the tumor-associated stroma send chemotactic signals (e.g., stromal cell-derived factor [SDF-1], CXCL12), which will recruit precursors of endothelial cells in the stroma.[17] VEGF is also released by cancer cells, TAMs, and fibroblasts in the tumor-associated stroma, which helps the endothelial cells mature into adult, functional endothelial cells that can make blood vessels.[22] Tumor cells clearly can produce VEGF via epidermal growth factor receptor (EGFR) signaling, but macrophages and myofibroblasts can as well. TAMs release powerful proangiogenic cytokines and growth factors, in addition to VEGF, such as TNFα, IL-8, and basic fibroblast growth factor (bFGF).[23] TAMs also express proteases such as urokinase-type plasminogen activator and the matrix metalloproteinases MMP-2, MMP-7, MMP-9, and MMP-12 that will make the path for the new blood vessel as it grows toward the tumor. Inflammatory cytokines promote tumorigenesis (malignant transformation) by stimulating tumor cell activation and cancer stem cell proliferation.[24]

A proangiogenic force, bFGF binds to its receptors on the endothelial cell. The endothelial cells start to proliferate. Angiopoietin-2 apparently destabilizes quiescent endothelial cells and may contribute to the new vessel sprouting. One of the endothelial cells becomes a tip cell, probably induced by VEGF, as discussed. As released enzymes dissolve holes in the basement membrane, the endothelial cells migrate out to the ECM. MMPs dissolve the ECM so the developing blood vessel tube can push its way through the tissue layers toward an area of the highest concentration of angiogenic factors (the tumor), which include bFGF, TGFβ, IL-8, angiopoietin, angiogenin, and PDGF.[17] Specific integrins help regulate angiogenesis and lymphangiogenesis. They help the endothelial cells migrate and survive during the process of new growth. They are also excellent targets for anticancer therapy.

Some TAMs have Tie2 expression, which gives them a proangiogenic ability. Tie2 is an RTK found on the developing vascular endothelial cells.[22,27] Tie receptors and their angiopoietin-1 and -2 ligands are important in vascular remodeling.[25] In particular, angiopoietin-1 and its receptor Tie2 play a significant role in regulation of capillary-like tubule formation and survival of endothelial cells.[26] Angiopoietins appear to be very important in angiogenesis. They modulate Tie2–TAM activity and help build efficient pericytes on the vessel walls. As the blood vessel normally develops, pericytes are attracted to the new vessel by PDGF/PDGFR; they are then tacked on in tight formation to the outside surface of the vessel like shingles to protect the vessel. The pericytes secrete angiopoietin-1, which binds to Tie2 (RTK) on endothelial cells, making the pericytes stick tightly to the vessel exterior. In cancer, the pericytes are fewer and are very loosely attached to the blood vessel exterior; in some cases, they may even be absent. This contributes to the leakiness of tumor blood vessels. Because cancer metastasizes by entering the blood or lymph vessels, these blood vessels with fenestrations (made by VEGF) and loose vessel exterior (few pericytes) help the tumor to metastasize. Interestingly, in inflammation, angiopoietin-1 stabilizes vessels, decreases leaking from the blood vessels, and decreases the number and size of gaps between adjacent endothelial cells.

Angiopoietin-2 was originally thought to be a Tie2 receptor antagonist, as it binds to Tie2 but does not always activate Tie2 receptor signaling. However, it does compete with angiopoietin-1, blocking angiopoietin-1 from binding to Tie2 and, in effect, turning it off. Angiopoietin-1 is expressed by pericytes and smooth muscle cells. In contrast, angiopoietin-2 is expressed by activated endothelial cells where active remodeling is taking place as it destabilizes endothelial cells.[28] In addition, it appears that angiopoietin-1 and -2 are both necessary for maturation of blood and lymph vessels.[29] Thus, there appears to be a critical balance between angiopoietin-1 and -2 in tumor angiogenesis.[30]

Once the tumor becomes invasive, breaching the basement membrane and entering the stroma, angiogenesis begins in earnest. In addition, as one wonders what the immune system is doing to halt tumor growth, it is important to note that VEGF has another role to play. Normally, when the body recognizes an antigen that should not be there, it calls in immature dendritic cells from the bone marrow and peripheral tissues to the antigen. The dendritic cell then engulfs the antigen, which activates the dendritic cell and causes it to differentiate into a mature dendritic cell. The mature dendritic cell presents the antigen to the immune system (in the lymph nodes, CD4 and CD8 T cells) so that any microorganisms with this antigen can be rounded up and killed. It is important in cancer that the dendritic cells not be allowed to mature, as they would otherwise find the antigens from cancer cells in the microenvironment that have died. VEGF and other factors made by the tumor recruit the immature dendritic cells and then prevent them from maturing; the immature dendritic cells then try to present the tumor antigens to the immune system and are ineffective. The failure of the dendritic cells gives the tumor with this antigen "immune privilege" so it will not be attacked by the immune system.[10]

In addition, tumors secrete VEGF that attracts via chemotaxis, bone marrow-derived cells, including hematopoietic and endothelial cell precursors that have VEGFR-1 receptors. In the metastatic niche, VEGFR-1–positive cells may migrate to the organ that will host the new metastatic cells and then attract bone marrow-derived cells that express VEGFR-1 to the new metastatic niche. They can begin making the stroma so that when the cells arrive, blood vessels will be ready to nourish the new tumor. In addition, endothelial progenitor cells expressing VEGFR-2 are then incorporated into the growing vascular bed to construct the blood vessels in the stroma and tumor.[10]

ANTIANGIOGENIC DRUG THERAPY

A powerful antiangiogenic drug was first proposed in 1971, but it was not until 2004, when bevacizumab (Avastin) was approved by the Food and Drug Administration (FDA) for treatment of patients with advanced colorectal cancer, that the patient and healthcare community became excited. Bevacizumab has changed the landscape of targeted therapy. Bevacizumab is a humanized monoclonal antibody (MAb) that targets VEGF, thereby preventing it from binding to its receptors VEGFR-1 and VEGFR-2. This prevents endothelial cell proliferation and angiogenesis, as well as the many other roles VEGF plays, including their role in chemotaxis of bone marrow-derived progenitor cells.[10] However, because all patients do not respond to bevacizumab, it suggests there are many more pathways involved besides the VEGF pathway. This finding has stimulated very exciting work, and there are over 300 antiangiogenic drugs being studied as of 2009.[3] Today, there are a number of other drugs that block angiogenesis, either directly (e.g., bevacizumab, sunitinib, and sorafenib) or indirectly by targeting the mammalian target of rapamycin (mTOR) pathway that is turned on by HIF. There are also the thalidomide analogues, which are immunomodulators and target the microenvironment.

Mancuso et al. showed that treatment with angiogenesis inhibitor drugs caused rapid (within hours) regression of tumor blood vessels by blocking VEGFR.[31] The fenestrations and vascular sprouts disappeared with loss of blood flow in 50–60% of tumor vessels. Within 1 week, 80% of tumor blood vessels had regressed. The 20% of remaining blood vessels normalized, appearing and functioning normally. The pericytes were not affected. However, the regressed blood vessels had left empty (blood vessel) sleeves of basement membrane. When the antiangiogenic drug was stopped, within 1 day, the endothelial sprouts grew into the empty sleeves of basement membrane, and within 1 week, the tumor was fully revascularized and vessels were fully functional. The pericytes remained unchanged and were once again loosely adhering to the tumor blood vessel exterior walls. Interestingly, when the antiangiogenic drug was reintroduced, the regrown blood vessels regressed to the same degree they did the first time. This suggests that antiangiogenic therapy needs to be continued for an unknown length of time, as the regressed blood vessels leave their empty sleeves of vascular basement membrane and together with remaining pericytes become a scaffold for rapid tumor revascularization.[32]

However, over time, tumors may become resistant to antiangiogenic drugs. It may be that after blocking the VEGF pathway for a period of time, with tumor cell proliferation and the development of new mutations, the cells develop or turn on other angiogenic signaling pathways, as was demonstrated by Batchelor et al.[33] Bergers and Hanahan suggest that there are two modes of resistance to antiangiogenic therapy[34]:

- Evasive resistance—Adaptation to circumvent the specific angiogenic blockade, such as (1) revascularization by upregulating proangiogenic signals, protecting the tumor vasculature from the drug by recruiting proinflammatory cells or increasing pericyte coverage so the drug cannot reach the endothelial cell; (2) a new invasiveness to find normal blood vessels it can share; or (3) increased metastatic seeding and tumor growth in lymph nodes and distant organs
- Intrinsic (preexisting) resistance—Related to stage of tumor progression, exposure to drugs, genomic or genotype that offers protection, or a microenvironment that is indifferent to the antiangiogenic drug(s)

In both cases, it appears that effective cancer antiangiogenic treatment must involve combination strategies targeting both angiogenesis as well as the resistance mechanisms.[34] Jain et al. suggest that an important area of research is in identifying biomarkers of response and resistance to angiogenic therapy.[35] Some studies have shown emergence of escape pathways, and these could be targeted along with the original target.

In addition, activation of the EGFR pathway stimulates the release of VEGF as we have discussed. Blocking EGFR also can turn off or downregulate VEGF, and there is some evidence that the reverse is also true.[36] This finding supports development of multitargeted tyrosine kinase inhibitors that can block both EGFR and VEGF, such as the investigational agents vandetanib (Zactima), BMS-690514, XL647, and AEE-788.[37]

As scientific research peels away more layers of the mystery of cancer biology, new pathways become targets. One such pathway is the Notch signaling pathway, which is very active and one of the few signaling pathways in embryogenesis (Figure 3-2). It is necessary for organ development and cell differentiation. The delta-like protein 4 (DLL4)–Notch signaling pathway is necessary for blood vessels to develop. The ligand of the Notch receptor is the DLL4, which binds to Notch. The notch receptor extends through the cell membrane, but when its ligand binds to it, it activates an enzyme that cuts the protein in two. The portion of the receptor in the cell cytoplasm sends the message to the cell nucleus to turn on (copy) genes in the cell's DNA. It actually is a negative regulator, decreasing endothelial cell sprouting and branching during tumor angiogenesis. This action results in improved flow and function of the newly formed blood vessel.[38] Another Notch ligand, Jagged1 is a very powerful proangiogenic regulator. It competes with DLL4 to bind to the Notch receptor to regulate angiogenesis.[39] If Notch signaling is blocked, there is increased tumor blood vessel formation, but the vessels do not work (are nonproductive). This results in decreased tumor perfusion and decreased tumor growth.[40] In addition, it appears cross-talk between the Notch pathway and the p53 and p63 (member of p53 family, active in development) pathways helps tumor

Figure 3-2   Notch signaling pathway.

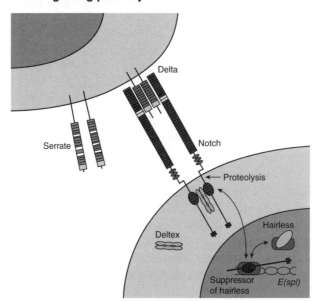

Notch signaling is important in cell proliferation, apoptosis, stem cell maintenance, cell fate determination, and angiogenesis. Notch1 dysregulation is found in more than 50% of patients with T-cell acute lymphoblastic leukemia. There is cross-talk with the Sonic Hedgehog (SHH) pathway and Wnt receptor signaling pathway.

Source: Data from Kim HT, Stevens J, Kaplan-Lefko P. Top NOTCH: Notch signaling in cancer. *Drug Development Res* 2008;69(6):319-328; Li J-L, Harris AL. Notch signaling from tumor cells: A new mechanism of angiogenesis. *Cancer Cell* 2005;8(1):1-3.

cell differentiation and survival, as cross-talk among them regulates response to external damage signals and control of stem cell differentiation.[41]

Tumor vasculature can be targeted via two distinct mechanisms, although some drugs may do both[42]:

- Angiogenesis-inhibiting agents, which prevent angiogenesis. Agents include bevacizumab, which targets VEGF; sunitinib and sorafenib, which target VEGFR; the multitargeted agent vandetanib; and other investigational agents, such as angiopoietin-inhibiting agents (e.g., AMG386), the multitargeted TKI258 (which blocks FGFR, VEGFR, and PDGFR), and Notch inhibitors.
- Vascular-disrupting agents (VDAs), all of which are investigational. These agents damage the already existing tumor vasculature.

Angiogenesis-inhibiting agents: This chapter will review the FDA-approved drugs bevacizumab (Avastin), sunitinib (Sutent), sorafenib (Nexavar), and the investigational agents vandetanib, and AMG 386. AMG 386 is a peptibody (peptide fused to the Fc protein of an antibody, or a peptide–Fc fusion protein) that selectively inhibits the interactions of angiopoietins-1 and -2 with Tie2. It has been shown to inhibit tumor endothelial cell proliferation and tumor growth as it blocks angiogenesis but not tumor cell proliferation.[43] Other drugs in the pipeline are VEGF traps (e.g., aflibercept, which is being developed by Regeneron Pharmaceuticals and Sanofi-Aventis), which are human, soluble decoys made from part of the immunoglobulin domain of the VEGFR-1 and part of the domain of VEGFR-2, together with the Fc domain of a human IgG_1 molecule. This combination brings the best attributes of high affinity for all forms of VEGF-A and PIGF, and also has antibody-dependent cellular cytotoxicity (ADCC) capabilities to recruit the immune effector cells to kill the cancer cells.[10]

Vascular-disrupting agents (VDAs): VDAs work differently from antiangiogenic drugs. VDAs shut down blood flow to the tumor by causing the collapse of the existing blood vessels around the tumor and killing tumor cells dependent on them. Not only do they selectively attack new tumor blood vessels, but they also attack the existing blood vessels while avoiding normal vessels.[44] These agents have synergy with chemotherapy, radiotherapy, and other antiangiogenic agents. While the center of the tumor, as it grows, is necrotic, the cells between the outside and the core are hypoxic; VDAs can kill the tumor blood vessels in the hypoxic layer but ignore the outer layer of oxygenated cells, which can be killed by radiotherapy or chemotherapy. This approach also leads to improved tumor perfusion, as the chaotic tumor blood vessels are destroyed.[44] It is hoped this group of agents will avoid drug-resistant mutations in the tumor endothelial cells or areas targeted. In the past, efforts to destroy tumor blood vessels included certain chemotherapy agents such as arsenic trioxide and vincristine, and biologic agents such as tumor necrosis factor (TNF). These agents can select blood vessels that are newly formed or abnormal. Studies have shown that damaging only a few tumor blood vessels results in the death of thousands of tumor cells.[44] Today, VDAs are focusing on small-molecule drugs, which selectively target proliferating endothelial cells. They can be divided into two types of VDAs:

- Tubulin-binding agents, which are thought to selectively depolymerize the endothelial cells' microtubules in the cytoskeleton, resulting in changes in the shape of the endothelial cell, formation of thrombi, and vascular collapse. Research with the tubulin-binding agents suggests they work because the tumor vessels have immature and insufficient pericytes. However, by themselves they cannot stop tumor growth and must be used together with chemotherapy or other conventional treatments.[45]
- Cytokine-inducing agents, which cause the release of cytokines. These agents, especially TNFα, disrupt established tumor vasculature and lead to hemorrhagic necrosis.[42]

An example of the tubulin-binding VDA is combrestastatin A4 phosphate (CA4P; fosbretabulin [Zybrestat, a product of OXiGENE]), which is being studied in combination with bevacizumab (Avastin). An example of cytokine-releasing VDA is ASA404 (5,6-dimethylxanthenone-4 acetic acid, or DMXAA [Vadimeza, a product of Novartis]), which is being studied in patients with non–small cell lung cancer (NSCLC) also receiving carboplatin and paclitaxel. ASA404 directly causes endothelial cell apoptosis and indirectly, through the effects of TNFα and nitric oxide, causes inhibition of blood flow in the tumor. Together these effects lead to extensive tumor necrosis.[46]

In summary, VDAs attack existing tumor vasculature selectively, ignoring normal vessels because the drug focuses on vessels with greater proliferation, fragility, irregular openings in the vessels, high vascular permeability, and high internal fluid pressure.[47] They are used together with conventional therapy such as chemotherapy.

HYPOXIA-INDUCIBLE FACTOR, mTOR, AND ANGIOGENESIS

A second important pathway that affects angiogenesis is the mTOR, so named because rapamycin was found to inhibit the molecule, and the mTOR molecule was a target of rapamycin. Unfortunately, rapamycin is very immunosuppressive and, therefore, has not been successful in anticancer strategies. Clearly, blocking mTOR complex 1 would turn off cell proliferation and survival, and the search has been underway for analogues (or "rapalogues") of rapamycin (sirolimus). Of note, mTOR is highly conserved, and all organisms possess it. In the embryo, if mTOR is lost, the embryo dies.[48] Figure 3-3 shows the mTOR signaling pathway.

mTOR plays a central role in angiogenesis, as it controls production of HIF proteins HIF1a and HIF1b. HIF is a critical transcription factor that allows the expression of genes whose products (proteins) are involved in angiogenesis, as well as cell proliferation, motility, adhesion, and survival—all qualities necessary for tumor progression.[50] HIF induces gene expression to produce VEGF (which stimulates endothelial cells to proliferate and migrate toward the tumor in a new tube) and angiopoietin-2 (which destabilizes existing blood vessels so they can develop the tube extension in concert with VEGF and then grow toward the tumor). Angiogenesis is tightly controlled. Hypoxia tips the balance toward angiogenesis to increase the oxygen delivered to tissues and is mediated by HIF, which is controlled by the von Hippel–Lindau (VHL) protein, a tumor suppressor. During hypoxia, HIF is released so new blood vessels can be stimulated, and when tissue is oxygenated, HIF is rapidly broken down. In the presence of very high levels of HIF, apoptosis occurs.[50] When tumors subvert the upstream signaling pathways, mTOR is activated, and high levels of HIF are produced; if VHL protein is mutated or lost, HIF is not broken down, and high levels persist. This

Figure 3-3   mTOR signaling in epithelial cells.

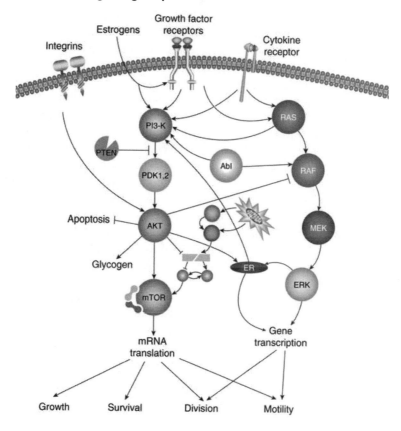

Modified from Novartis Oncology.[49]

way the tumor can get the proteins and essential nutrients it needs to continue to proliferate and have adequate energy even in hypoxic conditions, such as aerobic glycolysis.[51] Activated mTOR also upregulates VEGF-C, which is associated with lymphangiogenesis.[52]

This important cell-regulating pathway can be thought of as a Grand Central Station of many critical cell functions, such as sensing the environment and helping the cell respond to these changes (e.g., insufficient nutrients, stress), but it also regulates the key proteins that are involved in cell growth, movement, death (apoptosis), and division, as well as replication of DNA. One of the proteins that it controls is VEGF-A. mTOR controls the cells' response to hypoxia by transcribing VEGF-A in response to HIF-1α, as well as a number of other hypoxia-related proteins that tumors express.[49] We have already discussed the important role of VEGF-A (or just VEGF) in initiating and continuing the growth of new blood vessels to supply tumor growth beyond 1–2 mm. mTOR is considered a biologic switch. It senses the availability of nutrients (e.g., amino acids, glucose, and energy) that the cell will need to continue to survive. It processes growth signals from other cells, such as hormones or growth factors. It also processes and assesses the threat of stressors that may cause the cell to die, such as hypoxia, DNA damage, heat shock, and oxidative stress. It is like a large computer or trafficking center that decides what the cell should do based on the given variables and switches on or off the process of cell growth, motility, division, and death accordingly. If the cell does not have enough nutrients or energy to divide and the cell receives messages to divide, the cell will either stop cell division (e.g., restriction point R1 in the G_1 phase of the cell cycle), or it will turn on a process called autophagy, which allows the cell to break down some of its own internal cell organelles to free up the elements to make the required components the cell needs. If the cell senses hypoxia, the gene for VEGF-A is expressed, the gene is transcribed by mRNA, which carries the recipe for the protein to the ribosomes in the cytoplasm of the cell, and VEGF-A is made and released to start the mTOR signaling in the process of angiogenesis.

One may wonder, how does mTOR, a serine/threonine protein kinase found in the cytoplasm of the cell, get the messages to help it make the decisions about regulating cell growth, proliferation, motility, and survival, as well as making the proteins it needs to regulate these pathways? It gets the messages from receptors on the outside of the cell (upstream) such as insulin-like growth factors (IGF-1, IGF-2), EGFR, HER2, VEGF, and PDGF, as well as cytokine receptors on the cell surface. Nutrients also weigh in here—the presence or absence of amino acids and glucose, as well as the level of oxygen. Also important is the cell's adhesion status, which is given to it by integrins on the cell surface. In cancer, many of these receptors are overexpressed, turning on the mTOR machinery so that the cell proliferation and angiogenesis occur without interruption. Messages from inside the cell, such as from estrogen, can also turn on the mTOR machinery. Much like the signal transduction cascades already discussed, the message from outside the cell reaches the mTOR molecule by a series of bucket brigade-like steps, each involving phosphorylation of enzymes by protein kinases along the cascade. Again in cancer, as the proto-oncogenes are mutated to form oncogenes that drive cell division, and as tumor suppressor genes are silenced, mTOR can receive continuous signals to switch the cell machinery "on" (see Figure 3-3).

Many of the genes mutated in cancer are upstream of mTOR and are responsible for control of the mTOR pathway. The silencing of the tumor suppressor gene PTEN (phosphatase and tensin homologue) activates mTOR signaling. PTEN is often deleted from chromosome 10.

Mutations in the RAS signaling pathway: Normally, the *ras* gene is a proto-oncogene, and it codes for proteins that bring the message from the cell surface growth factor receptors to other protein messengers further down the signal cascade as part of the bucket brigade. It lies inside the cell surface, in the cytoplasm. Once RAS gets the message to help the cell grow or divide, the next step is raf; through phosphorylation, raf is activated, and it then sends the message downstream to MEK. MEK is phosphorylated and sends the message downstream to MAP kinases, which are also called the extracellular signal-regulated kinase or ERK pathway. As shown in Figure 3-4, ERK sends the message into the nucleus, resulting in gene transcription; thus, the proteins are made that make the cell undergo cell division and develop motility. However, there is much cross-talk with the RAS/ERK pathway, such as RAS with P13K (phosphoinositide 3-kinases), which then leads to stimulation of mTOR. RAF talks with Abl kinase, which talks to P13-K. Unfortunately, in many tumors, the RAS proto-oncogene is mutated, forming the ras oncogene, such as in cancers of the pancreas, colon, thyroid, and lung. This mutation results in increased signaling along this pathway (gain of function); the RAS oncogene is turned on and keeps sending messages to the cell nucleus instead of stopping after the message is delivered as happens in the normal cell.

Mutations in the P13K/AKT signaling pathway: Normally, P13K transduces (sends) the message it receives from activated receptors on the outside surface of the cell, or from RAS, downstream to the cell nucleus via mTOR. For example, it is involved in getting the message from the insulin-like growth factor (IGFR) to regulate glucose uptake in the cell. P13K signaling leads to cell growth, survival, proliferation, and motility through mTOR. P13K is mutated in many cancers, such as some colon, gastric, breast, ovarian, and lung cancers and glioblastoma. In addition, P13K also talks with PTEN, a tumor suppressor gene, which antagonizes P13K and thus can reverse its activity. PTEN is silenced (mutated) in many tumors as well. These tumors that have mutated PTEN include glioblastoma, prostate, and endometrial cancers. These mutations are thought to be linked to tumor insensitivity to insulin and the availability of nutrients (calories).[53] In the lab, if either a normal P13K or PTEN correction is made, then the tumor cell becomes dietary-restriction sensitive. PTEN mutation also allows cells to survive when they detach from the basement membrane (anchorage independence); in normal cells, detachment and migration to another area, except for certain leucocytes, is met with apoptosis. In patients with breast cancer who are HER2+, those with mutated PTEN (thus silencing PTEN) become resistant to trastuzumab.[54]

When P13K is activated, it is phosphorylated and sends the message to the next step in the bucket brigade. That molecule then phosphorylates and sends the message to AKT. AKT is also a serine/threonine kinase and is also known as protein kinase B (PKB). Once it receives the message to grow, survive, proliferate,

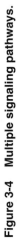

Figure 3-4   Multiple signaling pathways.

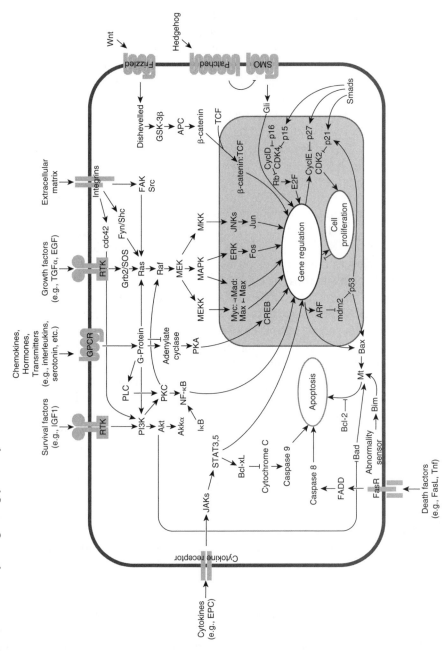

or move, it sends it along to the cell nucleus for action (e.g., gene transcription). There are three family members, and two are well known. Akt1 promotes survival of the cell by blocking apoptosis. It is very important in balancing the pro- and antiapoptotic forces in favor of cell survival.[55] It can induce protein synthesis as well. Akt2 is important in the insulin signaling pathway, as it pays attention to the glucose level in the cell and is able to induce glucose transport to make glycogen stores.

AKT is frequently mutated or activated (i.e., becomes an oncogene) in cancer, and high levels have been found in tumors of the gastrointestinal (GI) tract, prostate, and breast.[56] High levels of Bcl-2 may predict resistance to an mTOR inhibitor.[57]

mTOR and angiogenesis: Cancers that overexpress HIF-α are often aggressive, associated with a poor prognosis, and have mutations in the mTOR signaling pathways. When hypoxia activates mTOR signaling, hypoxic stress genes are turned on, and proteins like VEGF and PDGF are synthesized to relieve the hypoxia by providing new blood vessels. These ligands bind to their respective receptors on the endothelial cell and pericyte, begin proliferation and migration, and orchestrate the building of new tumor blood vessels.

mTOR inhibitors block angiogenesis by preventing the release of VEGF and PDGF, thus directly decreasing angiogenesis. In addition, mTOR inhibition blocks the growth and proliferation of both tumor and endothelial cells as the synthesis of necessary proteins is halted. This blocks tumor cell proliferation and makes tumor cells undergo apoptosis.

Immunomodulatory agents: As discussed, the microenvironment is very important in angiogenesis. It is unclear how the immunomodulatory drugs thalidomide and lenalidomide exert their antiangiogenic properties. These drugs inhibit proinflammatory cytokines, TNFα, IL-1β, and IL-6. One study by Dredge et al. showed that lenalidomide inhibited endothelial cell migration and Akt phosphorylation, leading to antiangiogenesis. However, it did not affect endothelial cell proliferation.[58]

NURSING CONSIDERATIONS AND DRUG INFORMATION

Nurses play an important role in the care of patients receiving antiangiogenic therapies. The antiangiogenic drugs include:

- MAbs directed against VEGF directly (bevacizumab) and indirectly (cetuximab, which has already been discussed)
- Small-molecule tyrosine kinase inhibitors (TKIs) such as the VEGFR inhibitors sorafenib and sunitinib, and indirectly by erlotinib
- mTOR inhibitors (temsirolimus, everolimus)
- Immunomodulatory drugs lenalidomide and thalidomide

Before discussing the drugs that are considered antiangiogenesis drugs, it is important to review common class effects such as hypertension, bleeding, risk of GI perforation, renal insufficiency, and, rarely, cardiac toxicity.

Hypertension

Hypertension appears to be related to the blocking of nitric oxide by antiangiogenesis drugs, although there are probably other factors involved. Nitric oxide is a potent vasodilator that helps control blood pressure by opposing vasoconstriction. Hypertension may arise because VEGF is necessary for the synthesis of the vasodilator nitric oxide. Normally, VEGF activates the endothelial cell to stimulate the production of nitric oxide synthase, which produces nitric oxide.[59,60] When VEGF is blocked, hypertension results from the inability of arteries to vasodilate, which leads to vasoconstriction, increased peripheral resistance, and hypertension; in addition, low nitric oxide levels are associated with reduced renal excretion of sodium, with resulting sodium and water retention.[61] Neutralizing VEGF (bevacizumab) or blocking its binding to VEGFR (sorafenib, sunitinib) reduces the production and release of nitric oxide, resulting in the gradual development of hypertension in many patients receiving antiangiogenesis agents. The incidence of grades 3 and 4 hypertension is about 8–18%.[62,63] Specifically, the incidence of hypertension with bevacizumab is 22% (60% when given with irinotecan, 5-FU, and leucovorin [IFL]), with 11% grade 3 or 4 and onset in 7–316 days (median 131 days).[63,64] Similarly for sorafenib, the incidence of hypertension is 24%, with 8% grade 3 or 4.[65] Hypertension developed within 3 weeks of starting therapy with sorafenib.[66] Hypertension occurs with sunitinib after 3–4 weeks of therapy.[67]

Many Americans have hypertension, especially those aged 60 years or older who are also at risk for developing cancer.[68] Risk for hypertension includes obesity, tobacco and alcohol use, physical inactivity, diabetes, arthrosclerosis, renal insufficiency, and a family history for this disease.[69] If a person with hypertension develops cancer and is treated with an antiangiogenesis drug, the risk of treatment-related hypertension may be increased. Recommended treatment of hypertension resulting from antiangiogenic therapy is left to the provider's discretion; however, most clinical trials exclude the use of drugs that are metabolized by the P450 microenzyme system to prevent drug interactions, especially with sorafenib and sunitinib.[68] Angiotensin-converting enzyme (ACE) inhibitors are chosen by many providers because they increase the level of nitric oxide,[70] while the American Diabetes Association recommends the use of angiotensin-receptor blockers (ARBs) if the patient has diabetes, proteinuria, and/or microalbuminuria.[71] The 2003 Seventh Report of the Joint National Committee on Prevention, Detection, Evaluation, and Treatment of High Blood Pressure (JNC 7) hypertension guidelines emphasize that for people older than 50 years, an elevated systolic blood pressure (SBP) > 140 mm Hg is a "more important risk factor" for cardiovascular disease (CVD) than an elevated diastolic blood pressure (DBP). The risk of CVD, beginning at a blood pressure of 115/75 mm Hg, doubles with each increment of 20/10 mm Hg, and interestingly, if a person is normotensive at age 55 years, the person has a 90% lifetime risk of developing hypertension.

Prehypertension is defined as having an SBP of 120–139 mm Hg, or a DBP of 80–89 mm Hg, and although it does not require antihypertensive medication, the person is strongly encouraged to change lifestyle parameters such as obesity, smoking, and exercise. Stage 1 hypertension is defined as an SBP of 140–159 or DBP 90–99; this person should be started on an antihypertensive medication such as a thiazide-type diuretic (for most people), or consider an ACE inhibitor, ARB, beta-blocker, calcium channel blocker (CCB), or a combination. Drug interactions need to guide drug selection. For patients also taking sunitinib, which is partially metabolized via the cytochrome P450 CYP3A4 microenzyme system, the drug is inhibited by the CCBs verapamil and diltiazem. Thus, the metabolism of sunitinib may be decreased, resulting in increased serum levels of drug and greater toxicity. If possible, both of these drugs should be avoided.[72] Stage II hypertension is defined as an SBP ≥ 160 and a DBP ≥ 100. It requires a two-drug antihypertensive regimen—usually a thiazide-type diuretic plus an ACE inhibitor or ARB or beta-blocker or a CCB. In addition, teaching to reduce risk factors in lifestyle habits, such as smoking cessation (which is difficult when a person is coping with cancer), is important.[73] JNC 8 is expected to be released for public comment in December 2009 and presented in its final form in the spring of 2010.

A hypertensive emergency is defined as marked hypertension and acute organ damage (e.g., unstable angina, myocardial infarction, acute pulmonary edema, eclampsia, stroke, encephalopathy, head trauma, aortic dissection, or life-threatening arterial bleeding). Such an emergency occurs rarely but is the rationale behind holding the antiangiogenic drug until hypertension is well controlled. Rarely, too, reversible progressive leukoencephalopathy syndrome (RPLS) may occur and is believed to be related to uncontrolled hypertension. Although the exact cause is still unknown, the syndrome appears to involve a rapid rise in blood pressure that overwhelms the brain's normal regulatory systems, leading to a dilation of cerebral arterioles with capillary leak (leakage, or vasogenic edema) in the posterior part of the brain (posterior parietal and occipital lobes) where the circulation has less sympathetic adrenergic innervations and is therefore less able to tolerate rapid rises in blood pressure.[74] Other causes of RPLS may be changes in endothelial function resulting in blood–brain barrier dysfunction.[59] Onset is 16 hours to 1 year after treatment with bevacizumab. Signs and symptoms are seizures, hypertension, headache, decreased level of consciousness, altered cognitive functioning, and visual loss including cortical blindness. Antiangiogenic drugs should be stopped until the syndrome is reversed and signs and symptoms are resolved; in most cases, the drug (e.g., bevacizumab) is not resumed. A review of the literature shows case reports of RPLS with bevacizumab, sorafenib, and sunitinib.[75–77]

Hypertension associated with these agents emerges over time, so it is very important to assess blood pressure prior to treatment, at least every 2 weeks with bevacizumab therapy, weekly for the first 6 weeks of sorafenib therapy, and every cycle (6 weeks) with sunitinib therapy.[78–81] In addition, blood pressure should be monitored more frequently in patients with preexisting hypertension or when patients are started on antihypertensive medications.[81]

Early identification of RPLS is very important, so nurses should assess for changes in blood pressure, cognition (e.g., confusion, or any changes in mental status), or other changes such as decreased vision or onset of seizure activity. Magnetic resonance imaging (MRI) of the brain is diagnostic. Prompt control of blood pressure along with drug cessation can reverse the process. Management includes control of blood pressure, where a 10–20% decrease in mean arterial pressure is usually sufficient to terminate the process.[74] If hypomagnesemia is present, it should be corrected. Seizures should be treated with anticonvulsants. Fortunately, most patients' symptoms resolve or improve within days, although some patients have ongoing neurologic issues.

Proteinuria

The glomeruli are made up of capillaries, and it appears that VEGF is necessary for glomerular endothelial repair; thus one hypothesis is that blocking VEGF may compromise the glomeruli endothelial cell integrity.[82] In addition, hypertension may be related to proteinuria, as VEGF is very important in normal renal function.[83]

Because most patients are asymptomatic, the incidence of proteinuria is not actually known, but in pivotal studies, almost a third of patients had it.[84] Assess urine for protein baseline and regularly during treatment. If the urine dipstick is ≥ 2+, a 24-hour urine for protein should be collected prior to the next cycle, and if urine protein is ≥ 2 g, delay the bevacizumab dose until urine protein has fallen to < 2 g. In this case, repeat the 24-hour urine for protein prior to each cycle. If the 24-hour urinary protein falls to < 1 g, resume monitoring with urine dipstick.[78] Proteinuria has occurred in patients receiving bevacizumab (incidence 36%), but it has not been reported in patients receiving sunitinib or sorafenib. This is probably due to the short half-lives of these drugs compared to bevacizumab (about 20 days).

Hemorrhage

Bleeding may occur with each of the agents, and the etiology is unclear. The incidence of bleeding for bevacizumab is 35% (epistaxis), with 4.7–5.4% hemorrhage; in metastatic colorectal cancer (mCRC), GI hemorrhage occurs in 24% (with IFL chemotherapy).[78] For sorafenib, hemorrhage including GI occurs in 15%.[80] For sunitinib, incidence of epistaxis is 30%, with 10% grade 3 or 4.[79] It is thought that endothelial cell defects contribute to bleeding, but given the increased incidence of thrombosis as well, there are probably many effects of VEGF that are not well understood.[59] Fatal hemoptysis has occurred when bevacizumab was studied in patients with squamous cell histology of NSCLC. For this reason, the drug is contraindicated in patients with squamous cell histology. In addition, the drug is contraindicated in patients with or having a history of hemoptysis of greater than one-half teaspoon of red blood.[78]

Epistaxis is the most common bleeding that occurs. Rarely, patients receiving bevacizumab may develop a perforated nasal septum.[78] Bleeding is also common with sunitinib and sorafenib. Teach patients that nosebleeds may occur and to apply pressure and hold head down for 15 to 20 minutes until the nosebleed resolves. If a nosebleed does not resolve, the patient should call his or her provider and go to the emergency department for evaluation. If bleeding occurs elsewhere, such as hematuria, black tarry stools, or frank blood, the patient should call his or her provider and go to the emergency department to be evaluated right away. If hemorrhage occurs, the patient should call 911 or an ambulance immediately.

GI Perforation

GI perforation may occur rarely with each of the agents. The pathophysiology is unclear, but VEGF is necessary for functioning of the intestinal villous capillaries.[85] It is also hypothesized that for CRCs as the tumor shrinks and pulls away from the mucosa, it may thin the area, resulting in increased risk of perforation.[86,87] Factors that appear to increase risk are tumor at the anastomotic site, abdominal carcinomatosis, bowel obstruction, intact colon or rectal tumor, history of pelvic/abdominal radiation, or recent colonoscopy.[86,87] In bevacizumab studies, it generally occurred during the first 60 days of treatment. In order to prevent GI perforation, bevacizumab should be held for at least the drug half-life (20 days) before elective surgery including colonoscopy. For major surgery, it may be prudent to wait up to 60 days for some surgical procedures such as hepatic metastatectomy, as complications have occurred up to 56 days after the last bevacizumab dose.[87] GI perforation occurs rarely with sorafenib and sunitinib. On patient assessment, the history is often significant for diffuse abdominal pain associated with fever, constipation, and/or vomiting; upon examination, the patient will have tachycardia, rebound tenderness of the abdomen, and peripheral vasoconstriction with cool extremities.[78,87] It is important that patients are taught to go to the emergency department right away if they develop severe abdominal pain, with or without constipation, nausea, fever, and vomiting. If the patient develops GI perforation, including fistula formation and/or intra-abdominal abscess, bevacizumab should be discontinued.[78]

Diarrhea as a class effect has not been fully elucidated.[88] VEGF is responsible for permeability, proliferation, migration, maintenance, and protection of endothelial cells. The GI gut mucosa is constantly injured by normal wear and tear of digestion, and ongoing healing and angiogenesis are required for gut mucosal reconstitution.[89] Thus, blockade of VEGF in intestinal mucosa may result in decreased healing of mucosal injury, resulting in increased release of enzymes, inability to reabsorb water, and diarrhea. The incidence of diarrhea is 34% (with IFL chemotherapy) with bevacizumab, 43% with sorafenib, and 58% with sunitinib.

Fortunately, patients are effectively managed with dietary modification, bulking and antidiarrheal medications, and adequate hydration.[90] Nursing assessment should focus on the patient's bowel elimination pattern baseline and with diarrhea, noting stool consistency, frequency, whether it contains mucus or blood, what makes it better or worse, and any associated symptoms that may further compromise the patient, such as nausea, vomiting, inability to take oral fluids, dizziness, or safety issues. In addition, note the patient's medication profile for stool softeners, laxatives, or chemotherapy that may increase the risk of diarrhea such as irinotecan and 5-FU, or any potentially interacting medications that might increase toxicity. Assess the patient's and family's knowledge about how to assess diarrhea, when to call the provider (i.e., if diarrhea continues for more than 24 hours, if patient has vomiting or fever, or if patient is unable to take oral fluids), dietary modifications including increased oral fluid intake, and patient self-administration of loperamide or other recommended antidiarrheal agent.

Dietary modifications include use of the bananas, rice, applesauce, and toast (BRAT) diet, although this diet should not be used for a long period of time because it is low in protein; avoidance of milk and dairy products, as the mucosal injury may make the patient temporarily lactose intolerant; increase in soluble fiber; avoidance of foods with insoluble fiber; increase in oral fluids to at least 8–10 large glasses of clear liquids a day, such as fat-free chicken broth and sports drinks; avoidance of caffeine, fried, spicy, or fatty foods, alcohol, and other foods that can cause gas; and consumption of small, frequent meals. Some patients find that medicinal fiber helps to increase bulk in the stool and slow peristalsis.[90] The goal of antidiarrheal medications is to reduce GI motility and secretion, and most patients have resolution of their diarrhea with loperamide. Because no evidence-based guidelines exist for the management of diarrhea associated with targeted therapies, the guidelines developed for chemotherapy-induced diarrhea are often very helpful.[91]

Hypothyroidism

Hypothyroidism may also be a class effect. The thyroid gland has many capillaries, and in animal models, VEGF inhibition results in regression of more than 50% of the thyroid capillaries in 3 weeks.[59] With all of the agents, it is important to assess baseline thyroid function tests and to monitor for signs and symptoms of hypothyroidism (i.e., increased sensitivity to cold, dry skin, hoarse voice, weight gain, myalgias and arthralgias, or depression), especially in patients receiving sunitinib. If hypothyroidism is confirmed, it is treated using standard medications.

Teratogenicity and Fetotoxicity

Teratogenicity and fetotoxicity result from inhibition of new blood vessel formation, as angiogenesis is critical to the development of the embryo and fetus. These agents are either pregnancy class C (bevacizumab) or D (sorafenib and sunitinib). Teach female patients of childbearing age to use effective contraception to avoid pregnancy; also if currently breastfeeding an infant, teach them not to breastfeed while receiving the drug. Effective birth control and avoidance of breastfeeding should continue for at least 2 weeks following cessation of sorafenib and for at least 20 days after stopping bevacizumab.

MAbs Directed Against VEGF

Drug: Bevacizumab (Avastin)

Indications: Bevacizumab (Avastin) is FDA indicated for the treatment of patients with:

- mCRC, with intravenous (IV) 5-FU–based chemotherapy for first- or second-line treatment
- Nonsquamous NSCLC, with carboplatin and paclitaxel for first-line treatment of unresectable, locally advanced, recurrent, or metastatic disease
- HER2-negative metastatic breast cancer, with paclitaxel, for patients who have not received chemotherapy (for metastatic disease)
  - Effectiveness based on progression-free survival
  - Not indicated for disease progression following anthracycline and taxane chemotherapy administered for metastatic disease
- Glioblastoma with progressive disease after prior therapy, as a single agent (Based on improved objective response rate)
- Metastatic renal cell cancer (mRCC) in combination with interferon-α

Class: Antiangiogenic agent

Mechanism of Action: In normal blood vessel development, VEGF binds to receptors on endothelial cells, turning on the cell surface receptors KDR and Flt-1, which then function as tyrosine kinases sending the message to the cells to proliferate and migrate. This leads to the establishment of new blood vessels (neovascularization) in tumors. Studies show that tumors that express VEGF tend to be more aggressive, more invasive, and more likely to metastasize. Bevacizumab binds to all human forms of VEGF-A, thus preventing it from binding to its receptors on the endothelial cells. This theoretically prevents one step in the process of angiogenesis from occurring. In addition, it appears that VEGF is necessary to maintain existing tumor blood vessels, and when blocked by bevacizumab, these blood vessels normalize, reducing tumor interstitial pressure, and allowing normal blood flow throughout the tumor. When given with chemotherapy, this theoretically results in increased chemotherapy penetrating the tumor and cell death. Bevacizumab may augment the body's antitumor immune response by helping dendritic cells function more effectively. Finally, bevacizumab is an IgG$_1$ MAb that theoretically recruits immune effector cells such as natural killer (NK) cells and macrophages, which attack tumor cells (ADCC), as well as stimulating complement-mediated killing of tumor cells.

Pharmacokinetics: Drug is humanized via recombinant technologies, resulting in a 93% human MAb. It is widely distributed throughout the body and has a terminal half-life of approximately 20 days (range 11–50 days). It appears to reach steady state in 100 days. Drug clearance varies by body weight, gender, and tumor burden. Men and patients with a large tumor burden have higher clearances than females, but this does not appear to decrease drug efficiency. Drug clearance has not been studied in patients with either renal or hepatic impairment, but it appears that there is minimal drug clearance by these organs. Concurrent administration of 5-fluourouracil, carboplatin, doxorubicin, cisplatin, or paclitaxel does not affect pharmacokinetics of the drug.

Dosage and Administration:
Administer initial dose over 90 minutes, second infusion over 60 minutes, and subsequent infusions over 30 minutes if initial and second infusions well tolerated. Administer in 0.9% normal saline ONLY. A nonrandomized study has been published that demonstrated that a shorter infusion time was safe at infusion rates of 0.5 mg/kg/min, or 10 minutes for the 5 mg/kg dose.[92] For CRC, dosage is 5 mg/kg IV every 2 weeks when combined with IFL.

- CRC: 10 mg/kg IV every 2 weeks when combined with FOLFOX
- NSCLC: 15 mg IV every 3 weeks when combined with carboplatin and paclitaxel (nonsquamous NSCLC)
- Breast cancer: 10 mg/kg IV every 2 weeks when combined with paclitaxel
- Glioblastoma: 10 mg/kg IV every 2 weeks
- mRCC: 10 mg/kg IV every 2 weeks with interferon-α

Dose Modifications:
- **Discontinue drug** for GI perforation (including fistula, intra-abdominal abscess), wound dehiscence and wound healing complications requiring medical intervention, serious hemorrhage (requiring medical intervention), severe arterial thromboembolic events, hypertensive crisis or hypertensive encephalopathy, RPLS, or nephrotic syndrome.
- **Interrupt drug and temporarily suspend** for at least 4 weeks prior to elective surgery, severe uncontrolled hypertension, moderate to severe proteinuria pending further evaluation, or severe infusion reaction.

Available as: Single-use vials contain 4 mL to deliver 100 mg, and 16 mL to deliver 400 mg per single-use vial. Use within 8 hours of opening. Store at 2–8°C (36–46°F). Protect from light. Do not freeze or shake.

Reconstitution and Preparation: Aseptically draw ordered dose. Further dilute in 100 mL 0.9% normal saline for injection. Administer over 90 minutes initial dose, 60 minutes second dose, and 30 minutes all subsequent doses if well tolerated.

Drug Interactions: Paclitaxel/carboplatin combination may decrease paclitaxel exposure after four cycles of treatment (day 63). Bevacizumab is incompatible with dextrose solutions.

Warnings and Precautions:

- **GI perforation:** May occur in 2.4% of patients. Typically presents with abdominal pain, nausea, emesis, constipation, and fever. Majority occur within the first 50 days of treatment. May be complicated by intra-abdominal abscess and fistula formation. Discontinue drug if this occurs.
- **Surgery and wound healing complications:** Discontinue bevacizumab at least 28 days prior to elective surgery, and do not initiate for at least 28 days after surgery and until the surgical wound has fully healed. Incidence is 15% compared to control of 4%.
- **Hemorrhage:** Severe or fatal hemorrhage, hemoptysis, GI bleeding, central nervous system (CNS) hemorrhage, and vaginal bleeding may occur. Do not give drug to patients with serious hemorrhage or recent hemoptysis ($\geq$ than half teaspoon). Typically bleeding is either minor hemorrhage, such as nosebleed (epistaxis), or serious hemorrhage, which may be fatal. Incidence of severe hemorrhage is up to 4.6%. Patients most likely to have serious hemorrhagic hemoptysis are those with squamous cell histology NSCLC, so the drug is contraindicated in this population.
- **Non-GI fistula formation:** Rare, occurring < 0.3% in clinical studies. Occurred during the first 6 months of therapy. Involved tracheaesophageal, bronchopleural, biliary, vaginal, and bladder. Discontinue drug if this occurs.
- **Arterial thromboembolic events (ATE):** Incidence of grade 3 or higher ATE was 2.6% compared to control of 0.8%. Risk is increased in patients with a history of arterial thromboembolism or age greater than 65 years. Discontinue drug if patient develops a severe ATE.
- **Hypertension:** The incidence of grade 3 or higher hypertension is 5–18%. Blood pressure should be monitored every 2–3 weeks during treatment, and if hypertension develops, it should be treated with appropriate antihypertensive therapy with appropriate monitoring. Temporarily suspend drug if hypertension is uncontrolled, but discontinue drug if patient develops hypertensive crisis or hypertensive encephalopathy. Continue to monitor blood pressure in these patients after drug discontinuation.

- **RPLS:** Rare, with an incidence of < 0.1% in clinical studies. Symptoms began from 16 hours to 1 year after initial dose of bevacizumab. Presenting symptoms may include headache, seizure, lethargy, confusion, blindness, and other visual and neurologic disturbances. Mild to moderate hypertension may be present. RPLS is confirmed by MRI. Discontinue drug if this occurs.
- **Proteinuria:** Nephrotic syndrome is rare, occurring in < 1% of patients in clinical trials, but may be fatal. Monitor urine protein. Discontinue drug if nephritic syndrome occurs. Temporarily suspend drug for moderate proteinuria. Pathology of renal dysfunction was thrombotic microangiopathy in selected patients. Monitor urine dipstick baseline and regularly during treatment. If dipstick is 2+ or greater, hold drug and collect 24-hour urine for protein. Suspend drug if 24-hour urine protein is ≥ 2 grams of protein per 24 hours, and resume when urine protein is < 2 grams. Discontinue drug if patient develops nephrotic syndrome (> 3.5 grams of protein per 24 hours, low serum albumin, high cholesterol serum levels, and peripheral edema). Manufacturer states postmarketing study showed poor correlation between urine protein/creatinine ratio and actual 24-hour urine protein measurement (Pearson correlation 0.39% [95% CI, 0.17–0.57]).[78]
- **Infusion reactions:** Although the drug is a humanized MAb, rarely, hypersensitivity reactions may occur. Stop drug for severe infusion reactions, and institute appropriate medical interventions. The incidence of infusion reactions is < 3% in patients receiving first dose, and severe reactions occur in 0.2% of patients. The reactions may be characterized by hypertension, hypertensive crisis associated with neurologic signs and symptoms, wheezing, oxygen (O_2) desaturation, chest pain, headaches, rigors, diaphoresis, symptomatic bronchospasm (grade 3).

Contraindications: None, but drug can cause fetal harm. Women of childbearing age should use effective contraception. Nursing mothers should either stop the drug or stop nursing.

Adverse Reactions (**bold** indicates most common, occurring in > 25% of patients):

Cardiovascular: **Hypertension**, deep vein thrombosis (DVT)

Pulmonary: **Dyspnea**

CNS/neurologic/ENT: **Headache**, rhinitis, taste alterations, lacrimation disorder

Dermatologic: Dry skin, exfoliative dermatitis, skin ulcer

GI: Rectal hemorrhage, anorexia, **stomatitis**, dyspepsia

Hematologic: **Epistaxis**, hemorrhage, GI hemorrhage, neutropenia, thrombocytopenia; increased risk of neutropenia, infection when combined with chemotherapy

Genitourinary: **Proteinuria**

Musculoskeletal: Pain

General: Weight loss, **asthenia**

Nursing Discussion:
Please refer to the section on class effects on pages 204–209 for a detailed discussion of the management of hypertension, epistaxis, risk of hemorrhage, and GI perforation.

Therapy continuation: The optimal duration of therapy is unknown. In metastatic CRC, bevacizumab is usually stopped upon progression and the chemotherapy agent is changed. Grothey et al. did a retrospective review of registry data and found that patients who had their bevacizumab continued after progression, but their chemotherapy stopped and a new regimen started, had significantly longer survival.[93] This finding is being studied in a prospective trial.

In the recent adjuvant NSABP-C08 study, patients were randomized to receive bevacizumab plus mFOLFOX6 chemotherapy, or mFOLFOX6 plus placebo. There was a transient benefit to the patients who received bevacizumab for 12 months, giving them a 40% risk reduction ($P = .0004$) 1 year after chemotherapy was initiated. The disease free survival (DFS) difference remained significant for 2.5 years (3–5%), but at 3 years' follow-up, there was no significant difference in DFS.[94] The AVANT study using XELOX instead of mFOLFOX6 should be completed with results available by 2010. Determining whether or not bevacizumab should be given for a longer period of time should aid in the design of future adjuvant studies.

Tyrosine Kinase Inhibitors, mTOR Kinase Inhibitors, and Immunomodulatory Thalidomide Analogues
Drug: Sorafenib (Nexavar, BAY 43-9006)

Indications: Sorafenib is indicated for the treatment of patients with:
- Unresectable hepatocellular cancer
- Advanced renal cell cancer

Class: Serine/threonine kinase inhibitor; multiple-targeted TKI; antiangiogenesis agent

Mechanism of Action: Drug inhibits a number of tyrosine kinases, including Raf kinase, an enzyme in the RAS pathway (RAS is mutated in about 20–30% of solid tumors), as well as RTKs VEGFR-2 and PDGFR-b, thus preventing endothelial cell proliferation and angiogenesis. First, sorafenib inhibits the signaling cascade in the RAS pathway, blocking uncontrolled cell growth from either excessive stimulation of the RAS pathway or through mutations of RAS and RAF proteins. In addition, sorafenib inhibits angiogenesis by preventing the message created when VEGF binds to its receptor VEGFR-2 from reaching the endothelial cell nucleus. Thus, the endothelial cells do not proliferate and migrate, and angiogenesis is prevented. It also inhibits the message that would be sent to the cell nucleus when the ligand PDGF attaches to its receptor PDGFR-b; PDGF is necessary for pericytes around the blood vessels to provide external structure during angiogenesis, and when they are not available, angiogenesis is stopped.

Pharmacokinetics: After oral administration, mean relative bioavailability is 38–49%, peak plasma levels are in 3 hours, and mean elimination half-life is 25–48 hours. Steady state plasma concentrations are reached in 7 days with multiple doses. When drug is given with a high-fat meal, bioavailability is reduced 29% compared to that in a fasted state. Drug is highly protein bound (99.5%). Drug is metabolized by the liver P450 microenzyme system specifically by CYP3A4, with glucuronidation mediated by UGT1A9. There are eight metabolites of the drug. Following oral dose, 96% of the drug is recovered in 14 days, with 77% of the dose excreted in the feces and 19% in the urine. Japanese patients may have a 45% lower systemic exposure. Patients with mild to moderate hepatic dysfunction may have sorafinib area under the curve (AUC) 23–65% lower than those with normal hepatic function.

Dosage and Administration: 400 mg orally twice daily (total daily dose of 800 mg) taken 1 hour before or 2 hours after a meal, until patient is no longer receiving clinical benefit from drug or toxicity is unacceptable.

When dose reduction is indicated, reduce to a single 400-mg PO dose daily; if further reduction is needed, change to 400 mg PO every other day.

Hand–foot syndrome (HFS): For grade 2 (painful erythema, swelling of hands or feet, or symptoms interfering with normal activities of daily living [ADLs]), observe (using topical emollients such as Eucerin cream) for 7 days. If symptoms do not improve, hold drug until symptoms resolve or decrease to grade 1 (numbness, dysesthesia, paresthesia, tingling, painless swelling, erythema, or discomfort in hands or feet; symptoms do not interfere with ADLs). If HFS recurs, withhold drug until skin toxicity resolves to grade 0 or 1 and then resume at 400 mg PO daily. Or, if this is the third occurrence, resume at 400 mg PO every other day. If skin toxicity recurs on reduced dose, stop drug and resume when grade 0 or 1 at an additional decrease in drug dose. If skin toxicity recurs a third time, discontinue drug. Also discontinue drug if life-threatening or disabling skin toxicity (grade 4) occurs.

Available as: 200-mg tablets, in bottles of 120 tablets. Drug is available through a restricted distribution program called REACH (Resources for Expert Assistance and Care Helpline; download form online at http://www.nexavar-us.com/scripts/pages/en/home/index.php, then fax back to REACH at 866-639-5181 for approval; or call 866-639-2827, 866-NEXAVAR). This program assists patients with reimbursement issues. Providers do not need to register to prescribe sorafenib, but patients must be registered to receive the drug. The drug is available only through specialty pharmacies, and REACH will identify options for patients.

Reconstitution and Preparation: None, as oral tablet. Store at room temperature, 59–86°F (15–30°C), in a dry place, away from children and pets. Use gloves when handling the tablets, and return any unused drug in the bottle to the dispensing pharmacy for disposal.

Drug Interactions:

- UGT1A1 (e.g., irinotecan) and UGT1A9 substrates: Caution, drug AUC increases when coadministered with sorafenib.
- Docetaxel: Caution, docetaxel AUC increases when coadministered with sorafenib. Doxorubicin: Caution, doxorubicin AUC increases when coadministered with sorafenib. Fluorouracil: Caution, fluorouracil AUC changes when coadministered with sorafenib.
- CYP2B6 and CYP2C8 substrates: Caution, substrate drugs will have higher systemic exposure, so potential for their toxicity is increased when coadministered with sorafenib.
- CYP3A4 inducers: Expected to increase metabolism of sorafenib, decrease the systemic sorafenib drug level in the blood, and possibly reduce sorafenib efficacy.
- **Warfarin:** If coadministered, monitor international normalized ratio (INR) regularly for changes in prothrombin time (PT), INR, or clinical bleeding episodes.

Warnings and Precautions:

- Cardiac ischemia and/or infarction may occur. Incidence was 2.7% compared to 1.3% in placebo group (mRCC), and 2.9% vs. 0.4% in the hepatocellular trial. Patients with unstable coronary artery disease or past myocardial infarction were ineligible for the clinical trials. Consider temporary or permanent discontinuation of sorafenib.
- Bleeding may occur; however, incidence of bleeding from any cause was lower in patients with hepatocellular cancer receiving sorafenib compared to placebo; it was higher in mRCC patients than placebo (15.3% vs. 8.2%). If bleeding necessitates medical intervention, consider discontinuation of sorafenib.
- Hypertension usually occurs early in the course of treatment, is mild-moderate, and is managed with standard antihypertensive therapy. Incidence was 9.4% in sorafenib group vs. 4.3% in placebo group. Monitor

blood pressure weekly during the first 6 weeks and periodically thereafter, and treat as required.

- Hand–foot skin reaction, usually grade 1 or 2, and rash are common. They usually occur during the first 6 weeks of treatment. Usual management includes topical therapies for symptomatic relief, temporary treatment interruption and/or dose modification, or in severe or persistent cases, permanent discontinuation of sorafenib (rarely needed).
- GI perforation occurs rarely (< 1%); if it occurs, sorafenib should be discontinued. Teach patients to seek emergency care if they experience severe abdominal pain, with or without constipation, nausea, vomiting, or any evidence of bleeding (beyond epistaxis).
- **Temporary interruption of Nexavar therapy is recommended in patients undergoing major surgical procedures. Drug should be resumed when wound is healed.**
- Caution is recommended when coadministering substances metabolized/eliminated predominantly by the UGT1A1 pathway (e.g., irinotecan). Use caution when coadministering with docetaxel, doxorubicin, or fluorouracil, as the AUC of these agents is increased when coadministering with sorafenib.
- Use caution when coadministering sorafenib with substrates of CYP2B6 and CYP2C8 (see Chapter 5).
- Use caution when coadministering CYP3A4 inducers (e.g., St. John's wort, phenytoin, carbamazepine, dexamethasone, rifampin); consider sorafenib dose increase if coadministration is necessary (see Chapter 5).
- Elevated serum lipase and decreased phosphate of unknown etiology may occur.

Contraindications:
- Patients with known hypersensitivity to the drug or its components.
- Drug may cause fetal harm; teach women of childbearing age to use effective contraception and not to become pregnant during treatment and for 2 weeks following drug discontinuance. Teach patient to advise physician right away if she thinks she may be pregnant.
- Drug should not be used in women who are breastfeeding.

Adverse Reactions (**bold** indicates most common, occurring in > 25% of patients):

Cardiovascular: Myocardial ischemia, myocardial infarction, hypertension

Pulmonary: Dyspnea, cough

CNS/Neurologic: Peripheral sensory neuropathy, headache

Dermatologic: **Rash/desquamation**, **HFS**, **alopecia**, dry skin, subungual (splinter) hemorrhages under fingernails

CNS/Metabolic: **Hypophosphatemia (35%**, with 11% grade 3 [1–2 mg/dL]), **elevated lipase (40%**, with 9% grade 3 or 4), **elevated amylase (34%), hypoalbuminemia (54%), INR elevation (42%)**

GI: **Diarrhea, abdominal pain, anorexia, nausea, weight loss**, GI perforation, vomiting, constipation, liver dysfunction, stomatitis, mucositis (which may be severe)

Hematologic: **Lymphopenia, thrombocytopenia** (4% grade 3 or 4), hemorrhage, epistaxis

Musculoskeletal: Joint pain, myalgia

General: **Fatigue**, weakness, **flu-like symptoms, fever**

Nursing Discussion:

Patient teaching: Teach patients drug self-administration, in the context of their current medication profile, to prevent drug interactions and to allow optimal drug absorption. If the patient is taking any over-the-counter (OTC) medications, assess them, and remind the patient not to take any histamine receptor-blocking agents (e.g., omeprazole, ranitidine) within 2 hours of taking sorafenib. Teach patient that lipase, amylase, and phosphorus blood tests will be repeated during therapy and that a plan to address any abnormalities will be made if they occur.

Skin reactions:
- *HFS/reaction* occurs in almost a third of patients, and is usually grade 1 or 2; it appears during the first 6 weeks of treatment. Hyperkeratosis (callus) formation is the usual presentation, especially on the soles of the feet. Teach patients that this reaction may occur and to keep the skin of the hands and feet, as well as areas of friction, hydrated with skin emollients such as Eucerin cream, and to avoid repetitive movements such as jogging. If the calluses are very thick, use of topical exfoliating products such as Kerasal (over the counter) or Keralac (prescription) will help thin the calluses.[90] Teach patients to assess skin areas and to report any pain, as painful skin erythema or edema that interferes with ADLs is considered grade 2. Topical agents are used for up to 7 days, but if there is no relief, the drug should be interrupted until it resolves to a grade 1 or 0 and then resumed at a reduced dose.
- *Subungual (splinter) hemorrhage* does not require treatment. Teach patient it occurs as a small amount of blood within the dermis of the nail bed in a layer of squamous cells that adhere to the undersurface of the nail.[90]
- *Rash, dry skin, and pruritus* may occur. Rash is macular or papular. Teach patient to use gentle soap to wash, followed by application of skin emollient cream to moisten the skin. If the scalp itches, suggest that the patient use antidandruff shampoos and conditioner.[90] Lotions containing

aloe vera or dimethicone will help to increase comfort. If the rash is severe, it may require assessment by a dermatologist along with dose interruption.

Hypertension: Teach patients to keep a diary if they are found to have hypertension, and to record their values with each measurement. In addition, the patient can record blood pressure medication self-administration. If patients are interested and able, teach them to monitor their own blood pressure at home and to call if the blood pressure goal is not maintained. Help them develop a realistic plan to optimize their nonpharmacologic management of lifestyle changes, such as smoking cessation if that is an issue.

Diarrhea: Review the patient's normal bowel regimen, and remind him or her to stop taking stool softeners or laxatives. Other important teaching points include[90]:

- Diet modifications, adequate fluid intake, and self-administration of loperamide
- Calling the nurse or physician if diarrhea persists > 24 hours or is refractory to loperamide
- Diet modification with increased bulking agents, such as Benefiber, which may increase stool consistency and reduce the number of stools; minimization of gas-producing foods such as beans; avoidance of carbonated beverages, fried foods, or spicy foods
- Use of antacids and acidophilus products such as some yogurts and cheese

Mucositis: Assess the oral mucosa baseline and at each visit. Teach the patient to self-assess the oral mucosa daily, to practice effective oral hygiene, and to report any pain in the oral mucous membranes or other areas. Pain may be present despite only mild erythema on physical exam. Assess ability to chew and swallow, as this may be impacted. Teach patient to call the nurse or physician if any difficulty swallowing is present, or if unable to take in adequate fluid (at least 1–2 quarts per day, taken as a full glass every 1–2 hours when awake) or food.

Drug: Sunitinib (Sutent)

Indications: FDA approved for the treatment of:
- GI stromal tumor (GIST) after disease progression on imatinib mesylate
- Advanced renal cell carcinoma (based on response rate and response duration)

Class: Multitargeted TKI

Mechanism of Action: Drug has both anti-tumor and antiangiogenesis activity, and inhibits multiple RTKs that are involved in tumor growth, angiogenesis, and metastatic cancer progression. It inhibits PDGF receptors (alpha and beta); VEGFR-1, -2, and -3; stem cell factor receptor (KIT), fms-like tyrosine kinase-3

(FLT-3), colony-stimulating factor receptor type 1 (CSF-1R), and the glial cell line–derived neurotrophic factor receptor (RET).

Pharmacokinetics: After oral ingestion, maximal plasma concentrations are reached within 6 to 12 hours, regardless of food intake. Drug and primary metabolite bind to plasma protein 90–95%. Drug is metabolized by the cytochrome P450 enzyme CYP3A4 to produce its primary metabolite, which is then itself metabolized by CYP3A4. Terminal half-lives of sunitinib and its primary metabolite are 40–60 hours and 80–110 hours, respectively. Drug is primarily excreted via the feces.

Dosage and Administration:
- 50 mg PO daily × 4 weeks, followed by 2 weeks off, in a 6-week cycle.
- Dose escalation or reduction in 12.5-mg increments.
- Consider dose reduction in patients with severe hepatic dysfunction.
- Dose reduce or temporarily hold dose if left ventricular ejection fraction (LVEF) decreases 20–50% from baseline without signs of heart failure; when LVEF returns to baseline, resume at reduced dose. If patient develops signs/symptoms of congestive heart failure (CHF), promptly discontinue drug. All patients should receive a baseline determination of LVEF (e.g., echocardiogram or gated blood pool scan). Patients with a history of cardiac events, or at risk for them, should receive periodic evaluation of LVEF during sunitinib therapy.
- Discontinue drug if patient develops CHF.
- Dose reduce or temporarily hold dose if patient develops severe hypertension (SBP > 200 mm Hg, DBP > 110 mm Hg); when blood pressure returns to baseline, resume at reduced dose.
- If signs/symptoms of pancreatitis present, discontinue drug and provide supportive care.
- If RPLS (with signs and symptoms of hypertension, headache, decreased alertness, altered mentation, or loss of vision) occurs, temporarily stop drug and control hypertension; when signs/symptoms resolve, resume therapy.

Available as: 12.5-mg (orange/orange), 25-mg (caramel/orange), and 50-mg (caramel/caramel) capsules. Store at room temperature, 59–86°F (15–30°C), in a dry place, away from children and pets. Use gloves when handling the tablets, and return any unused drug in the bottle to the dispensing pharmacy for disposal.

Reconstitution and Preparation: None (oral tablet)

Drug Interactions:
- CYP3A4 inhibitors (e.g., atazanavir, clarithromycin, diltiazem, indinavir, itraconazole, ketoconazole, nefazodone, nelfinavir, ritonavir, saquinavir,

telithromycin, verapamil, voriconazole, grapefruit or grapefruit juice) increase plasma level of sunitinib. Do not give together, or dose reduce sunitinib if used concurrently.

- CYP3A4 inducers (e.g., barbiturates, carbamazepine, dexamethasone, modafinil, nafcillin, phenobarbital, phenytoin, rifabutin, rifampin, rifapentine, St. John's wort) decrease plasma level of sunitinib by 23–46%. Do not give together, or increase dose of sunitinib if given concurrently.
- Drugs that prolong the QT interval on electrocardiogram (ECG), such as atypical antipsychotics (e.g., olanzapine, risperidone), droperidol, erythromycin, fluoroquinolone antibiotics, procainamide, quinidine, prochlorperazine, should be avoided.

Warnings:
- Drug is fetotoxic. Teach women of childbearing potential to use effective birth contraception.
- Drug may cause a decrease in the pumping ability of the left ventricle of the heart as evidenced by a decline in LVEF to below the lower limit of normal. Monitor patients for signs and symptoms of CHF, and discontinue drug promptly if they appear. Interrupt or reduce drug dose if LVEF falls 20–50% below baseline.
- Prolonged QT intervals and torsade de pointes (unusual ventricular tachycardia) have been observed in < 0.1% of patients. Use cautiously in patients at risk for developing QT interval prolongation (e.g., those with congenital risk, those taking medications that prolong the QT interval) or in patients receiving concomitant drugs that are CYP3A4 inhibitors (as the serum level of sunitinib will be increased with greater risk of toxicity, including torsades de pointes). Assess baseline ECGs and monitor during treatment. Monitor serum magnesium and potassium frequently, and replete electrolytes as needed.
- Hypertension may occur (incidence 30% with 10% grade 3). Treat with standard antihypertensive medications.
- Hemorrhage may occur, including tumor-related hemorrhage in patients with GIST, or in clinical trials with other solid tumors (e.g., patients with squamous cell NSCLC). Incidence is 30%, and most common hemorrhage was epistaxis, with less common rectal, gingival, upper GI, genital, and wound bleeding. If patients have bleeding, follow serial complete blood counts (CBCs), along with physician exam, and monitor patients very closely during treatment.
- Thyroid dysfunction may occur in 3–4% of patients. Assess baseline thyroid function tests, and correct with thyroid standard therapy prior to beginning sunitinib therapy. Repeat thyroid function tests as needed if patient develops signs/symptoms of hypo- or hyperthyroidism. Manage with standard medical practice.

- Adrenal hemorrhage may rarely occur; monitor adrenal function, especially in cases of stress such as surgery, trauma, or severe infection.
- CBC, platelet count, and serum chemistries, including phosphate, should be performed baseline and prior to each cycle. Baseline LVEF should be determined, and if at risk, the patient should have testing repeated periodically during treatment. Baseline ECG showing QT interval should be documented and, if at risk, repeated periodically during therapy.

Contraindications: None

Adverse Reactions (**bold** indicates most common, occurring in > 25% of patients):

Cardiovascular: **Hypertension**, decreased LVEF, peripheral edema, prolonged QT interval, venous thromboembolism, periorbital edema

Pulmonary: Dyspnea (mild), cough

CNS/Neurologic: Headache, dizziness, peripheral neuropathy, seizures, RPLS, increased lacrimaton

Dermatologic: **Rash, HFS, skin discoloration**

CNS/Metabolic: Hypothyroidism, adrenal insufficiency, increased serum lipase, increased serum amylase, increased uric acid, hypokalemia, hypernatremia

GI: **Diarrhea, nausea (moderate risk), mucositis/stomatitis (may be severe), vomiting, dyspepsia, abdominal pain, constipation, anorexia, increased LFTs (liver transaminases, alkaline phosphatase**, total bilirubin, and indirect bilirubin), altered taste (glossodynia), flatulence, dehydration, oral pain

Hematologic: **Neutropenia, thrombocytopenia, anemia (in GIST patients, with recovery in 2-week rest period prior to the next cycle), bleeding**, rare severe hemorrhage, epistaxis, grade 3 or 4 neutropenia, grade 3 or 4 anemia

Genitourinary: Increased serum creatinine

Musculoskeletal: **Arthralgia**, limb pain, myalgia, back pain

General: **Fatigue, asthenia**, fever

Nursing Discussion:

Patient Teaching: Teach patients drug self-administration, in the context of their current medication profile, to prevent drug interactions. Teach patients self-administration of prescribed antiemetic agents and to call if experiencing persistent nausea and/or vomiting > 24 hours, or if unable to keep fluids or food down.

Skin Reactions:

- *HFS/reaction* occurs in about 21% of patients, usually grade 1 or 2, but may be severe. It appears during the first 6 weeks of treatment and may be preceded by a tingling sensation. Hyperkeratosis (callus) formation may occur on the soles of the feet. Teach patients that this may occur and to keep the skin of the hands and feet, as well as areas of friction, hydrated with skin emollients such as Eucerin cream, and to avoid repetitive movements such as jogging. Affected areas may desquamate and be very painful. Teach patients to assess skin areas and to report any pain, as painful skin erythema or edema that interferes with ADLs is considered grade 2. Topical agents are used for up to 7 days, but if there is no relief, the drug should be interrupted until it resolves to a grade 1 or 0, then resumed at a reduced dose.

- *Subungual (splinter) hemorrhage* does not require treatment. Teach patient it occurs as a small amount of blood within the dermis of the nail bed in a layer of squamous cells that adhere to the undersurface of the nail.[90]

- *Rash, dry skin, and pruritus* may occur. Rash is macular or papular. Teach patient to use gentle soap to wash, followed by application of skin emollient cream to moisten the skin. If the scalp itches, suggest that the patient use antidandruff shampoos and conditioner.[90] Lotions containing aloe vera or dimethicone will help to increase comfort. If the rash is severe, it may require assessment by a dermatologist, along with dose interruption.

- *Skin color* may change, turning a yellow color within 1 week of starting therapy; other skin toxicities usually begin 3–4 weeks after starting therapy.

- *Reversible zebra hair color* (reversible hair depigmentation) occurs during therapy, then normal hair color returns during the 2-week break; the repeated cycles result in alternating white, then normal color hair, similar to a zebra pattern; in males, may be visible in facial hair 2–3 weeks and in scalp hair 5–6 weeks after beginning the drug.

- *Alopecia* occurs in about 5–12% of patients.

Hypertension: Teach patients to keep a diary if they are found to have hypertension and to record their values with each measurement. In addition, patients can record their blood pressure medication self-administration. If patients are interested and able, teach them to monitor their own blood pressure at home and to call if the blood pressure goal is not maintained. Help them develop a realistic plan to optimize their nonpharmacologic management of lifestyle changes, such as smoking cessation if that is an issue.

Diarrhea: Review the patient's normal bowel regimen, and remind him or her to stop taking stool softeners or laxatives. Other important teaching points include[90]:

- Diet modifications, adequate fluid intake, and self-administration of loperamide

- Calling the nurse or physician if diarrhea persists > 24 hours or is refractory to loperamide
- Diet modification with increased bulking agents, such as Benefiber, which may increase stool consistency and reduce the number of stools; minimization of gas-producing foods such as beans; avoidance of carbonated beverages, fried foods, or spicy foods
- Use of antacids and acidophilus products such as some yogurts and cheese

Mucositis: Assess the oral mucosa baseline and at each visit. Teach the patient to self-assess the oral mucosa daily, to practice effective oral hygiene, and to report any pain in the oral mucous membranes or other areas. Pain may be present despite only mild erythema on physical exam. Assess ability to chew and swallow, as this may be impacted. Teach patient to call the nurse or physician if pain or any difficulty swallowing is present, or if unable to take in adequate fluid (at least 1–2 quarts per day, taken as a full glass every 1–2 hours when awake) or food. Pain may be severe and require IV hydration as well as IV opioids.

Drug: Temsirolimus (Torisel)

Indications: Treatment of advanced renal cell cancer

Class: **mTOR kinase inhibitor**

Mechanism of Action: Drug binds to the intracellular protein FKBP-12, and the protein–drug complex inhibits mTOR (or FKBP-12) kinase that is responsible for cell division. mTOR is also responsible for sensing the nutrients in the cell's environment and for organizing actin, trafficking of the membrane, insulin secretion, protein degradation, protein kinase C signaling, and tRNA synthesis. Inhibition of the kinase makes the cell think it is starving, and it stops growing (arrests cell growth in G_1 phase of the cell cycle). This reduces the levels of HIF and VEGF. As more is learned about the function of this pathway, it appears that rapamycin and mTOR inhibitors affect only some of mTOR functioning.

Pharmacokinetics: The drug is metabolized by the P450 microenzyme system in the liver (CYP3A4) into five metabolites. Sirolimus is the active metabolite. Metabolites are primarily excreted in the feces (82% within 14 days). Mean half-lives of temsirolimus and sirolimus were 17.3 hours and 54.6 hours, respectively.

Dosage and Administration: 25 mg IV over 30–60 minutes weekly until tumor progression or intolerable toxicity. Premedicate with 25–50 mg diphenhydramine 30 minutes before temsirolimus dose.

- Hold for absolute neutrophil count (ANC) < 1000 cells/mm^3, platelet count < 75,000 cells/mm^3, or grade 3 or higher toxicity (National Cancer Institute-Common Toxicity Criteria of Adverse Events [NCI-CTCAE]). Once toxicity has resolved to grade 2 or less, drug may be restarted at a dose reduced by 5 mg/week, to a dose no lower than 15 mg/week.

- Check CBC weekly and chemistries every other week.
- Drug should be stored in bottles (glass, polypropylene) or plastic IV bags (polypropylene, polyolefin), and administer through a polyethylene-lined administration set with an in-line polyethersulfone filter with a pore size less than 5 microns.
- After premedication, administer IV over 30–60 minutes once a week via an infusion pump if possible.
- Do not use bags or tubing containing the plasticizer di-2-ethylhexyl phthalate (DEHP), which may leach from the polyvinylchloride (PVC) infusion bags or sets into IV solution and be administered into the patient.
- Use personal protective equipment when preparing and administering drug.

Available as: Temsirolimus 25 mg/mL vial with an overfill of 0.2 mL; accompanying diluent vial has a deliverable volume of 1.8 mL.

Reconstitution and Preparation:
- Before preparation, store in the refrigerator at 2–8°C (36–46°F) and protect from light.
- During preparation, protect from excessive room light and sunlight. Inspect product for particulate matter and decolorization before administration.
- Step 1: Inject 1.8-mL diluent into vial that together with an overfill of 0.2 mL results in a 10-mg/mL solution. Withdraw 3 mL (including overfill).
- Invert vial to mix, and allow air bubbles to subside. This vial is stable for 24 hours at controlled room temperature.
- Step 2: Withdraw ordered drug amount from vial (prepared in step 1), and inject rapidly into a 250-mL container (glass, polyolefin, polyethylene) of 0.9% sodium chloride injection. Invert bag or bottle to mix but do not shake, as this will cause foaming. Do not use PVC IV sets or bags, as drug may leach phthalates (DEHP) from the PVC infusion sets or IV bag. Drug contains polysorbate 80, which increases the rate of DEHP extraction from PVC tubing or bags.
- Drug must be used within 6 hours of adding the diluted drug to the IV bag.

Drug Interactions:
- Strong CYP3A4 inhibitors (ketoconazole, itraconazole, clarithromycin, atazanavir, indinavir, nefazodone, nelfinavir, ritonavir, saquinavir, telithromycin, voriconazole, grapefruit juice): Avoid coadministration. If coadministration is necessary, decrease temsirolimus dose to 12.5 mg weekly; when interacting drug is discontinued, allow a 1-week washout period, then resume dose prior to giving interacting drug. Do not coadminister with grapefruit or grapefruit juice.
- Strong CYP3A4 inducers (dexamethasone, phenytoin, carbamazepine, rifampin, rifabutin, rifampacin, phenobarbital, St. John's wort): Avoid concomitant use. If drug must be coadministered with temsirolimus, increase

temsirolimus dose to 50 mg weekly; when interacting drug is discontinued, resume dose before giving interacting drug. Do not coadminister with St. John's wort.

- ACE inhibitors (e.g., lisinopril) may cause angioneurotic edema.
- Calcineurin inhibitors (e.g., cyclosporine) may increase risk of hemolytic uremic syndrome. Use together cautiously, and monitor patient closely.
- Live attenuated vaccines increase risk of serious infection. Do not coadminister.
- Vaccines decrease immune response and efficacy.
- Sunitinib: Concomitant use increases toxicity. Use together cautiously, if at all, and monitor patient for toxicity closely, especially erythematous maculopapular rash, cellulitis, and gout requiring hospitalization.

Contraindications: None. However:

- Use cautiously if at all in patients with known hypersensitivity to temsirolimus, its metabolites, or polysorbate 80.
- Drug should not be administered to pregnant or breastfeeding women; both men and women of childbearing age should be taught to use effective contraception measures during treatment and for 3 months after the drug has been discontinued.

Warnings and Precautions:

- Patients may develop a hypersensitivity reaction to temsirolimus, characterized by anaphylaxis, dyspnea, flushing, and chest pain. If this occurs, stop the drug immediately and treat with an antihistamine and other measures as needed. Observe the patient for 30–60 minutes depending upon the severity of the reaction. The physician may wish to restart the drug at a slower rate over 60 minutes, following premedication with an H_1 antihistamine if not already given and/or an H_2-receptor antagonist (e.g., ranitidine 50 mg or famotidine 20 mg IV).
- Hyperglycemia and hyperlipemia are likely and may require treatment. Monitor glucose and lipid profiles, and manage with standard medical care. Some patients will require initiation of insulin and/or an oral hypoglycemic agent. Teach patient signs and symptoms of hyperglycemia and to report them right away.
- Infections may result from immunosuppression, including opportunistic infections.
- Monitor for interstitial lung disease (ILD) symptoms (e.g., cough, dyspnea, hypoxia, fever) or indicative radiographic changes (e.g., infiltrates). If ILD is suspected, discontinue temsirolimus and consider use of corticosteroids and/or antibiotics. Teach patient to report any new or worsening pulmonary symptoms.

- Bowel perforation may occur. Evaluate fever, metabolic acidosis, abdominal pain, bloody stools, diarrhea, and/or acute abdomen promptly. Teach patient to report any new or worsening abdominal pain right away.
- Renal failure, sometimes fatal, has occurred. Monitor renal function at baseline and while on temsirolimus.
- Drug is likely to cause increases in serum triglycerides and cholesterol. Assess baseline and monitor regularly during therapy.
- Due to abnormal wound healing, use temsirolimus with caution in the perioperative period.
- Live vaccinations and close contact with those who received live vaccines should be avoided.
- Women of childbearing potential should be advised to use effective contraceptive to avoid pregnancy.
- Patients with CNS tumors (primary or metastatic) and/or receiving anticoagulant therapy may be at increased risk of developing intracerebral bleeding. Monitor these patients very closely.
- Monitor baseline: Renal and hepatic function tests, CBC/platelets, fasting blood glucose, serum electrolytes, lipid profile, chest x-ray
- Monitor weekly during treatment: CBC/platelets
- Monitor every 2 weeks during therapy: Fasting blood glucose, serum electrolytes
- Monitor regularly during treatment: Renal and hepatic function tests, chest x-ray

Adverse Reactions (**bold** indicates most common, occurring in > 25% of patients):

Cardiovascular: Hypertension, chest pain

Pulmonary: ILD, pharyngitis, rhinitis, dyspnea, cough, upper respiratory infection (URI)

CNS/Neurologic: Pain, headache, insomnia, depression, conjunctivitis, increased lacrimation

Dermatologic: **Rash, edema,** dry skin, nail disorder, acne, impaired wound healing

CNS/Metabolic: **Hyperglycemia/glucose intolerance, hyperlipidemia, hypertriglyceridemia,** hypokalemia

GI: **Mucositis, nausea, anorexia, elevated alkaline phosphatase, hypophosphatemia, elevated aspartate aminotransferase (AST),** weight loss, diarrhea, constipation, abdominal pain, vomiting, dysgeusia, bowel perforation

Hematologic: **Anemia, lymphopenia, thrombocytopenia, leucopenia,** epistaxis, venous thromboembolism, pulmonary embolus, decreased neutrophil and platelet count

Genitourinary: **Elevated serum creatinine**, urinary tract infection (UTI)

Musculoskeletal: Back pain, myalgias, arthralgias

General: **Asthenia, hypersensitivity reactions**, pyrexia, chills

Nursing Discussion:

Drug has shown increased efficacy in the management of mantle cell lymphoma at a dose of 250 mg/m^2 once weekly.

Hypersensitivity reactions may occur, but incidence is reduced with premedication with diphenhydramine. Stop the infusion right away if the patient has a reaction, monitor vital signs and O$_2$ saturation for at least 30–60 minutes, depending on the severity of the reaction. Discuss with midlevel practitioner or physician the addition of an H$_2$ antagonist 30 minutes prior to resuming the infusion to prevent further hypersensitivity. Ensure that medications necessary for the management of hypersensitivity/anaphylaxis are readily available (e.g., epinephrine, antihistamines, corticosteroids). Assess baseline vital signs and monitor frequently during the infusion. Be prepared to provide emergency support as necessary (including IV saline, epinephrine, antihistamines, bronchodilators). If reaction is mild, when symptoms resolve, resume the infusion at 50% of the rate of the previous infusion (e.g., over 60 minutes), as directed by the physician or midlevel practitioner.

Patients will be immunosuppressed and are at risk for infections, including opportunistic infections. In addition, the incidence of decreased neutrophils was 19% (grade 3 or 4, 5%), platelets 40% (1%), hemoglobin 94% (20%), and lymphocytes 53% (16%). Grade 3 or 4 neutropenia occurred in 7% of patients, thrombocytopenia in 5%, and anemia in 9% of patients in clinical trials comparing doses 75–250 mg weekly. Assess baseline blood counts and platelets. Teach patient to report fever and signs/symptoms of infection or bleeding right away. Assess medication profile and OTC medications taken. Teach patient to avoid OTC medications containing nonsteroidal anti-inflammatory drugs (NSAIDs) or aspirin. Teach patient to talk to nurse or physician before beginning any OTC medications.

Patients are at risk for altered nutritional status related to mucositis, nausea, anorexia, diarrhea, hyperglycemia, hypertriglyceridemia, and bowel perforation. In clinical studies, mucositis affected 70% of patients, nausea 43%, diarrhea 27%, and anorexia 40% of patients. Bowel perforation occurs rarely but may be fatal. Presentation includes fever, abdominal pain, metabolic acidosis, bloody stools, diarrhea, and/or acute abdomen. The incidence of hypercholesteremia is 87%, triglyceridemia 83%, and hyperglycemia 89%; in terms of grade 3 and 4 toxicities, hyperglycemia occurred in 17% of patients, hypophosphatemia 13%, and hypertriglyceridemia in 6% of patients. mTOR is involved in insulin signaling, which possibly explains the hypertriglyceridemia and hyperglycemia. Assess serum triglycerides, cholesterol, and glucose baseline and during treatment with the drug. Teach the patient to report any new or worsening abdominal pain or bloody stools right away and to come to the emergency department for immediate evaluation. Premedicate with antiemetics. Encourage small, frequent meals of cool, bland foods and increased fluid intake. Assess oral mucosa prior to drug administration and instruct patient to report changes. Teach patient oral hygiene measures and self-assessment. Teach patient to notify physician/nurse if experiencing excessive thirst or any increase in volume or frequency of urination. Notify physician or midlevel provider of any abnormalities and discuss implications and management.

Alterations in skin integrity may occur. Maculopapular rash is the most common toxicity, affecting 47%; acne occurs in 10%, nail disorder in 14%, dry skin in 11%, and pruritus in 19%. Assess patient skin integrity, including nails baseline and regularly during treatment. Teach patient self-assessment and local comfort measures, including the use of water-based emollients. Teach patient to report skin changes; if self-care is ineffective, discuss plan with physician or midlevel practitioner, especially if severe.

Asthenia affects 51% of patients in clinical studies (depression 4%), but at the higher dose of 250 mg every week, 5% had grade 3 and 4 depression. In the context of advanced renal cell cancer, much may be contributed by the underlying tumor. Assess baseline comfort, mental status, and activity tolerance, and reassess during treatment, asking patients to identify what activities they are now unable to do, sleep habits, and also emotional state. Discuss alternating rest and activity periods and the possibility of other family members or friends assisting with energy-consuming responsibilities to increase energy reserve. Assess baseline alertness and sleep patterns. Assess other drugs taken, especially those with sedating qualities, and alcohol ingestion. Instruct patient to avoid alcohol and to take drug at bedtime. Assess degree of drowsiness and dizziness for safety of patient. If significant, teach measures to ensure safety.

Drug: Everolimus (Afinitor)

Indications: Treatment of patients with advanced renal cell carcinoma after failure of treatment with sunitinib or sorafenib

Class: mTOR inhibitor

Mechanism of Action: mTOR is an intracellular serine/threonine kinase protein that regulates cell proliferation and angiogenesis. It is found in the cytoplasm and turns on and off the translation of signals that tell the cell's protein factory (ribosomes) to make proteins. Proteins control all the cell functions. Proteins that activate mTOR are growth signals from EGF, IGF, and VEGFs. Proteins that stop mTOR activity are tuberous sclerosis complex-1 and -2, and if there are not enough nutrients to support more cells, mTOR activity is blocked. As an mTOR inhibitor, everolimus interferes with the central regulation of tumor cell division, metabolism, and angiogenesis. Blocking this important protein results in cell cycle arrest and cell death. mTOR is also a very important component of the P13K/AKT signaling pathway that is often dysregulated in solid tumors, as it plays a role in cell cycle regulation, and it also suppresses apoptosis.[95]

Specifically, everolimus binds to an intracellular protein, FKBP-12, a protein-folding chaperone, and this inhibits mTOR kinase activity. Everolimus also reduces the activity of downstream effectors of mTOR that are involved in protein synthesis, inhibits the expression of HIF-1, and reduces expression of VEGF. Through these actions, everolimus reduces cell proliferation, angiogenesis, and glucose uptake.[96]

Pharmacokinetics: Peak serum concentrations are achieved 1–2 hours after oral dosing, with steady state reached within 2 weeks with once-daily dosing. mTOR inhibition is complete after a 10-mg oral daily dose. In clinical studies, a high-fat meal reduced AUC by 16%, but the manufacturer recommends the dose be given without regard to meals. Plasma binding is about 74%. Drug is a substrate of CYP3A4 and PgP (P-glycoprotein). Everolimus is mainly metabolized by CYP3A4 in the liver and to some extent in the intestinal wall and is a substrate for the multidrug efflux pump PgP. It is metabolized into six metabolites that have less activity than the intact drug. The mean elimination half-life of everolimus is 30 hours, with 80% of drug excreted in the feces and 5% in the urine. Moderate hepatic dysfunction (Child-Pugh class B) doubles the AUC, so dose should be reduced in these patients. Oral clearance of the drug is 20% higher in black patients than in Caucasian; Japanese patients had, on average, a higher drug exposure than non-Japanese. The implications of ethnic differences are unknown.

Dosage and Administration: 10 mg PO daily with or without food. Teach patient not to chew or crush the tablet.
- Dose reduce to 5 mg PO daily to manage severe and/or intolerable adverse reactions, and/or interrupt dose.
- Administer 5 mg PO daily for patients with moderate hepatic impairment.
- If coadministered with a strong CYP3A4 inducer, consider increasing dose from 10 mg PO daily to 20 mg PO daily in 5-mg increments; if the strong CYP3A4 drug is discontinued, the everolimus dose should be changed to the original dose prior to initiation of the strong CYP3A4 inducer.

Available as: 5-mg and 10-mg tablets in blister packs.

Reconstitution and Preparation: None, oral tablet. Store at room temperature 59° to 86° F (15° to 30° C), in a dry place, away from children and pets. Use gloves when handling the tablets, and return any unused drug in the bottle to the dispensing pharmacy for disposal.

Drug Interactions:

- Everolimus is a substrate of CYP3A as well as a substrate and moderate inhibitor of PgP multidrug efflux pump. It is also a competitive inhibitor of CYP3A4 and a mixed inhibitor of CYP2D6.
- Coadministration with strong or moderate CYP3A4-inhibitors or PgP (e.g., amprenavir, aprepitant, atazanavir, clarithromycin, delavirdine, diltiazem, erythromycin, fluconazole, fosamprenavir, grapefruit juice, indinavir, itraconazole, ketoconazole, nafazodone, nelfinavir, ritonavir, saquinavir, telithromycin, verapamil, voriconazole) is not recommended unless the benefit outweighs the risk. These drugs will significantly increase the serum levels of everolimus and should NOT be used together.
- Coadministration with strong CYP3A4 inducers (e.g., carbamazepine, dexamethasone, phenobarbital, phenytoin, rifabutin, rifampicin) is not recommended, but if needed, the dose of everolimus should be increased from 10 mg daily to 20 mg daily, using 5-mg increments.
- Grapefruit and grapefruit juice can interfere with the CYP3A4 metabolic pathway; do not take while receiving everolimus.
- St. John's wort can increase the metabolism of everolimus and thus lower drug serum levels; do not use together.
- Inhibitors of PgP (e.g., ketoconazole, quinidine, erythromycin, verapamil, probenecid, cimetidine) may decrease the efflux of everolimus from intestinal cells and increase everolimus blood concentrations; thus, they should be avoided. Do NOT coadminister.
- Everolimus is a competitive inhibitor of CYP3A4 and of CYP2D6 microsomal pathways so that drugs metabolized via these pathways may have higher serum levels; if the drug has a narrow therapeutic window, monitor for side effects or decrease dose of interacting drug.

Warnings:

- Noninfectious pneumonitis: Incidence is 14%, with 4% severe. Monitor for clinical signs and symptoms (e.g., hypoxia, pleural effusion, cough, dyspnea) or radiologic changes. Fatal cases have occurred. If the patient has few or no symptoms, continue everolimus without dose alteration. If symptoms are moderate, interrupt therapy until symptoms improve; then reintroduce everolimus at 5 mg daily. If symptoms are severe, discontinue everolimus, and use corticosteroids until clinical symptoms resolve. Then if desired, reinitiate therapy at a reduced dose of 5 mg daily depending on the clinical circumstance.
- Localized and systemic infections (e.g., pneumonia, other bacterial infections, aspergillosis, candidiasis) may occur. If patient has a preexisting invasive fungal infection prior to starting everolimus, the patient should receive complete treatment before everolimus is initiated. Drug is

immunosuppressive and increases the risk of infections, some fatal. Monitor for signs and symptoms, and treat promptly. If the patient develops an invasive fungal infection while on everolimus treatment, discontinue the drug, and treat with appropriate antifungal therapy.

- Oral ulceration occurs in 44% of patients. Stomatitis with ulceration is common but is most often grade 1 and 2 (NCI-CTCAE). Teach patient self-assessment and systematic oral cleansing after meals and at bedtime with a cleanser such as sodium bicarbonate or normal saline gargles. Avoid mouth rinses that contain alcohol or peroxide. Antifungal rinses should not be used unless a fungal infection has been diagnosed.
- Laboratory test alterations: Elevations of serum creatinine, blood glucose, and lipids (hyperlipidemia, hypertriglyceridemia) may occur. Ensure that patients with baseline elevated glucose or lipids have these corrected with appropriate medication prior to starting everolimus therapy. Decreases in hemoglobin, neutrophils, and platelets may also occur. Monitor renal function, blood glucose, lipids, and hematologic parameters baseline prior to treatment and periodically thereafter.
- Vaccinations (e.g., intranasal influenza, measles, mumps, rubella, oral polio, bacillus Calmette-Guérin, yellow fever, varicella, and typhoid): Avoid live vaccines and close contact with those who have received live vaccines.
- Drug is fetotoxic and is pregnancy category D. Women of childbearing age should use effective contraception, avoiding pregnancy during therapy and for 8 weeks following the end of treatment. Women should not breastfeed while receiving the drug.

Contraindications: Hypersensitivity to everolimus or other rapamycin derivatives
- Women should avoid pregnancy.
- Nursing women should discontinue drug or nursing.
- Patients with Child-Pugh hepatic impairment should not receive the drug.

Adverse Reactions (**bold** indicates most common, occurring in > 25% of patients):

Cardiovascular: **Peripheral edema**, chest pain, hypertension, tachycardia, CHF

Pulmonary: **Cough**, dyspnea, pneumonitis, pleural effusion, pharyngolaryngeal pain, rhinorrhea

CNS/Neurologic: Headache, insomnia, dizziness, paresthesia, eyelid edema, conjunctivitis

Dermatologic: **Rash**, pruritus, dry skin, HFS, nail disorder, erythema, onychoclasis, skin lesion, acneiform dermatitis

CNS/Metabolic: **Hypercholesterolemia, hypertriglyceridemia, hyperglycemia, hypophosphatemia**

GI: **Stomatitis**, **diarrhea**, dehydration, abdominal pain, nausea, vomiting, mucosal inflammation, epistaxis, anorexia, dysgeusia, dry mouth, dysphagia, hemorrhoids, weight loss, exacerbation of or new-onset diabetes mellitus, increased liver function tests (LFTs)

Hematologic: **Infections**, **anemia**, **lymphopenia**, hemorrhage, decreased neutrophils and platelets

Genitourinary: Renal failure, increased serum creatinine

Musculoskeletal: Pain in extremity, jaw pain

General: **Asthenia**, **fatigue**, pyrexia, chills

Nursing Discussion:
Increased risk for local and systemic infections: Everolimus is immunosuppressive and increases risk for opportunistic infections. Infections may be localized or systemic and include pneumonia, other bacterial infections, and invasive fungal infections (e.g., aspergillosis, candidiasis). Incidence is approximately 37%, with 7% grade 3, and 3% grade 4. Cough occurs in 30% of patients, pyrexia in 20%, and dyspnea in 24%. In addition, some patients may experience neutropenia (14%). Assess baseline white blood cells (WBC), lymphocyte, and neutrophil counts, and monitor frequently during therapy. Assess skin integrity and potential for infection, and teach patient measures to prevent infection (e.g., keeping skin intact, avoiding sources of infection, good hand washing). Teach patient to report any signs/symptoms of infection (e.g., redness, heat, exudate on skin, T > 100.5°F, cough, sputum production, dysuria). Assess for signs/symptoms of infection during therapy and at each visit. If the patient is receiving therapy for a preexisting invasive fungal infection, therapy should be completed before starting therapy with everolimus. If during everolimus therapy, a diagnosis of systemic fungal infection is made, discontinue everolimus and treat with appropriate antifungal therapy.

   Nutritional issues are related to stomatitis, hyperglycemia, hypertriglyceridemia, hypophosphatemia, anorexia, nausea, vomiting, and diarrhea. In clinical studies, oral mucositis (e.g., stomatitis, mouth ulcers) affected 44% of patients (compared with 7% placebo). In general, this is grade 1 or 2. Hyperglycemia, hypercholesteremia, and hypophosphatemia have been reported. mTOR is involved in insulin signaling, which possibly explains the hypertriglyceridemia and hyperglycemia. Drug can also increase serum creatinine. Anorexia occurs in 25% of patients. Diarrhea occurs in about 30% of patients, nausea in 26%, and vomiting in 20%. Assess baseline nutritional status and appetite. Assess fasting serum triglycerides, cholesterol, phosphate, glucose, blood, urea, nitrogen, and serum creatinine baseline and during treatment with the drug. Teach the patient to report signs/symptoms of hyperglycemia (polyuria, polydipsia, polyphagia). Discuss with physician correction of lipids, triglycerides, and glucose if baseline tests are abnormal prior to beginning everolimus therapy.

Assess oral mucosa prior to drug administration, as well as ability to eat and drink, and at each visit; instruct patient to self-assess and report changes, including the appearance of white patches (candida), pain, and inability to eat or drink. Teach patient oral hygiene measures and self-assessment. If oral mucositis is painful or candida is present, discuss prescription of topical analgesics and anticandidiasis oral treatment. Discuss appropriate antiemetic (e.g., prochlorperazine) and antidiarrheal (e.g., loperamide) medicines if patient develops these symptoms. Teach patient to notify physician/nurse if oral ulcers occur or if excessive thirst or any increase in volume or frequency of urination occurs. In addition, call nurse or physician for diarrhea, nausea, or vomiting that does not resolve within 24 hours with recommended OTC medicines. Notify physician of any abnormalities and discuss implications and management.

Skin issues are related to rash, pruritus, and dry skin and increase the risk of losing skin integrity.

Rash has been reported in 29% of patients. In addition, pruritus was reported in 14% and dry skin in 13% of patients in clinical trials. In addition, HFS may occur in 5% of patients, as well as nail disorders and dermatitis. Assess patient skin integrity, including nails baseline and regularly during treatment. Teach patient self-assessment and local comfort measures, including the use of water-based emollients. Teach patient to report skin changes and if self-care is ineffective to discuss plan with physician, especially if severe.

Fatigue, asthenia, and risk of activity intolerance: Asthenia, weakness (affects 33% vs. 23%), fatigue 31% and anemia (92% overall, with 12% grade 3 and 1% grade 4; compared to placebo: overall 79%, with 5% grade 3). Assess baseline CBC, Hgb, comfort, and activity tolerance, and reassess during treatment, asking patient to identify what activities can now be performed, sleep habits, and also emotional state. Discuss alternating rest and activity periods and the possibility of other family members or friends assisting with energy-consuming responsibilities to increase energy reserve. Teach patient to report increasing fatigue and signs of severe anemia (shortness of breath, chest pain/angina, headaches). Monitor hemoglobin/hematocrit; discuss transfusion with physician if signs/symptoms develop or hematocrit falls below 25 mg/dL. Teach patient about diet high in iron.

Drug: Thalidomide (Thalomid)

Indications:

- Treatment of patients with newly diagnosed multiple myeloma in combination with dexamethasone
- Treatment of patients with erythema nodosum leprosum (acute treatment of moderate to severe cutaneous manifestations and maintenance and suppression of cutaneous recurrence)
- Pregnancy is an absolute contraindication.

Class: Inhibitor of TNFα, antiangiogenesis agent, immunomodulatory agent

Mechanism of Action: Drug has immunomodulatory, anti-inflammatory, and antiangiogenic properties. Drug probably decreases TNFα production and modifies some cell surface adhesion molecules involved in leukocyte migration. It is hypothesized that drug may modulate VEGF by inhibiting neovasculature and thus have an antiangiogenesis effect in malignant tumors.

Pharmacokinetics: Well absorbed after oral administration. Mean peak serum level is reached at 4–5 hours. Elimination half-life is 4–12 hours, with drug found in the plasma after 24 hours. NOT metabolized using P450 hepatic enzyme system and has low renal excretion.

Dosage and Administration:
- Multiple myeloma: In combination with dexamethasone in 28-day treatment cycles. Thalidomide 200 mg PO daily with water, preferably at bedtime, at least 1 hour after a meal. Give dexamethasone 40 mg PO days 1–4, 9–12, 17–20, every 28 days.
- Dose modification: If constipation, oversedation, or peripheral neuropathy, patient may benefit by either temporarily discontinuing the drug or continuing at a lower dose and then readjusting once side effects abate.

Available as: 50-mg, 100-mg, 150-mg, and 200-mg capsules. Drug is available only through the drug manufacturer Celgene's STEPS program (System for Thalidomide Education and Prescription Safety). Patients must be willing and able to comply with the mandatory contraceptive measures for all women of childbearing age and for all men; women must comply with mandatory pregnancy testing, and both men and women must participate in patient surveys. Providers must give patients specific oral and written information about the risks of fetal exposure, and patients must document their understanding to either use effective contraception or abstain from heterosexual sexual contact.

Reconstitution and Preparation: Oral, given at bedtime. Store at room temperature, 59–86°F (15–30°C), in a dry place, away from children and pets. Use gloves when handling the tablets, and return any unused drug in the bottle to the dispensing pharmacy for disposal.

Drug Interactions:
- Women taking hormonal contraception as well as barbiturates, glucocorticoids, phenytoin, or carbamazepine have decreased efficacy of the hormonal contraception and must use barrier contraception as well.
- CNS depressants: Barbiturates, alcohol, chlorpromazine, reserpine, and opioids cause increased sedation.
- Dexamethasone and antineoplastic agents: Combined use increases risk of thrombotic events.
- Neurotoxic medications (e.g., antiretroviral medication, cisplatin, dapsone phenytoin): Increased risk of peripheral neuropathy.

Contraindications: Pregnant women. Pregnancy tests must be routinely negative (with a sensitivity at least 50 mIU/mL) within 24 hours prior to beginning therapy in women of childbearing age. Contraception is mandatory in men and women.

Warnings and Precautions:

- Drug can cause severe, life-threatening birth defects.
- Drug can be only prescribed through the STEPS program.
- Female patients of childbearing age must have a negative pregnancy test performed within 24 hours of starting the drug, then weekly for the first month of treatment, then at 4-week intervals in women with regular menstrual cycles, or every 2 weeks if menstrual cycles are irregular. Pregnancy testing and counseling should occur if a patient misses her period or if there is abnormal menstrual bleeding.
- Drug increases the risk in multiple myeloma patients of venous thromboembolic events, such as DVT or pulmonary embolism (PE). Risk is increased when drug is combined with dexamethasone (22%). Patients should be taught to seek medical care right away if they develop shortness of breath, chest pain, or arm or leg swelling.
- Drug causes somnolence and drowsiness. Patients should be taught not to drive a car or operate heavy or complex machinery while taking the drug, or until they are aware of its effect on them. Patients should also be taught not to take other CNS-depressing medications or to drink alcohol.
- Peripheral neuropathy occurs and may be permanent. Patients should be taught to report the onset of numbness and tingling in the hands or feet, and should be seen by their physicians for a neurologic exam monthly for the first 3 months of treatment. Electrophysiologic testing of the sensory nerve action potential (SNAP) should be considered baseline and every 6 months to detect early changes. The drug should be discontinued at the first signs/symptoms of peripheral neuropathy, and reinstituted when signs/symptoms resolve. Use other neurotoxic drugs cautiously if at all.
- Drug causes dizziness and orthostatic hypotension, so patients should be taught to sit upright for a few minutes before standing.
- Neutropenia may occur; drug should not be started if ANC is < 750/mm^3; if during treatment the ANC falls to < 750/mm^3, the treatment plan should be reevaluated; if it persists, the drug should be held.
- Drug can cause an increase in HIV viral load. Patients who are HIV positive should have their viral loads assessed baseline, then the first and third months after starting the drug, then every 3 months thereafter.
- Thalidomide is found in the serum of patients and in the semen of men taking the drug. Patients should be taught to use protective precautions when handling the drug, such as using gloves, not removing the capsule from the blister pack until just before taking it, and washing hands with

soap and water before and after self-administration of the drug. Pregnant caregivers should not handle the capsules.

- Patients should be counseled not to donate blood or sperm (in the case of male patients) while taking the drug.
- Teach patient to stop drug if a rash develops and to be evaluated. Drug should be discontinued if rash is exfoliative, bullous, or purpuric (Stevens-Johnson syndrome [SJS] or toxic epidermal necrolysis).

Adverse Reactions (**bold** indicates most common, occurring in >25% of patients):

Cardiovascular: **Edema**, bradycardia, orthostatic hypotension

Pulmonary: URI, pneumonia, pharyngitis, sinusitis

CNS/Neurologic: **Tingling of the extremities**, **somnolence**, **peripheral sensory neuropathy**, **lightheadedness**, **dizziness**, confusion, anxiety/agitation, motor neuropathy, seizures, nervousness, vertigo, syncope

Dermatologic: **Dry skin**, **rash**, severe rash, rare SJS, toxic epidermal necrolysis

CNS/Metabolic: Hypocalcemia, hypokalemia, hyperglycemia (with dexamethasone)

GI: **Constipation**, weight gain, very low risk of nausea and vomiting, diarrhea, dry mouth, abnormal LFTs

Hematologic: **Neutropenia**, DVT, PE

Genitourinary: Renal insufficiency, hematuria, impotence

Musculoskeletal: Pain, back pain

Reproductive: Fetal malformations, with highest risk in early pregnancy between 34 and 50 days after the last menstrual cycle[97]

General: **Fatigue**, rare hypersensitivity (characterized by fever, erythematous macular rash, chills, tachycardia, hypotension, eosinophilia), increased HIV viral load (HIV RNA)

Nursing Discussion:
Drug is teratogenic and a single dose can cause birth defects. Drug is found in the serum of patients taking the drug and is excreted in semen. It can cross the placenta and will cause fetal malformations. Assess reproductive status, sexual activity, and birth control measures used for both men and women. Instruct male patients to use barrier contraception and women to use both barrier and hormonal contraception. Women of childbearing age must have a negative pregnancy test baseline to begin the drug, and pregnancy test should be repeated every 2 weeks for 2 months, then every month. Instruct patient to continue contraception 1 month after drug is discontinued. Physicians, patients,

and pharmacists must participate in Celgene's STEPS program. In addition, patients must be counseled about contraception, monthly pregnancy testing, and emergency contraception.

Peripheral neuropathy occurs in about 25% of patients (range 10–50%). If drug is discontinued at the first sign of neuropathy, symptoms are reversible. Neuropathy is a distal axonal degeneration affecting long and large diameter motor and sensory axons in hands and feet. Initially, there is numbness of toes/feet, described often as a "tightness around the feet." There may be decreased sensitivity to light touch, pinprick (sensory loss) in hands and feet, muscle cramps, symmetrical sensorimotor neuropathy, painful paresthesias in hands and feet, distal hypoesthesia, proximal weakness in lower limbs, slight postural tremor, leg cramps, and absent ankle jerks. If treatment is continued, there is permanent paresthesias of feet and hands, which progresses proximally. Increased risk of occurrence with increased age (> 70 years old) and high total doses > 14 g (40–50 g). Assess baseline neurologic status, especially presence of peripheral neuropathy. Teach patient to stop drug and report immediately dysesthesias, numbness, and/or muscle cramps. Perform assessment for peripheral neuropathy at every visit.

Drowsiness and orthostatic hypotension can threaten patient safety. Drug has nonbarbiturate sedative qualities, and drowsiness is the most frequent side effect. Tolerance to daytime drowsiness occurs over several weeks of use. Drowsiness and dizziness are more frequent at doses of 20–400 mg/day than at lower doses. HIV-infected patient studies reported drowsiness, dizziness, and mood changes 33–100% of the time. Assess baseline alertness and sleep patterns. Assess other drugs taken, especially those with sedating qualities, and alcohol ingestion. Instruct patient to avoid alcohol and to take drug at bedtime. Assess degree of drowsiness and dizziness and safety of patient. If risk appears significant, teach measures to ensure safety. Tell patient that tolerance develops over 2–3 weeks.

Rash can occur. Pruritic, erythematous macular rash may appear over trunk and back 2–13 days after initiation of therapy. There is an increased incidence in patients with HIV infection with low CD4 counts. Drug rechallenge often results in immediate reaction of rash, tachycardia, and fever. Rash resolves with drug discontinuation. Teach patient to self-assess for rash, and instruct to discontinue drug and report rash to nurse or physician immediately. If necessary, manage symptomatic itching with antihistamines.

Mild constipation occurs in 3–30% of patients. Instruct patient to prevent constipation by using stool softeners and mild laxatives if needed (e.g., Milk of Magnesia), and to use bulk (e.g., psyllium). In addition, teach dietary interventions (e.g., increased fiber, 3 quarts/day of fluids), and mild exercise. Instruct patient to report constipation unresponsive to these interventions.

Drug: Lenalidomide (Revlimid)

Indications: FDA approved for the treatment of patients with:

- Transfusion-dependent anemia due to low- or intermediate-1-risk myelodysplastic syndromes associated with a deletion 5q cytogenetic abnormality with or without additional cytogenetic abnormalities
- Multiple myeloma, in combination with dexamethasone, who have received at least one prior therapy

Class: antiangiogenesis agent, immunomodulatory agent, thalidomide analogue

Mechanism of Action: Exact mechanisms not fully known. Drug has antineoplastic, immunomodulatory, and antiangiogenic properties. Induces G_0/G_1 growth arrest and apoptosis, and increases expression of genes found on 5q locus, including genes involved in cell adhesion. Inhibits COX-2 expression, stimulates T-cell proliferation, as well as the anti-inflammatory cytokines interleukin (IL)-2, IL-10, and interferon-γ. Decreases the secretion of proinflammatory cytokines that mediate tumor cell growth and survival (TNFα, IL-1β, and IL-6); stimulates host natural killer cell immunity. Induces cell cycle arrest and apoptosis of multiple myeloma cells.

Pharmacokinetics: Rapidly absorbed after oral administration, with maximal plasma concentrations occurring 0.6–1.5 hours after dose in normal subjects, and 0.5–4.0 hours in patients with multiple myeloma. Coadministration with food reduces maximal plasma concentration by 36%. In patients with multiple myeloma with mild renal impairment, AUC exposure was 57% higher than in healthy volunteers. Drug has 30% protein binding. Two-thirds of the drug is excreted unchanged in the urine. Elimination half-life of the drug is 3 hours. Patients with moderate to severe renal insufficiency had a threefold increase in half-life and a 65–75% decrease in drug clearance compared to healthy patients. Patients requiring hemodialysis had a 4.5-fold increase in half-life and an 80% reduction in drug clearance, with about 40% of the drug removed during dialysis.

Dosage and Administration:

- **Myelodysplastic syndrome:** 10 mg PO daily with water, in a single dose. Patients should not break, chew, or open the capsules.
- **Multiple myeloma:** 25 mg PO daily, given with water as a single dose on days 1–21 of repeated 28-day cycles. Patients should not break, chew, or open the capsules. The recommended dose of dexamethasone is 40 mg/day on days 1–4, 9–12, and 17–20 of each 28-day cycle for the first 4 cycles of therapy and then 40 mg/day PO on days 1–4 every 28 days. Dosing is continued or modified based on clinical outcome.
- Teach patients to store at room temperature 59–86°F (15–30°C), in a dry place, away from children and pets. Use gloves when handling the tablets, and return any unused drug in the bottle or blister pack to the dispensing pharmacy for disposal.

- Monitor CBC/differential, platelets, and renal function closely, with dose modifications made for thrombocytopenia, neutropenia, and creatinine clearance < 60 mL/min.

Dose modifications:

Starting dose adjustment for renal impairment (creatinine clearance < 60 mL/min.)

Myelodysplastic syndrome: Thrombocytopenia WITHIN 4 wk of starting 10 mg daily	
If baseline $\geq$ 100,000/mm^3, when	
Platelets fall to < 50,000/mm^3	Interrupt lenalidomide treatment.
Platelets return to $\geq$ 50,000/mm^3	Resume lenalidomide at 5 mg daily.
If baseline < 100,000/mm^3 when	
Platelets fall to 50% of baseline value	Interrupt lenalidomide treatment.
If baseline $\geq$ 60,000/mm^3 and returns to $\geq$ 50K	Resume lenalidomide at 5 mg daily.
If baseline < 60,000/mm^3 and returns to $\geq$ 30K	Resume lenalidomide at 5 mg daily.
Thrombocytopenia develops AFTER 4 wk of starting at 10 mg daily, when	
Platelets < 30,000/mm^3 or < 50,000/mm^3 and platelet transfusions	Interrupt lenalidomide treatment.
Return to $\geq$ 30,000/mm^3 (without hemostatic failure)	Resume lenalidomide at 5 mg daily.
If thrombocytopenia develops during treatment at 5 mg daily, when	
Platelets < 30,000/mm^3 or < 50,000/mm^3 and platelet transfusions	Interrupt lenalidomide treatment.
Return to $\geq$ 30,000/mm^3 (without hemostatic failure)	Resume lenalidomide at 5 mg every other day.

(continues)

Myelodysplastic syndrome: Thrombocytopenia WITHIN 4 wk of starting 10 mg daily (continued)	
Neutropenia develops WITHIN 4 weeks of starting treatment at 10 mg daily, when neutrophils (ANC)	
Fall to $< 750/\text{mm}^3$	Interrupt lenalidomide treatment.
Returns to $\geq 1000/\text{mm}^3$	Resume lenalidomide at 5 mg daily.
If baseline ANC $< 1000/\text{mm}^3$, when ANC	
Falls to $< 500/\text{mm}^3$	Interrupt lenalidomide treatment.
Returns to $\geq 500/\text{mm}^3$	Resume lenalidomide at 5 mg daily.
If neutropenia develops AFTER 4 weeks of starting at 10 mg daily	
$< 500/\text{mm}^3$ 7 days or more, or if ANC $< 500/\text{mm}^3$ but is associated with fever ($\geq 38.5°C$)	Interrupt lenalidomide treatment.
Returns to $\geq 500/\text{mm}^3$	Resume lenalidomide at 5 mg daily.
Patients with neutropenia during treatment at 5 mg daily, when	
$< 500/\text{mm}^3$ 7 days or more, or if ANC $< 500/\text{mm}^3$ but is associated with fever ($\geq 38.5°C$)	Interrupt lenalidomide treatment.
Returns to $\geq 500/\text{mm}^3$	Resume lenalidomide at 5 mg every other day.
MULTIPLE MYELOMA grade 3 or 4, on dose of 25 mg daily, when	
Thrombocytopenia: platelets drop to $< 30,000/\text{mm}^3$	Interrupt lenalidomide treatment; follow CBC weekly.
Platelets return to $\geq 30,000/\text{mm}^3$	Resume lenalidomide at 15 mg daily.
For each subsequent drop $< 30,000/\text{mm}^3$	Interrupt lenalidomide treatment.
Return to $\geq 30,000/\text{mm}^3$	Resume lenalidomide at 5 mg less than the previous dose; do not dose below 5 mg daily.

Myelodysplastic syndrome: Thrombocytopenia WITHIN 4 wk of starting 10 mg daily (continued)	
Neutropenia: ANC falls to < 1000/mm³	Interrupt lenalidomide treatment, add G-CSF, and follow CBC weekly.
Returns to ≥ 1000/mm³ and neutropenia the only toxicity	Resume lenalidomide at 25 mg daily.
Returns to ≥ 1000/mm³ but other toxicity	Resume lenalidomide at 15 mg daily.
For each subsequent drop < 1000/mm³	Interrupt lenalidomide treatment.
Return to > 1000/mm³	Resume lenalidomide at 5 mg less than the previous dose. Do not dose below 5 mg daily.

Renal Function	Multiple Myeloma	Myelodysplastic Syndrome
Moderate impairment: 30–60 mL/min	10 mg every 24 hr	5 mg every 24 hr
Severe impairment: < 30 mL/min, not requiring dialysis	15 mg every 48 hr	5 mg every 48 hr
End-stage renal disease: < 30 mL/min, requiring dialysis	5 mg once daily; on dialysis days, dose is taken after dialysis	5 mg 3 times a week following each dialysis

From Celgene.[98]

Available as: 5-, 10-, 15-, and 25-mg capsules in bottles of 30 or 100 (for 5- and 10-mg caps); 21 or 100 (for 15-mg caps); and 25 or 100 (for 25-mg caps), under a restricted distribution program, RevAssist, which is similar to the STEPS program for thalidomide; prescribers and pharmacists must be registered with the program. Patients must meet all the conditions of the RevAssist program (see the following Pregnancy section).

Pregnancy test results must be verified by the prescriber and the pharmacist prior to dispensing the prescription.

Reconstitution and Preparation: None (oral)

Pregnancy

Before prescribing lenalidomide: Females of childbearing potential (defined as sexually mature females who have not had a hysterectomy or have not been postmenopausal for at least 24 consecutive months [i.e., had a menstrual period within the last 24 months] or had a bilateral oopherectomy) should have:

- Two negative pregnancy tests (sensitivity of at least 50 mIU/mL). The first test should be performed within 10–14 days and the second test within 24 hours prior to the dose being prescribed. The drug prescription for a woman of childbearing potential must not be issued by the prescriber until the prescriber has confirmed that the pregnancy tests are negative.
- Females of childbearing potential must start two measures of effective contraception at least 4 weeks before lenalidomide is started, unless the female instead chooses continuous abstinence from heterosexual sexual contact. One highly effective contraception measure must be used, such as intrauterine device, hormonal contraception, tubal ligation, or partner's vasectomy.
- Male patients must agree to always use a latex condom during any sexual contact with females of childbearing potential, even if they have had a vasectomy.

Once treatment has started and during dose interruptions: Female patients of childbearing potential should have *weekly pregnancy tests for the first 4 weeks of taking the drug, then repeat pregnancy testing every 4 weeks in females with regular menstrual periods*, and every 2 weeks if their periods are irregular or if there is any abnormal menstrual bleeding. The drug should be discontinued during pregnancy testing/evaluation, and pregnancy test results must be validated by the prescriber and pharmacist before dispensing any prescription for lenalidomide.

Female patients of childbearing age must be able and willing to carry out their responsibility, and agree to the following: Patients will not become pregnant while taking the drug. They will comply with the mandatory use of contraceptive measures, pregnancy testing, patient registration, and completion of patient surveys. They must receive both verbal and written instructions about the risks of taking lenalidomide when pregnant, risk to the fetus, and risk of possible failure of contraception. They must use two reliable forms of contraception simultaneously.

- Contraception with two effective measures must begin 4 weeks before lenalidomide is started and continue during therapy, during periods of interruption, and for 4 weeks after treatment is ended.
- The parent or legal guardian of females 12–18 years old must read the educational materials and agree to the requirements.

Male patients must be able and willing, and agree (in writing) to their responsibilities: Always use effective latex condom contraception when having sexual intercourse with women of childbearing potential, even if the male patient has had a vasectomy. Register for the RevAssist program and complete the patient survey. He must understand that it is unknown if the drug is excreted in the semen. The parent or legal guardian of males 12–18 years old must read the educational materials and agree to the requirements.

Drug Interactions:

- Dexamethasone increases drug activity and also increases risk for DVT and PE.
- Abatacept or anakinra cause increased risk for serious infection.
- Drugs that reduce contraception efficacy should be avoided. These drugs include antibiotics, carbamazepine, griseofulvin, HIV-protease inhibitors, phenytoin, rifamycin. If taking one of these agents, patient should consider using two highly effective contraception strategies that do not include hormonal contraception.
- Bone marrow suppressive agents cause additive bone marrow suppression.

Contraindications:

- Drug is pregnancy category X because it is teratogenic and fetotoxic. Contraindicated in pregnant women or those who may become pregnant because they are not using the two required forms of birth control or are not continually abstaining from reproductive heterosexual sexual intercourse.
- Drug should not be used in mothers who are breastfeeding.
- Drug should not be used by patients who developed a grade 4 rash from thalidomide, as potentially fatal angioedema, SJS, or toxic epidermal necrolysis (TEN) may occur.
- If a woman does become pregnant while receiving lenalidomide, stop the drug immediately and have her evaluated by an obstetrician/gynecologist experienced in reproductive toxicity. Report any suspected fetal exposure to the FDA MedWatch at 1-800-FDA-1088 and also to Celgene at 1-888-423-5436.

Warnings and Precautions:

- Drug is a teratogen and is likely to be fetotoxic. Drug must not be used during pregnancy.
- Drug is associated with significant neutropenia and thrombocytopenia (80% incidence) in patients with del 5q myelodysplastic syndrome (MDS). Incidence of grade 3 or 4 neutropenia was 48%, and grade 3 or 4 thrombocytopenia was 54%. Median time to onset of grade 3 or 4 neutropenia was 42 days (range 14–411 days), and median time to recovery was 17 days (range 2–170 days). Median time to grade 3 or 4 thrombocytopenia

was 28 days (range 8–290), with recovery 22 days (range 5–224 days). Blood counts should be assessed weekly in patients with del 5q MDS for 8 weeks, then at least monthly. In multiple myeloma patients, blood counts should be monitored every other week for the first 12 weeks, then monthly. Patients may require dose adjustments based on their CBC/platelet counts.

- Risk for DVT and PE is increased in patients with multiple myeloma receiving combination therapy. Teach patients to seek emergency care if they develop shortness of breath, chest pain, or arm or leg swelling. Providers may choose to administer concomitant anticoagulation, such as one 81- or 325-mg aspirin daily, based on the individual patient's underlying risk factors.
- Angioedema, SJS, and TEN may rarely occur. If grade 2 or 3 rash develops, interrupt or discontinue lenalidomide. If angioedema develops, drug must be discontinued. If grade 4 rash, exfoliative rash, or bullous rash develops, or if SJS or TEN is suspected, discontinue drug and do not resume.
- Tumor lysis syndrome (TLS) may occur in patients with a high tumor burden, as drug is antineoplastic and sensitive tumor cells will lyse with the initial treatment. Patients should receive adequate prehydration, and have adequate urinary output. Ensure that patients receive TLS precautions and that they are monitored closely.
- Laboratory tests:
  - Del 5q MDS: CBC with differential; platelet count should be assessed weekly for the first 8 weeks of lenalidomide therapy, then at least monthly to monitor for cytopenias.
  - Multiple myeloma: CBC with differential; platelet count should be assessed every other week for the first 12 weeks, then monthly.
  - Consider baseline thyroid function tests (total thyroxine).

Adverse Reactions (**bold** indicates most common, occurring in > 25% of patients):

Cardiovascular: Peripheral edema, hypertension, palpitations, chest pain, DVT and PE in patients also receiving dexamethasone

Pulmonary: Nasopharyngitis, cough, dyspnea, pharyngitis, URI, pneumonia

CNS/Neurologic: Dizziness, headache, insomnia, hypoestesia, depression, peripheral neuropathy

Dermatologic: **Pruritus**, **rash**, dry skin, night sweats, sweating

CNS/Metabolic: Hypothyroidism, hypokalemia, hypomagnesemia

GI: **Diarrhea**, constipation, low-risk nausea, vomiting; abdominal pain, anorexia, increased AST, dry mouth, dysgeusia

Hematologic: Thrombocytopenia, neutropenia requiring dosage adjustment in 80% of patients, epistaxis, anemia, ecchymoses

Genitourinary: UTI, dysuria

Reproductive: Teratogenicity

General: Fatigue, fever, rigors

Nursing Discussion:
Drug is selectively designed to be more potent (10,000 times) and to have a different adverse event profile than thalidomide.

Drug is teratogenic, and a single dose can cause birth defects. Critical period is in early pregnancy, between 34 and 50 days after the last menstrual period. It can cross the placenta and will cause fetal malformations. Assess reproductive status, sexual activity, and birth control measures used for both men and women. Instruct male patients to use latex condom contraception and women to use both barrier and hormonal contraception. This should be practiced for 4 weeks prior to starting the drug. Women of childbearing age must have two negative pregnancy tests baseline to begin the drug, and pregnancy testing should be repeated every week for the first month, then every month. Pregnancy testing should be performed every 2 weeks in women with irregular menstrual cycles. Pregnancy testing and counseling should be performed if a patient misses her period or if there is any abnormality in menstrual bleeding. If pregnancy occurs, drug must be discontinued immediately. The patient should be referred to an obstetrician/gynecologist experienced in reproductive toxicity to receive further evaluation and counseling. Instruct patient to continue contraception 1 month after drug is discontinued. Physicians, patients, and pharmacists must participate in drug manufacturer Celgene's RevAssist program. In addition, patients must be counseled about contraception, monthly pregnancy testing, and about emergency contraception.

Serious infection can occur. Significant neutropenia and thrombocytopenia required dose adjustments in 80% of patients in initial dose, and 34% required second dose adjustment in the pivotal study of MDS patients. Grade 3 or 4 neutropenia developed in 48% of patients, with a median time to onset of 42 days, and recovery in 17 days. Grade 3 or 4 thrombocytopenia developed in 54% of patients, with a median time to onset of 28 days, and recovery in 22 days. Anemia occurred in 11% of patients. Assess baseline CBC, WBC, differential, and platelet count prior to chemotherapy, then weekly for the first 8 weeks of treatment, then monthly. Assess for signs/symptoms of infection or bleeding. Teach patient the signs/symptoms of infection or bleeding and to report these immediately; also teach patient self-care measures to minimize risk of infection and bleeding. Measures include avoidance of crowds, proximity to people with infections, and OTC aspirin-containing medications. Discuss need for blood product support or growth factors with physician or midlevel practitioner. Drug should be used in combination with another agent that does not cause bone marrow suppression, like bortezomib (Velcade) rather than chemotherapy.

Comfort and safety may be threatened. Itching develops in 42% of patients, rash in 36%, and dry skin in 14%. Pruritus may be limited to the scalp and occur within 1 week of treatment. Fatigue is experienced by 31% of patients, peripheral edema by 20%, arthralgias by 21%, back pain by 21%, and muscle cramps by 18%. About 20% of patients reported dizziness or headache. Assess patient's baseline comfort, and teach patient that these symptoms may occur. Assess skin integrity baseline and during therapy. Teach symptom management strategies to minimize discomfort. Teach patient to notify nurse or physician if fatigue, rash, itching, or leg cramps are severe or do not resolve with local management. Teach patient to change position slowly and to report severe dizziness. Teach patient to report leg cramps or new onset of shortness of breath or chest pain, and evaluate for DVT or PE.

Constipation may occur, while other patients may develop diarrhea. Diarrhea occurs in about 49% of patients, while constipation affects about 23%. Nausea affects about 23% of patients, and vomiting 10%. Dysgeusia occurs in 6% of patients, hypokalemia in 10%, anorexia in 10%, and hypomagnesemia in 6%. Assess baseline nutrition, electrolytes, and bowel elimination pattern. Teach patient that nausea, rarely vomiting, diarrhea, or, less commonly, constipation may occur. Teach patient self-care strategies to minimize symptoms and to report them if they do not resolve. Teach patient self-administration of antiemetics or antidiarrheals as prescribed and to notify provider if diarrhea persists for dose interruption. Teach patient dietary modification if diarrhea, constipation, nausea, or vomiting occur (e.g., the BRAT diet for diarrhea), and to increase oral fluids to prevent dehydration. Assess electrolytes' baseline and periodically during treatment. If patient has diarrhea, instruct patient to manage with loperamide, diet modification, and increased fluid intake. If constipation, instruct patient to use stool softeners, mild laxatives if needed (e.g., Milk of Magnesia), and bulk (e.g., psyllium). In addition, teach dietary interventions (e.g., increased fiber, fluids of 3 quarts/day) and mild exercise. Instruct patient to report diarrhea or constipation unresponsive to these interventions.

Investigational Antiangiogenic Agents

Drug: Midostaurin (PKC412, investigational)

Class: Multitargeted kinase inhibitor

Mechanism of Action: Potent inhibitor of the FLT-3 RTK, which is commonly mutated in patients with acute myeloid leukemia (AML; about 33%) and confers a poor prognosis. Other targets that are important in AML development are also blocked: VEGFR-2, PDGFR, c-KIT. Finally, the drug inhibits the PgP-mediated multidrug resistance gene, MDR, which causes lack of response to many chemotherapeutic agents. In addition, it inhibits protein kinase C-alpha, a serine/threonine PKC. These multiple effects result in increased apoptosis and decreased cell proliferation of tumor cells.

Pharmacokinetics: Unknown

Dosage and administration: Per protocol. However, the following dosages are being studied: 50–100 mg PO twice to three times daily.

Reconstitution and Preparation: Oral. Administer about the same time each day.

Drug Interactions: Unknown, may increase the sensitivity of FLT-3–mutated AML cells to daunorubicin and cytarabine.

Adverse Reactions (**bold** indicates most common, occurring in > 25% of patients):

   Cardiovascular: **May prolong QT interval**

   CNS/Neurologic: **Headache**

   GI: **Nausea, diarrhea, increased LFTs, diarrhea**

   General: **Fatigue**

Drug: Neovastat (investigational)

Class: Angiogenesis inhibitor made from cartilaginous spine of dogfish shark.

Mechanism of Action: Appears to inhibit VEGD signaling, to inhibit MMPs, and to induce apoptosis. Differs from OTC shark cartilage, which is made primarily from shark fins.

Pharmacokinetics: Unknown

Reconstitution and Administration: Available orally in liquid form, taken twice daily, per protocol

Drug Interactions: Unknown

Adverse Reactions: Well tolerated without reported side effects. Clinical trials in patients with lung or ovarian cancer and multiple myeloma, with or without chemotherapy, are ongoing (NCI, others).

Drug: Pomalidomide (Actimed, CC-4047, investigational)

Class: Immunomodulatory agent, antiangiogenic agent

Mechanism of Action: Third-generation thalidomide analogue with multiple mechanisms of action that modulate the microenvironment of the cancer cell and stop the growth of blood (angiogenesis inhibition), modulation of levels of key proinflammatory and regulatory cytokines, and immune cell costimulation (T cells, NK cells), and may kill cancer cells. Immunologic modulation probably due to inhibition of TNFα. Drug is as potent an antiangiogenic drug as thalidomide but is 4–5 times more potent an anti-inflammatory agent (against monocytes), stimulator of T-cell/NK-cell costimulation, and inhibitor of T-regulatory cells, and is 4 times more effective in ADCC.

Pharmacokinetics: Unknown

Dosage and administration: Per protocol; given in combination with dexamethasone (multiple myeloma) or prednisone (myelofibrosis); studies in relapsed multiple myeloma are 2 mg PO daily days 11–28 of a 28-day cycle, with dexamethasone 40 mg PO daily on days 1, 8, 15, and 22 of each cycle; aspirin 325 mg PO daily given for DVT prophylaxis.

Reconstitution and Preparation: Oral

Adverse Reactions (**bold** indicates most common, occurring in > 25% of patients):

> ***Cardiovascular:*** **Atrial fibrillation**
>
> ***GI:*** **Diarrhea**
>
> ***Hematologic:*** **Neutropenia, thrombocytopenia**
>
> ***General:*** **Drug is a thalidomide analogue so probably is teratogenic, requiring close monitoring of pregnancy testing, and male and female compliance with contraception measures.**

Drug: Vandetanib (D6474, Zactima, investigational)

Class: Multitargeted TKI, blocking both angiogenesis and EGF-stimulated tumor growth, progression, and angiogenesis.

Mechanism of Action: Vandetanib is a potent, selective inhibitor of multiple tyrosine kinases; it blocks VEGFR-2 and EGFR-1 tyrosine kinases. This blocks both the proliferation of cells (EGFR-1) and the primary endothelial cell receptor, preventing new blood vessel formation. It also blocks RET kinase, which may be important in certain tumors.

Pharmacokinetics: Unknown

Dosage, Reconstitution, and Administration: Vandetanib doses being studied are 100–300 mg/daily orally, in combination with docetaxel, pemetrexed, or alone, per protocol.

Drug Interactions: Unknown

Adverse Reactions (**bold** indicates most common, occurring in > 25% of patients):

> ***Cardiovascular:*** May prolong QT interval
>
> ***CNS/Neurologic:*** Headache
>
> ***Dermatology:*** Rash

GI: Nausea, diarrhea, vomiting, anorexia, stomatitis, increased LFTs

Hematology: Bleeding

General: Flu-like symptoms, fatigue

Drug: Vatalanib (PTK787/ZK222584, investigational)

Class: Angiogenesis inhibitor; protein kinase inhibitor

Mechanism of Action: Drug is a potent inhibitor of all known VEGF tyrosine kinases (VEGFR-1, -2, -3) that are expressed on endothelial cells; also inhibits c-KIT and PDGFR.

Metabolism: Rapidly absorbed in 1–2 hours following oral ingestion; half-life of 4–5 hours.

Dosage, Reconstitution, and Administration: Vatalanib is being studied at 50–1500 mg/day; probably requires multiple dosing per day given half-life of every 4–5 hours. Per protocol.

Adverse Reactions:

Cardiovascular: Hypertension

CNS/Neurologic: Dizziness

Hematology: Thrombosis, bleeding

General: Fatigue

Drug: Axitinib (AG-013736, investigational)

Class: Small-molecule multi-TKI of angiogenesis, c-KIT

Mechanism of Action: Potent and selective inhibitor of VEGFR-1, -2, and -3 on the endothelial cells lining blood vessels, as well as PDGFR-b and cKIT (CD117). VEGFR inhibition prevents the blood vessel from sending capillary tubes to the tumor so angiogenesis does not occur.

Pharmacokinetics: Unknown

Dosage and Administration: Per protocol, being studied with gemcitabine in advanced pancreatic cancer; it is also being studied in renal cell carcinoma and breast cancer. One dose being studied is a starting dose of 5 mg orally twice daily.

Reconstitution and Preparation: Oral, per protocol

Drug Interactions: Unknown

Adverse Reactions (**bold** indicates most common, occurring in > 25% of patients):

Cardiovascular: **Hypertension**

CNS/Neurologic: **Hoarseness**

GI: **Diarrhea, bowel perforation**

General: **Fatigue**

Nursing Discussion: Drug is investigational. All issues relating to prior discussion of angiogenesis inhibitors will apply.

REFERENCES

1. Folkman J. Tumor angiogenesis: Therapeutic implications. *N Engl J Med.* 1971;285(21): 1182-1186.

2. Kerbel, RS. Tumor angiogenesis. *N Engl J Med.* 2008;358(19):2039-2049.

3. Understanding angiogenesis. Angiogenesis Foundation Web site. http://www.angio.org/ understanding/process.php. Updated June 23, 2009. Accessed October 1, 2009.

4. Friedl P, Gilmour D. Collective cell migration in morphogenesis, regeneration, and cancer. *Nat Rev Mol Cell Biol.* 2009;10:445-457.

5. Gerhardt H, Golding M, Frutttiger M, et al. VEGF guides angiogenic sprouting utilizing endothelial tip cell filopodia. *J Cell Biol.* 2003;161:1163-1177.

6. Eaves CJ. SDF-1 tells stem cells to mind their P's and Z's. *J Clin Invest.* 2005;115(1):27-29.

7. Muller A, Homey B, Soto H, et al. Involvement of chemokine receptors in breast cancer metastases. *Nature.* 2001;410(6824):50-56.

8. Jain RK, Booth MF. What brings pericytes to tumor vessels? *J Clin Invest.* 2003;112:1134-1136.

9. Loureiro RM, D'Amore PA. Transcriptional regulation of vascular endothelial growth factor in cancer. *Cytokine Growth Factor Rev.* 2005;16(1):77-89.

10. Ellis LM, Hicklin DJ. VEGF-targeted therapy: mechanisms of anti-tumor activity. *Nat Rev Cancer.* 2008;8:579-591.

11. Kawakami T, Tokunaga T, Hatanaka H, et al. Neuropilin 1 and 2 co-expression is significantly correlated with increased vascularity and poor prognosis in non small cell lung carcinoma. *Cancer.* 2001; 95(10):2196-2200.

12. Patan S. Vasculogenesis and angiogenesis. *Cancer Treat Res.* 2004;117:3-32.

13. Morabito A, DeMaio E, Di Maio M, Normanno N, Perrone F. Tyrosine kinase inhibitors of vascular endothelial growth factor receptors in clinical trials: current status and future directions. *Oncologist.* 2006;11:753-764.

14. Folkman J. What is the evidence that tumors are angiogenesis dependent? *J Natl Cancer Inst.* 1990;82:4-6.

15. Uzzan B, Nicholas P, Cucherat M, Perret GY. Microvessel density as a prognostic factor in women with breast cancer: a systemic review of the literature and meta-analysis. *Cancer Res.* 2004;64(9):2941-2955.

16. Hlatky L, Hahnfeldt P, Folkman J. Clinical application of antiangiogenic therapy: microvessel density, what it does and doesn't tell us. *J Natl Cancer Inst.* 2002;94:883-893.

17. Weinberg RA. Mechanisms of malignant progression. *Carcinogenesis.* 2008;29(6):1092-1095.

18. Li J-L, Harris AL. Notch signaling from tumor cells: a new mechanism of angiogenesis. *Cancer Cell.* 2005;8:1-3.

19. Zeng Q, Li S, Chepeha DB, et al. Crosstalk between tumor and endothelial cells promotes tumor angiogenesis by MAPK activation of Notch signaling. *Cancer Cell.* 2005;8(1):13-23.

20. Dufraine J, Funahashi Y, Kitajewski J. Notch signaling regulates tumor angiogenesis by diverse mechanisms. *Oncogene*. 2008;27:5132-5137.

21. Rizzo P, Osipo C, Foreman K, Golde T, Osborne B, Miele L. Rational targeting of Notch signaling in cancer. *Oncogene*. 2008;27:5124-5131.

22. DePalma M, Venneri MA, Galli R, et al. Tie2 identifies a hematopoietic lineage of proangiogenic monocytes required for tumor vessel formation and a mesenchymal population of pericyte progenitors. *Cancer Cell*. 2005;8;211-226.

23. Avraamides CJ, Garmy-Susini B, Varner JA. Integrins in angiogenesis and lymphangiogenesis. *Nat Rev Cancer*. 2008;8:604-617.

24. Sansone P, Storci G, Tavolari S, et al. IL-6 triggers malignant features of mammospheres from human ductal breast carcinoma and normal mammary gland. *J Clin Invest*. 2007;117:3988-4002.

25. Eklund L, Olsen BR. Tie receptors and their angiopoietin ligands are context-dependent regulators of vascular remodeling. *Exp Cell Res*. 2006;312:630-641.

26. Hayes AJ, Huang WQ, Mallah J, Yand D, Lippman ME, LI L-Y. Angiopoietin-1 and its receptor Tie-2 participate in the regulation of capillary-like tubule formation and survival of endothelial cells. *Microvasc Res*. 1999;58:224-237.

27. Martin V, Liu D, Fueyo J, Gomez-Manzano C. Tie2: a journey from normal angiogenesis to cancer and beyond. *Histol Histopathol*. 2008;23:773-780.

28. Rasmsauer M, D'Amore PA. Contextual role for angiopoietins and TFGβ1 in blood vessel stabilization. *J Cell Sci*. 2007;120:1810-1817.

29. Lewis CE, De Palma M, Naldini L. Tie2-expressing monocytes and tumor angiogenesis: regulation by hypoxia and angiopoietin. *Cancer Res*. 2007;67:8429-8432.

30. Shim WSN, Ho IAW, Wong PEH. A TIE(d) balance in tumor angiogenesis. *Mol Cancer Res*. 2007;5:655-665.

31. Mancuso MR, Davis R, Norberg SM, et al. Rapid vascular regrowth in tumors after reversal of VEGF inhibition. *J Clin Invest*. 2006;116:2610-2621.

32. McDonald DM. Tumor blood vessel dynamics during and after angiogenesis inhibition. *FASEB J*. 2008;22:88.1. [Meeting abstract 22/1/88.1]

33. Batchelor TT, Sorensen AG, di Tomaso E, et al. AZD2171 a pan-VEGF receptor tyrosine kinase inhibitor, normalizes tumor vasculature and alleviates edema in glioblastoma patients. *Cancer Cell*. 2007;11:83-95.

34. Bergers G, Hanahan D. Modes of resistance to anti-angiogenic therapy. *Nat Rev Cancer*. 2008;8:592-603.

35. Jain RK, Duda DG, Willett CG, et al. Biomarkers of response and resistance to antiangiogenic therapy. *Nat Rev Clin Oncol*. 2009;6:327-338.

36. Harari PM, Allen GW, Bonner JA. Biology of interactions: antiepidermal growth factor receptor agents. *J Clin Oncol*. 2007;25:4057-4065.

37. Pennell, NA, Lynch TJ, Jr. Combined inhibition of the VEGFR and EGFR signaling pathways in the treatment of NSCLC. *Oncologist*. 2009;14(4):399-411.

38. Gridley T. Notch signaling in vascular development. *Development*. 2007;134:2709-2718.

39. Benedito R, Roca C, Sorensen I, et al. The Notch ligands Dll4 and Jagged 1 have opposing effects on angiogenesis. *Cell*. 2009;137(6):1124-1135.

40. Reinacher-Schick A, Pohl M, Schmiegel W. Drug insight: antiangiogenic therapies for gastrointestinal cancers: focus on monoclonal antibodies. *Nat Clin Pract Gastroenterol Hepatol*. 2008;5(5):250-267.

41. Dotto GP. Crosstalk of Notch with p53 and p63 in cancer growth control. *Nat Rev Cancer*. 2009;9:587-595.

42. Horsman MR, Siemann DW. Pathophysiologic effects of vascular-targeting agents and the implications for combination with conventional therapies. *Cancer Res.* 2006;66(24):11520-11536.

43. Herbst RS, Hong D, Chap L, et al. Safety, pharmacokinetics and antitumor activity of AMG 386, a selective angiopoietin inhibitor in adult patients with advanced solid tumors. *J Clin Oncol.* 2009;27:3557-3565.

44. Gridelli C, Rossi A, Maione P, et al. Vascular disrupting agents: a novel mechanism of action in the battle against non-small cell lung cancer. *Oncologist.* 2009;14:612-620.

45. Kanthou C, Tozer GM. Microtubule depolymerizing vascular disrupting agents: novel therapeutic agents for oncology and other pathologies. *Int J Exp Pathol.* 2009;90(3):284-294.

46. ASA404. Novartis Oncology Web site. http://novartisoncology.com/research-innovation/pipeline/asa404.jsp. Accessed October 1, 2009.

47. Tozer GM, Kanthou C, Baguley BC. Disrupting tumour blood vessels. *Nat Rev Cancer.* 2005; 5:423-435.

48. Bjornsti MA, Houghton PJ. The TOR pathway: a target for cancer therapy. *Nat Rev Cancer.* 2004; 4:335-348.

49. Novartis Oncology. Exploring the essential role of mTOR in cancer cells. Basel, Switzerland: Novartis Oncology; 2005.

50. Semenza GL. Targeting HIF-1 for cancer therapy. *Nat Rev Cancer.* 2003;3:721-731.

51. Shaw RJ, Cantley LC. Ras, PI(3)K and mTOR signaling controls tumour cell growth. *Nature.* 2006;441:424-430.

52. Kobayashi S, Kishimoto T, Kamata S, et al. Rapamycin, a specific inhibitor of the mammalian target of rapamycin, suppresses lymphangiogenesis and lymphatic metastasis. *Cancer Sci.* 2007;98:726-733.

53. Kalaany NY, Sabatini DM. Tumours with PI3K activation are resistant to dietary restriction. *Nature.* 2009;458:725-731.

54. Nagata Y, Lan K-H, Zhou X, et al. PTEN activation contributes to tumor inhibition by trastuzumab, and loss of PTEN predicts trastuzumab resistance in patients. *Cancer Cell.* 2004;6(2):117-127.

55. Nicholson KM, Anderson NG. The protein kinase B/AKT signaling pathway in human malignancy. *Cell Signal.* 2002;14:381-395.

56. Chan S. Targeting the mammalian target or rapamycin (mTOR): a new approach to treating cancer. *Br J Cancer.* 2004;91:1420-1424.

57. Majumder PK, Febbo PG, Bikoff R, et al. mTOR inhibition reverses AKT-dependent prostate intraepithelial neoplasia through regulation of apoptotic and HIF-1 dependent pathways. *Nat Med.* 2004;10:1013-1023.

58. Dredge K, Horsfall R, Robinson SP, et al. Orally administered lenalidomide (CC-5013) is antiangiogenic in vivo and inhibits endothelial cell migration and Akt phosphorylation in vitro. *Microvasc Res.* 2005;69:56-63.

59. Kamba T, McDonald DM. Mechanisms of adverse effects of anti-VEGF therapy for cancer. *Br J Cancer.* 2007;96(17):1788-1795.

60. Zachary I. Signaling mechanisms mediating vascular protective actions of vascular endothelial growth factor. *Am J Physiol.* 2001;280:C1375-C1386.

61. Granger JP, Alexander BT. Abnormal pressure-naturiuresis in hypertension: role of nitric oxide. *Acta Physiol Scand.* 2000;168:161-168.

62. Saltz LB, Clarke S, az-Rubio E, et al. Bevacizumab in combination with oxaliplatin-based chemotherapy as first-line therapy in metastatic colorectal cancer: a randomized phase III study. *J Clin Oncol.* 2008;26:2013-2019.

63. Saltz LB, Lenz HJ, Kindler HL, et al. Randomized phase II trial of cetuximab, bevacizumab, and irinotecan compared with cetuximab and bevacizumab alone in irinotecan-refractory colorectal cancer: the BOND-2 study. *J Clin Oncol.* 2007;25:4557-4561.

64. Yang JC, Haworth L, Sherry RM, et al. A randomized trial of bevacizumab, an antibody against vascular endothelial growth factor antibody for metastatic renal cancer. *N Engl J Med.* 2003;349(5):427-434.

65. Motzer RJ, Hutson TE, Tomczak P, et al. Sunitinib versus interferon alfa in metastatic renal cell carcinoma. *N Engl J Med.* 2007;356:115-124.

66. Hutson T, Figlin R, Kuhn J, Motzer RJ. Targeted therapies for metastatic renal cell carcinoma: an overview of toxicity and dosing strategies. *Oncologist.* 2008;13(10):1084-1096.

67. Faivre S, Delbaldo C, Vera K, et al. Safety, pharmacokinetic and antitumor activity of SU11248, a novel oral multitarget tyrosine kinase inhibitor, in patients with cancer. *J Clin Oncol.* 2006;24(1):25-35.

68. Musini VM, Tejani AM, Bassett K, Wright JM. Pharmacotherapy for hypertension in the elderly. *Cochrane Database of Systematic Reviews* 2009, Issue 2. Art. No.: CD000028. DOI: 10.1002/14651858.CD000028.pub2

69. Whitworth JA. World Health Organization (WHO) International Society of Hypertension Writing Group: 2003 World Health Organization (WHO) International Society of Hypertension (ISH) statement on the management of hypertension. *J Hypertens.* 2002;21:1983-1992.

70. Dincer M, Altundag K. Angiotensin-converting enzyme inhibitors for bevacizumab-induced hypertension. *Ann Pharmacother.* 2006;40:2278-2279.

71. American Diabetes Association. Hypertension management in adults with diabetes. *Diabetes Care.* 2004;20:S65-S67.

72. Wang Y-H, Jones DR, Hall SD. Differential mechanism-based inhibition of CYP3A4 and CYP3A5 by verapamil. *Drug Metab Disposition.* 2005; 33:664-671.

73. Chobanian AV, Bakris GL, Black HR, et al. The seventh report of the Joint National Committee on Prevention, Detection, Evaluation, and Treatment of High Blood Pressure, the JNC 7 report. *JAMA.* 2003;289(19):2560-2571.

74. Garg RK. Posterior leukoencephalopathy syndrome. *Postgrad Med J.* 2001;77:24-28.

75. Glusker P, Recht L, Lane B, et al. Reversible posterior leukoencephalopathy syndrome and bevacizumab. *N Engl J Med.* 2006;354:980-982.

76. Kapiteijn E, Brand A, Kroep J, Gelderblom H. Sunitinib induced hypertension, thrombotic microangiopathy, and reversible posterior leukencephalopathy syndrome. *Ann Oncol.* 2007;18:1745-1747.

77. Vaughn C. Reversible posterior leukoencephalopathy syndrome in cancer. *Curr Oncol Rep.* 2008;10(1):86-91.

78. Avastin [package insert]. South San Francisco, CA: Genentech, Inc; July 2009.

79. Sutent [package insert]. New York: Pfizer Laboratories; February 2007.

80. Nexavar [package insert]. Wayne NJ: Bayer Healthcare Pharmaceuticals, Inc; 2009.

81. Veronese ML, Mosenkis A, Flaherty KT, et al. Mechanisms of hypertension associated with BAY 43-9006. *J Clin Oncol.* 2006;24:1329-1331.

82. Ostendorf T, Kunter U, Eitner F. VEGF mediates glomerular endothelial repair. *J Clin Invest.* 1999;104:913-923.

83. Martel CL, Presant CA, Ebrahimi B, et al. Bevacizumab-related toxicities: association of hypertension and proteinuria. *Comm Oncol.* 2006;3:90-93.

84. Zhu X, Wu S, Dahut W, Parikh CR. Risks of proteinuria and hypertension with bevacizumab, an antibody against vascular endothelial growth factor: a systematic review and meta-analysis. *Am J Kidney Dis.* 2007;49(2):186-193.

85. Kamba T, Tam BY, Hashizume H, et al. VEGF-dependent plasticity of fenestrated capillaries in the normal adult microvasculature. *Am J Physiol Heart Circ Physiol.* 2006;290:H560-H576.

86. Hurwitz H, Fehrenbacher L, Novotny W, et al. Bevacizumab plus irinotecan, fluorouracil, and leucovorin for metastatic colorectal cancer. *N Engl J Med.* 2004;350:2335-2342.

87. Saif MW, Elfiky A, Salem RR. Gastrointestinal perforation due to bevacizumab in colorectal cancer. *Ann Surg Oncol.* 2007;14:1860-1869.

88. Keefe DM, Gibon RJ. Mucosal injury from targeted anti-cancer therapy. *Support Care Cancer.* 2007;15:483-490.

89. Gardner-Thorpe J, Grikscheit TC, Ito H, et al. Angiogenesis in tissue-engineered small intestine. *Tissue Eng.* 2003;9(6):1255-1261.

90. Wood LS. Managing the side effects of sorafinib and sunitinib. *Comm Oncol.* 2006;558-562.

91. Benson AB, Ajani JA, Catalano RB, et al. Recommended guidelines for the treatment of cancer treatment-induced diarrhea. *J Clin Oncol.* 2004;22:2918-2926.

92. Reidy DL, Chung KY, Timoney JP, et al. Bevacizumab 5 mg/kg can be infused safely over 10 minutes. *J Clin Oncol.* 2007;25:2691-2695.

93. Grothey A. Biological therapy and other novel therapies in early stage disease: Are they appropriate? *Clin Cancer Res.* 2007;13:6909s-6912s.

94. Wolmark N, Yothers G, O'Connell MJ, et al. A phase III trial comparing mFOLFOX6 to mFOLFOX6 plus bevacizumab in stage II or III carcinoma of the colon: results of NSABP Protocol C-08. *J Clin Oncol.* 2009;27:18s. [suppl; abstr LBA4]

95. Fingar DC, Richardson CJ, Tee AR et al. mTOR controls cell cycle progression through its cell growth effectors S6K1 and 4E-BP1/Eukaryotic translation initiation factor 4E. *Mol Cell Biol.* 2004;24(1):200-216.

96. Afinitor [package insert]. East Hanover, NJ: Novartis Pharmaceuticals Corp; April 2009.

97. Beckwith MC, Tyler LS. *Cancer Chemotherapy Manual.* St. Louis, MO: Walters Kluwer Health; 2008.

98. Revlimid [package insert]. Summit, NJ: Celgene Corporation; Jan 2009.

CHAPTER 4

Targeting the Microenvironment: Bone Metastasis, Apoptosis, DNA Repair, and Mitosis

BONE METASTASIS

The microenvironment is critical to cancer's successful transformation, invasion, and metastasis, just as the seed needs fertile soil. Angiogenesis appears to be a key process during all phases of malignant growth. This process and the corresponding agents are discussed in Chapter 3. In particular, the immunomodulatory thalidomide derivative agents exert their effect on the microenvironment. While much has been learned about the multiple signaling pathway in cancer formation and invasion, there remain many questions about metastasis. One exciting advance has been in the understanding of bony metastasis from patients with advanced breast and prostate cancers and multiple myeloma. Unfortunately, bony metastasis can compromise quality of life through limitation of mobility (e.g., related to pathological bone fractures), pain, and life-threatening hypercalcemia.[1] Also, it is a frequent occurrence and may affect up to 70% of patients with breast or prostate cancer.[2] The process for each of these malignancies will be reviewed. Although the discussion will be simplified, it is important to remember that the process is very complex; for example, women with estrogen-positive breast cancer have frequent metastases to bone, while women with estrogen-negative breast cancer more commonly have visceral metastases, such as to the liver.[3] In addition, tumors in the lung or colon or renal cell cancer also metastasize to the bone.[4]

To review the basic physiology of bones, normal remodeling of the bone is constant during one's life, with osteoclasts breaking down bone cells (called resorption) and osteoblasts building new bone cell. To help keep these terms straight, it may help to think of the *c* in osteoclast as representing "catabolism" (meaning breakdown) and the *b* in osteoblast as representing "buildup." Systemic as well as local factors control this process.

Osteoclasts are stimulated and regulated by systemic and local factors:

- *Systemic factors*: The hormones parathyroid hormone-related peptide (PTHrP), 1,25-dihydroxyvitamin D_3, and thyroxine (T_4) stimulate the process by inducing the marrow stromal cells and the osteoblasts to express receptor activator of nuclear factor-kB ligand (RANKL, also known as osteoclast differentiation factor).[1] RANKL is also important in the immune system, as it helps dendritic cells to survive (survival factor) and helps to regulate thymus-dependent or T-lymphocyte–immune function. RANKL has been shown to have an important role in cell migration to the bone and in tissue-specific metastatic behavior of cancer cells.[5]

- *Local factors*: Osteoblasts secrete interleukin-6 (IL-6), IL-1, prostaglandin-Es, and colony-stimulating factors (CSFs), which lead to the formation of osteoclasts. Epidermal growth factor (EGF) and tumor necrosis factor (TNF) also stimulate osteoclastic activity, as can thymocyte-dependent lymphocytes (T-cells), which produce IL-17, thus stimulating the osteoclastic process.

Osteoclasts come from monocyte-macrophage precursors. Stromal cells in the bone microenvironment, as well as osteoblasts, produce macrophage CSF and RANKL. RANKL is released by activated T cells and is expressed on the surface of osteoblasts and stromal cells.[1] The systemic factors increase (upregulate) the expression of RANKL on the marrow stromal cells and osteoblasts. RANKL initiates osteoclastogenesis and differentiation of osteoclasts by binding to the RANK receptor on the osteoclast precursors. Within the cell, the message gets sent to the nucleus of the osteoclast by the nuclear factor-kB (NF-kB) and Jun-N-terminal kinase (JNK) pathways. NF-kB is a transcription factor that turns on or off genes that control cell proliferation and survival. In many cancers, NF-kB is dysregulated and it turns on unlimited tumor cell proliferation and survival. JNKs are members of the mitogen-activated protein kinase (MAPK) family and are responsible for interacting with stimuli from outside the cell (mitogens) and regulating gene expression as well as subsequent cell division, differentiation, proliferation, and survival or death (apoptosis). JNKs are also known as stress-activated protein kinases. Thus, as the message reaches the cell nucleus, it turns on the cellular genes to transform the cell into an osteoclast and to make sure the osteoclast survives.

The formation and activation of osteoclasts is tightly regulated. Local and systemic factors can halt the production of osteoclasts. Systemically, corticosteroids and T-cell–released IL-4, IL-18, and IF-gamma, together with locally produced TGFβ and osteoprotegerin (a cytokine called osteoclastogenesis inhibitory factor, a member of the TNF superfamily) inhibit the differentiation of macrophages into osteoclasts; osteoprotegerin works by binding to RANKL on osteoblast/stromal cells and osteoclast precursor cells.[6] Thus, much like a scale, the balance or ratio of RANKL to osteoprotegerin regulates both the formation and activity of the osteoclasts.[1]

The osteoclasts act on the trabecular bone surface to break down the bone minerals and matrix. They release proteases (enzymes) that dissolve the matrix, and this process also releases an acid that removes the minerals,[1] leaving small holes in the bone trabecula (framework of bone on the surface) where the bone has been removed. Once they have done their job, the osteoclasts undergo programmed cell death (apoptosis).

The osteoblasts then come along and fill the holes with new bone that still must be mineralized or calcified. Mesenchymal stem cells produce the osteoblasts, and differentiation of the osteoblast into an adult osteoblast depends upon a transcription factor called Runx-2 (also known as core-binding factor-α1 [CBFA1]). CBFA1 turns on the known genes necessary for osteoblast differentiation.[1] Bone morphogenetic proteins (BMPs) are growth factors and cytokines that stimulate the growth and development of osteoblasts. Systemic and local factors again control osteoblastic proliferation and differentiation.[1] Factors that increase osteoblastic proliferation and differentiation are:

- Systemic factors: parathyroid hormone; prostaglandins; cytokines; and platelet-derived growth factor (PDGF)
- Bone matrix-released growth factors: bone morphogenetic proteins (BMPs); insulin-like growth factor (IGF); fibroblast growth factor (FGF); vascular endothelial growth factor (VEGF); prostate-specific antigen (PSA), which increases osteoblast proliferation; and endothelin-1, which increases osteoblast differentiation and proliferation.

Corticosteroids cause the osteoblast to undergo apoptosis; thus, they block new bone formation.[1] The new bone has to be protected, so a lining of cells is laid over it. Old bone is replaced systematically so that building and breakdown are always balanced and the integrity of the human skeleton is intact (Figure 4-1). Normally, as women age, their bone buildup lags behind bone breakdown, and they are at risk for osteoporosis, a disease in which osteoclast action is greater than osteoblast activity. This risk intensifies as the woman reaches menopause at age 45–55 years[7] and increases a woman's likelihood of osteoporosis and bone fracture. In hormonal breast cancer treatment with ***selective estrogen receptor modulators***, women are at risk of losing bone density and are therefore advised to take calcium and vitamin D and to exercise regularly. Drugs like Fosamax slow the breakdown phase to help maintain bone mass.

The spectrum of bony metastases are anchored by osteolytic lesions on one end and osteoblastic lesions on the other, but in fact, patients may have both types. In general, patients with breast cancer have primarily osteoblastic lesions with about 15–20% osteolytic, while patients with prostate cancer have largely osteoblastic lesions.[8] Patients with multiple myeloma have only osteoblastic bone lesions. Bone scans show the osteoblastic process (active bone formation).[1]

Process of Metastasis to Bone

Roodman describes a process that depends upon both tumor and microenvironment-produced molecules, highlighting the importance of the "seed and soil" analogy.[1] The long bones containing red bone marrow receive high blood flow,

Figure 4-1   Process of bone building and breakdown.

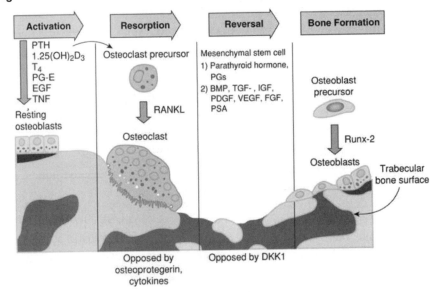

Data from Loberg RD, Logothetis CJ, Keller ET, Pienta KJ. Pathogenesis and treatment of prostate cancer bone metastases: Targeting the lethal phenotype. *J Clin Oncol.* 2005;23(32):8232-8241; Logothetis CJ, Lin SH. Osteoblasts in prostate cancer metastasis to bone. *Nat Rev Cancer* 2005;5(1):21-28; Roodman GD. Mechanisms of bone metastasis. *N Engl J Med.* 2004;350(16):1655-1664.

which makes it easy for embolized cells to find their way to bone. Breast, prostate, and myeloma tumor cells are able to make adhesion substances that allow the tumor cells to stick to the marrow stromal cells and surrounding matrix. Once the tumor cell adheres to the bone, the tumor cells ramp up the production of factors that turn up angiogenesis and bone resorption, as well as tumor proliferation.

Breast Cancer

Breast cancer cells can induce the osteoclasts to secrete PTHrP, TNFα, IL-1, IL-6, IL-8, and IL-11, which in turn tell the osteoblasts to release RANKL.[4] PTHrP and parathyroid hormone (PTH) both bind to the PTH receptor and effect the same physiologic results. PTHrP is produced by 92% of breast tumors metastatic to bone.[9] The tumor cells also produce prostaglandin E_2 and macrophage CSF.[1] All these factors increase the expression of RANKL, which directly affects osteoclast precursors to make osteoclasts.

There are many inactive growth factors in the bone matrix that become activated by the process of bone resorption. Once the osteoclasts begin the bone resorption process, the destroyed matrix releases growth factors that in turn drive the tumor (growth) as well as turn up bone destruction. This process is mediated by the released growth factors from the destroyed matrix: BMPs, IGF-1, TGFβ, FGFs, and PDGF. The stimulated breast cancer cells release more PTHrP, and the vicious cycle is heightened.[10]

Of course, calcium is released when the bone matrix is destroyed, thus raising the patient's serum calcium. Elevated calcium levels in turn stimulate breast cancer cell growth as well as the production of PTHrP. This occurs because there is an extracellular calcium-sensing receptor (CaR) that normally senses elevated calcium levels in the parathyroid and kidney, which then respond to correct the imbalance. However, in cancers of the breast, it appears the CaR actually stimulates the release of PTHrP from the tumor, along with the other osteoclast-driving growth factors, which drives further bone resorption and further release of calcium, resulting in the well-known hypercalcemia of malignancy.[11]

Additionally, it appears that breast cancer cells that produce osteolytic lesions in bone have increased levels of Wnt/beta-catenin signaling and expression of dickkopf1 (DKK1) (an antagonist to Wnt/beta-catenin that also inhibits osteoblast differentiation and osteoprotegerin expression, thus increasing osteoclast activity). Bu et al. suggest that breast-cancer–produced Dkk1 is an important link between primary breast cancers and secondary osteolytic bone metastases.[12] Although most breast cancer bony metastases are osteolytic lesions, some are also osteoblastic, or both. Again, both systemic and local factors are released, driving the formation of unstable bone. Systemic factors are PTH, prostaglandins, and cytokines as well as lymphocyte-produced PDGF, which together with the locally (bone matrix) produced BMPs, TGFβ, IGFs, and FGFs, drive the osteoblastic process.[1] It is thought that osteoblastic lesions occur as a result of endothelin-1 stimulation. Similarly, there is a vicious cycle: As the tumor cells release or induce endothelin-a, osteoblastic bone remodeling forms unstable bone, and the osteoblasts release growth factors such as more endothelin-1, PDGF, and urokinase (made by osteoblasts in the bone microenvironment). This then stimulates breast cancer cell growth and release of systemic factors, which together with local factors, drive the osteoblastic cycle around again.

Prostate Cancer

Prostate cancer bony metastases are primarily osteoblastic. Prostate cancer cells secrete osteoblast-stimulating factors (e.g., PDGF, IGFs, Wnt family ligands that turn on the signaling pathway for osteoblastic activity, endothelin-1, BMPs, urokinase-type of plasminogen activator.[1,4] PSA is able to break (cleave) the PTHrP molecule, so this may be a way osteoclastic activity is turned off. In addition, it appears to activate osteoblastic growth factors that are released from the bone matrix during bone building (osteoblastic activity): IGF-1, IGF-2, and TGFβ. However, although there is no evidence of increased osteoclast activity pathologically in the bone, it appears that bone resorption does occur, either before osteoblastic activity or after, as bone-resorptive (osteoclastic) markers are increased in patients with bony metastases (serum C-terminal telopeptide of type I collagen and tartrate-resistant acid phosphatase), and it appears that blocking osteoclastic activity decreases skeletal events in patients with metastatic prostate cancer with bony metastases.[1,13,14]

Multiple Myeloma

In multiple myeloma, osteoclasts accumulate next to myeloma cells on bone-resorbing surfaces, and it is the osteoclasts, not the tumor cells, that destroy the bone matrix.[1] It appears that IL-1, IL-6, macrophage inflammatory protein-1α (MIP-1α, a chemotactic cytokine also called CCL3), and RANKL are the culprits in ramping up the osteoclasts.[1] RANKL is produced in large measure by the myeloma cells. MIP-1α is produced by activated macrophages and induces the synthesis and release of the proinflammatory cytokines IL-1, IL-6, and TNFα. It is elevated in about 70% of patients with multiple myeloma, and it is not only important in increasing bone destruction and myeloma cell survival, but also enhancing the ability of myeloma cells to stick to the bone surface.[15] It does this by upregulating the myeloma cells' expression of β1 integrins ("grappling hooks") so that the cell can adhere to the bone surface; once this happens, the communication between the marrow stromal and myeloma cells amplifies the production of IL-6, RANKL, and MIP-1α.[1] Of course, this increases the vicious cycle of bone breakdown.

Just how osteoblast formation and differentiation is inhibited is less clear and is probably multifactorial. TNFα released by the myeloma cells can prevent growth and differentiation of osteoblasts, as can DKK1, which is expressed on myeloma cells.[1] DKK1 is an antagonist of the Wnt-signaling pathway, which is the principal pathway that brings the message to the cell nucleus to activate the genes that will move the precursor cell into an osteoblast. Giuliani et al. showed that myeloma cells block RUNX2/CBFA1 activity in the bone marrow osteoblast progenitor cells, thus inhibiting osteoblast formation and differentiation.[16] Because bone scans can pick up only osteoblastic density, and because there is none in multiple myeloma (osteolytic without any osteoblastic response), the bone scan may appear normal despite the presence of osteolytic lesions.[1]

Targets include:

- RANKL, by increasing the level of osteoprotegerin with recombinant osteoprotegerin to turn off or downregulate RANKL, or to block RANKL by a monoclonal antibody (MAb) targeted against RANKL
- Prevention of the osteoclast from adhering to the bone surface so it is not able to perform bone resorption, or inhibition of the proteases released by the osteoclast so it cannot make holes in the bone (e.g., cathepsin K)
- RUNX2/CBFA1 to prevent the block by myeloma cells so that osteoblast formation and differentiation can occur

- Endothelial-1 (ET-1), as it activates the ET_A-receptor, which facilitates prostate cancer progression (proliferation, avoidance of apoptosis, invasion) as well as new bony metastases; ET-1 also mediates the interaction of prostate tumor cell with bone microenvironment (osteoblast, osteoclast, stroma)[17]

Currently, two bisphosphate drugs are approved by the Food and Drug Administration (FDA) for the treatment of malignant hypercalcemia and the treatment of patients with bony metastases. The first approved was pamidronate (Aredia) for the treatment of patients with osteolytic lesions related to either breast cancer metastases or multiple myeloma. The second was zoledronic acid (Zometa), which is indicated for the treatment of patients with multiple myeloma; patients with documented bone metastases from solid tumors, in conjunction with standard antineoplastic therapy; and patients with prostate cancer that has progressed after treatment with at least one hormonal therapy. There is evidence that women treated with these agents have decreased skeletal events or increased disease-free survival.[18–20]

Further exploration into the mechanism of bone metastasis has revealed a dramatic story involving RANKL. As discussed, RANKL activates bone osteoclasts so that they start to break down bone. In cancer, there is a vicious circle of tumor-released factors that stimulate osteoclast activity, mediated by RANKL; breakdown of the bone matrix releases growth factors that stimulate both tumor growth and continued bone breakdown. Amgen has submitted an application to the FDA for consideration of denosumab (Prolia), an investigational RANKL inhibitor, for the treatment and prevention of bone loss in patients undergoing hormone ablation therapy for either prostate or breast cancer, and for treatment and prevention of postmenopausal osteoporosis in women.[21] Denosumab, is a fully human MAb that targets RANKL, by mimicking osteoprotegerin, which is a soluble decoy receptor for RANKL that blocks ligand binding to RANKL so it does not become activated and the message (signaling) is not sent to start differentiation and activation of the osteoclast.[5,22] In addition to being critical for osteoclast differentiation, function, and survival, when RANKL is released in large amounts from the bone marrow, it attracts cancer cells that express its receptor, RANK, to the bone where they can develop a metastatic site, and the microniche is well prepared to encourage strong metastatic growth.[5,23]

Denosumab has shown to be superior to the existing bisphosphonate drugs. In a large (N = 2049) international phase III, randomized, double-blind clinical trial comparing denosumab with zoledronic acid in the treatment of bone metastases in patients with advanced breast cancer, the group receiving denosumab had significantly longer time to first on-study skeletal-related events (SRE, e.g., fracture, radiation to bone, surgery to bone, or spinal cord compression [hazard ratio 0.82]) and longer time to the first and subsequent SREs (hazard ratio 0.77). The primary end point was to evaluate if denosumab was noninferior to zoledronic acid in the prevention of first on-study SRE, and the second end point was to see if denosumab was superior to zoledronic acid in terms of first on-study SRE as well as subsequent SREs. Both end points were met.[24] In prostate cancer, denosumab was effective in reducing N-telopeptide urine levels (marker of osteoclast activity) in patients who previously had received intravenous (IV) bisphosphonates.[24,25] Prostate cancer patients represented 45% of the total; the remainder was made up of patients with bony metastasis from other solid tumors and multiple myeloma. At week 25, 69% of the denosumab-treated patients continued to have urine N-telopeptide levels < 50 compared to 31% of the patients treated with IV bisphosphonates.

In addition to therapeutic benefit in reducing skeletal events from bony metastases, denosumab offers benefit to the many women and men who develop bone loss from endocrine therapy. Women with breast cancer receive aromatase inhibitors for 5 years. Although this treatment is intended to block estrogen effects, it also enhances and accelerates bone loss. While treatment with tamoxifen has been shown to benefit bone, the aromatase inhibitors, such as the third-generation anastrozole, letrozole, and exemestane, increase bone loss beyond that seen naturally after age 30 years.[26] Denosumab offers a benefit to these patients as well. Ellis et al., in the phase III HALT breast cancer study, showed that denosumab 60 mg administered every 6 months subcutaneously to women receiving adjuvant aromatase inhibitor therapy (N = 252) increased bone mineral density (BMD) in the lumbar region by an average 5.5% over that of patients receiving placebo at 12 months; at 24 months, BMD increased an average of 7.6% over placebo. Increases were also seen in total hip (4.7%), femoral neck (3.5%), trochanter (5.9%), and radius (6.1%).[27] Increases in lumbar spine BMD were apparent within 1 month of therapy and were not influenced by length of time on aromatase inhibitor therapy. The overall adverse effects were similar to placebo. Similarly, the phase III HALT prostate cancer study (N = 1400) of men with prostate cancer undergoing androgen deprivation therapy (ADT) met both its first and second end points by demonstrating significant increases in BMD in the lumbar spine compared to placebo at 2 years and also showing half the incidence of SREs (e.g., fractures) compared to placebo at 3 years, respectively.[28,29] Men with prostate cancer who survive at least 5 years with prostate cancer and have received ADT are estimated to have a 19.4% incidence of bone fracture, compared to 12.6% for those who did not receive ADT.[30]

PHARMACOLOGIC MANAGEMENT

Drug: Zoledronic acid (Zometa)

Indications: Zoledronic acid is FDA indicated for the treatment of patients with hypercalcemia of malignancy, and patients with multiple myeloma or documented bone metastases from solid tumors, in conjunction with standard antineoplastic therapy. Prostate cancer should have progressed after treatment with at least one hormonal therapy.

Class: Bisphosphonate (drug class that inhibits osteoclast activity in the bone)

Mechanism of Action: Inhibits bone resorption. Specifically, it inhibits tumor-related osteoclast activity in bone (bone breakdown), promotes apoptosis of osteoclasts, and, when it binds to bone, blocks dissolution of minerals (hydroxyapatite) in bone, thus preventing calcium release from bone, as well as osteoclastic resorption of cartilage. By inhibiting osteoclast activity and the release of calcium from the bones that is caused by tumor-related stimulatory factors, it stops hypercalcemia of malignancy. A single dose of the drug results in decreased serum calcium and phosphorus, and increased excretion of urinary calcium and phosphorus. It does not inhibit bone formation or bone mineralization. Drug is very rapidly taken up in the bone but very slowly released. Drug appears to inhibit endothelial cell proliferation and to inhibit the beta fibroblast growth factor (βFGF)-mediated angiogenesis. The drug is 100–850 times more potent than pamidronate.

Pharmacokinetics: Drug is primarily eliminated intact via the kidney. It has a long terminal half-life in plasma of 167 hours, and drug may remain in bone up to 5 years with prolonged low plasma concentrations. Rapid injection results in 30% increase in serum drug concentration and renal damage.

Dosage and Administration:

- *Hypercalcemia of malignancy*: 4 mg as a single IV dose given over no less than 15 minutes; 4 mg retreatment after a minimum of 7 days; also given IV over at least 15 minutes
- *Multiple myeloma and bone metasatases from solid tumors*: 4 mg as a single-dose IV over no less than 15 minutes every 3–4 weeks for patients with a creatinine clearance of > 60 mL/min
- Dose reduce for patients with renal impairment:
  - Baseline creatinine clearance 50–60 mL/min, 3.5 mg
  - Baseline creatinine clearance 40–49 mL/min, 3.3 mg
  - Baseline creatinine clearance 30–39 mL/min, 3.0 mg
- If serum creatinine prior to dose shows renal deterioration, dose should be held:
  - Baseline normal serum creatinine: increase of 0.5 mg/dL
  - Baseline abnormal serum creatinine: increase of 1.0 mg/dL
  - Resume drug only if serum creatinine returns to within 10% of baseline, then initiate at same dose as that prior to dose interruption
- Coadminister oral calcium supplements of 500 mg and a multivitamin containing 400 IU of vitamin D daily.

Available as: 4 mg/5 mL single-dose vials

Reconstitution and Preparation:

- Reconstitute drug by adding 5 mL sterile water for injection USP so that 4 mg = 5 mL. If the patient is receiving a reduced dose, withdraw the appropriate volume.
- Further dilute in 100 mL 5% dextrose injection USP or 0.9% sodium chloride injection USP. DO NOT use any other IV solution such as lactated Ringer solution.
- If not used immediately, it may be refrigerated at 2–8°C (36–46°F) for up to 24 hours, but administration must be completed within 24 hours of the initial dilution.

Drug Interactions: None known. However, the following drugs should be coadministered with caution, if at all:

- Aminoglycoside antibiotics: may have an additive effect to lower serum calcium for prolonged periods
- Loop diuretics: may increase risk of hypocalcemia
- Nephrotoxic drugs: additive nephrotoxicity
- Thalidomide: may increase risk of renal dysfunction

Contraindications: Hypersensitivity to any component of zoledronic acid (Zometa)

Warnings:

- Patients receiving should **not** be receiving Reclast, as they are both zoledronic acid.
- Ensure adequate rehydration of patients with hypercalcemia of malignancy prior to administering zoledronic acid, and monitor electrolytes baseline and during treatment. Replete calcium, phosphorus, and/or magnesium if hypocalcemia, hypophosphatemia, or hypomagnesemia occurs.
- Patients with renal dysfunction are at increased risk of renal toxicity. Never administer more than a 4 mg dose, and ensure the drug is administered over at least 15 minutes, no shorter. Monitor serum creatinine prior to each dose. Also, monitor patients very closely if they are receiving other potentially nephrotoxic drugs. Patients should be evaluated for albuminuria at least every 3–6 months; if this is unexplained (e.g., defined as > 500 mg/24 hours of urinary albumin), the drug should be held until a thorough workup can occur.[31]
- Osteonecrosis of the jaw may occur. Preventive dental exams should be performed prior to beginning zoledronic acid. Avoid invasive dental procedures during treatment with zoledronic acid. Risk factors that appear to increase risk are underlying disease (breast cancer or multiple myeloma) and dental status (dental extraction, periodontal disease, local trauma including poorly fitting dentures).

- Zoledronic acid can cause fetal harm. Patients should use effective contraception and avoid pregnancy.
- Severe bone, joint, and muscle pain may occur and be incapacitating, and may occur 1 day or several months after the first drug dose; discontinue the drug if severe symptoms develop, as most patients had symptom relief after drug cessation.
- Rarely, bronchoconstriction may occur in patients with asthma who also have aspirin sensitivity; monitor these patients closely.
- There is little known about use of zoledronic acid in patients with hepatic insufficiency.

Adverse Reactions (**bold** indicates most common, occurring in >25% of patients):

Cardiovascular: Hypotension, hypertension, bradycardia

Pulmonary: Dyspnea, coughing, bronchoconstriction

CNS/Neurologic: Insomnia, anxiety, confusion, agitation, headache, paresthesia, hypoesthesia, blurred vision, dizziness

Dermatologic: Alopecia, dermatitis, rare uveitis and episcleritis (ocular inflammation), increased sweating

CNS/Metabolic: Hypophosphatemia, hypokalemia or hyperkalemia, hypomagnesemia, hypernatremia, decreased weight

GI: **Nausea**, **constipation**, diarrhea, abdominal pain, **vomiting**, anorexia, dyspepsia, stomatitis, sore throat, dehydration

Hematologic: **Anemia**, neutropenia, thrombocytopenia

Genitourinary: Urinary tract infection (UTI), renal dysfunction, proteinuria, hematuria

Musculoskeletal: Skeletal pain, myalgia, back pain, pain in limb, arthralgia

General: **Fatigue**, **fever**, weakness, edema of lower limbs, rigors, hypersensitivity reactions, osteonecrosis of the jaw, aggravation or progression of malignancy

Nursing Discussion:

Osteonecrosis of the jaw (ONJ): ONJ is emerging as a significant adverse effect of bisphosphonate therapy (Table 4-1). The incidence is 1–10%, although prospective trials are being conducted to confirm the actual risk factors and incidence.[32] Risk factors for ONJ include head and neck radiotherapy, periodontal disease, dental procedures involving bone surgery, areas without teeth in the jaw, trauma from poorly fitting dentures, thrombosis, underlying malignancy, anemia, chemotherapy, corticosteroids, and systemic or regional infection.[33]

Table 4-1　Staging and Recommendations for Treatment of Bisphosphonate-Related Osteonecrosis of the Jaw

Stage	Recommended treatment
At risk: No apparent necrotic bone in patients who have been treated with either oral or IV bisphosphonates	Teach patient about risk and close need for monitoring; no treatment indicated
Stage 0: No clinical evidence of necrotic bone, but nonspecific clinical findings and symptoms	Systemic management, including the use of analgesics and antibiotics
Stage 1: Exposed and necrotic bone in patients who are asymptomatic and have no evidence of infection	Antibacterial mouth rinse, clinical follow-up on a quarterly basis, patient education, and review of indications for continued bisphosphate therapy
Stage 2: Exposed and necrotic bone associated with infection, as evidenced by pain and erythema in the region of exposed bone with or without purulent discharge	Symptomatic treatment with oral antibiotics, oral antibacterial mouth rinses, pain control, and superficial debridement to relieve soft-tissue irritation
Stage 3: Exposed and necrotic bone in patients with pain, infection, and one or more of the following: exposed and necrotic bone extending beyond the region of the alveolar bone; pathologic fracture; extra-oral fistulae; oral-antral or oral-nasal communication; or osteolysis extending to the inferior border of the mandible of the sinus floor	Antibacterial mouth rinse, antibiotic therapy and pain control, and surgical debridement/resection for longer-term palliation of infection and pain

Data from the American Association of Oral and Maxillofacial Surgeons (www.aaoms.org).

Christodoulou et al. have identified an increased risk in patients receiving both bisphosphonates and antiangiogenic factors.[34] Ruggiero et al. recommend the following antimicrobials for the patient who develops ONJ[33]:

- Antibacterials: penicillin VK (500 mg every 6–8 hours for 7–10 days, then twice daily for maintenance); amoxicillin (500 mg every 8 hours for 7–10 days then twice daily for maintenance); if allergic to penicillin, clindamycin (150–300 mg four times daily), erythromycin ethylsuccinate (400 mg three times daily), or azithromycin (500 mg orally (PO) × 1 on day 1, then 250 mg PO daily on days 2–5)

- Antifungals if needed: nystatin oral suspension (5–15 mL four times daily or 100,000 IU/mL); Mycelex Troche (clotrimazole) (10 mg three times daily for 7–10 days), or fluconazole (200 mg initially, then 100 mg daily)
- Antivirals if needed: acyclovir (400 mg twice daily), valacyclovir HC (500 mg to 2 grams twice daily)

Teach patients that they should:

- Keep teeth and gums healthy, and schedule an appointment for a dental exam and cleaning prior to starting bisphosphonate therapy. Any necessary dental work should be completed prior to starting therapy, and the dentist should discuss this with patient's oncologist prior to the work beginning. It is preferable, if possible, to perform root canals rather than having a tooth extracted.
- Tell their dentist to check and adjust dentures to make sure they fit properly.
- Tell their oncologist about any bleeding of the gums, pain, or unusual problems in the mouth or involving the teeth.
- Maintain a dental hygiene regimen that includes brushing teeth and tongue after every meal and using a soft toothbrush at bedtime; gently floss once a day; rinse mouth often with water to keep it moist; avoid mouthwashes with alcohol.
- Assess the mouth, lips, and teeth daily and immediately report any sores, bleeding, or changes as well as any pain to their dentist or oncology team.
- In the rare event of ONJ, report any of the following right away to their dentist and doctor or nurse[35]:
  - Pain, swelling, or infection of the gums
  - Loose teeth
  - Poor gum healing
  - Numbness or feeling of heaviness of the jaw

Key points in the nursing care of the patient receiving zoledronic acid:
- Patients should have an oral examination and preventive dentistry completed before starting bisphosphonate therapy and periodically during treatment if high risk or symptoms arise. Patients should avoid dental work while receiving bisphosphonate therapy and should be taught to report any problems to the nurse and physician.
- Serum creatinine must be monitored prior to each treatment and abnormal values discussed with physician, as risk must be weighed against benefit. Risk factors for deteriorating renal function and possibly renal failure are (1) impaired renal function and (2) multiple cycles of bisphosphonate therapy. Patients should be evaluated for albuminuria at least every 3–6

months; if it is unexplained (e.g., defined as > 500 mg/24 hours of urinary albumin), the drug should be held until a thorough workup can occur.[36]

• Teach patients to use effective birth control measures.

Determination of true calcium:

In reviewing normal calcium homeostasis, calcium is found primarily in bone. As such, 99% of the body's calcium is in the form of insoluble crystals, giving the human skeleton strength and durability. The remaining 1% is distributed between the body's intracellular and extracellular fluids: 45% is ionized in the serum, 45% is bound by protein, and 10% is found in insoluble complexes. The ionized fraction of calcium is necessary for excitation of nerves, voluntary skeletal muscle, cardiac muscle, and involuntary muscles in the gut. If the body has too much ionized calcium, there is decreased excitability of these tissues. For instance, symptoms of early hypercalcemia (calcium of 10–12 mg/dL) are fatigue, lethargy, constipation, anorexia, nausea and vomiting, and polyuria. Later symptoms, when the calcium is > 12 mg/dL, are altered mental status, coma, decreased deep tendon reflexes, increased cardiac contractility, and oliguric renal failure. In contrast, if there is too little ionized calcium in the body, there is increased excitability of nerves and muscle. The body attempts to regain more calcium to raise the level of ionized calcium by "raiding" the bone matrix.

Because 45% of the calcium outside of bone is bound to albumin, it is important to correct the value of ionized calcium in the serum if the albumin is low (normally bound calcium is now free in the serum, and the serum level may actually be higher than the laboratory value). The formula to determine ionized serum calcium, corrected for low serum albumin is:

$$\text{Corrected serum calcium} =$$
$$\text{measured total serum calcium (mg/dL)} + (4.0 - \text{serum albumin [g/dL]}) \times 0.8$$

For example, a patient has a serum calcium of 10.0 mg/dL but has a serum albumin of 2.2 (normal is 3.5–5.5 g/dL). The corrected serum calcium is:

$$10.0 \text{ mg/dL} + (4.0 - 2.2) \times 0.8 = 10.0 + 1.8 \times 0.8 = 11.44$$

Thus, a serum calcium level that appears normal may be abnormal (high) in the presence of a low serum albumin level.

Drug: Pamidronate (Aredia)

Indications: Indicated for the treatment of hypercalcemia of malignancy, in conjunction with adequate hydration, as well as prevention of osteolytic lesions in breast cancer and multiple myeloma

Class: Bisphosphonate (drug class that inhibits osteoclast activity in the bone)

Mechanism of Action: Drug adsorbs to calcium phosphate (hydroxyapatite) crystals in bone, and may block dissolution of the bone matrix, thus preventing the release of calcium from degraded bone. Drug also appears to inhibit osteo-clast activity in bone (bone breakdown). Does not inhibit bone formation or bone mineralization.

Pharmacokinetics: Drug is not metabolized and is excreted unchanged by the kidneys with 46% +/– 16% excreted within 120 hours. Drug remains in bone for up to 5 years.

Dosage and Administration:

- **Adult (hypercalcemia of malignancy):**
  - *Moderate hypercalcemia* (corrected serum calcium 12–13.5 mg/dL): 60–90 mg as IV infusion over 2–24 hours (> 2-hour infusion is associated with increased risk of renal toxicity, especially in patients with preexisting renal dysfunction)
  - *Severe hypercalcemia* (corrected serum calcium > 13.5 mg/dL): 90 mg as continuous infusion over 2–24 hours (like "moderate," increased renal toxicity with infusion > 2 hours)
  - *If retreatment required*: Wait a minimum of 7 days between treatments
- **Osteolytic lesions of multiple myeloma:** 90 mg in 500 mL sterile 0.45% or 0.9% sodium chloride USP, or 5% dextrose injection USP, administered over a 4-hour period monthly
- **Osteolytic bone metastasis of breast cancer:** 90 mg in 250 mL sterile 0.45% or 0.9% sodium chloride USP, or 5% dextrose injection USP, administered over a 2-hour period every 3–4 weeks
- Assess serum creatinine prior to each dose, and hold drug if there is a worsening of renal function as defined by a 0.5 mg/dL increase above normal baseline serum creatinine in patients with normal baseline creatinine, and an increase of 1.0 mg/dL above baseline if the baseline was abnormal.

Available as: 30-mg and 90-mg vials

Reconstitution and Preparation: Reconstitute by adding 10 mL sterile water for injection USP to each vial, resulting in a 30 mg/10 mL or 90 mg/10 mL concentration. The appropriate drug dose should then be added to the appropriate drug bag, based on disease being treated, and administered. Reconstituted drug may be stored under refrigeration for up to 24 hours at 2–8°C (36–46°F).

Drug Interactions: None known

Contraindications: Patients with known hypersensitivity to pamidronate or other bisphosphonates

Warnings:
- **Deterioration in renal function:** Drug may rarely cause renal insufficiency. Assess serum creatinine baseline and before each treatment, and perform periodic urinalyses for protein. Hold the drug for increased serum creatinine or proteinuria. Saline hydration to maintain urinary output of

2 L/day should be maintained during treatment for hypercalcemia. Patients should be evaluated for albuminuria at least every 3–6 months; if it is unexplained (e.g., defined as >500 mg/24 hours of urinary albumin), the drug should be held until a thorough workup can occur.[31]

- The drug has not been studied in patients with a creatinine clearance <30 mL/min, or patients with a serum creatinine >3.0 mg/dL.
- **Drug is fetotoxic:** Patients of childbearing age should use effective contraception.
- **Osteonecrosis of the jaw:** The drug may rarely cause ONJ, often in conjunction with a dental procedure such as tooth extraction. Patients should have an oral examination and preventative dentistry completed before starting bisphosphonate therapy and periodically during treatment if high risk or symptoms arise. Patients should avoid dental work while receiving bisphosphonate therapy.

Adverse Reactions (**bold** indicates most common, occurring in >25% of patients):

Cardiovascular: Hypertension, edema

Pulmonary: **Cough**, dyspnea, sinusitis, upper respiratory infection

CNS/Neurologic: Anxiety, **headache**, insomnia

GI: **Constipation, diarrhea, nausea,** anorexia, dyspepsia, abdominal pain, vomiting

Hematologic: **Anemia**, granulocytopenia, thrombocytopenia

Musculoskeletal: **Myalgias**, arthralgias, skeletal pain

Genitourinary: UTI, renal dysfunction

General: Asthenia, **fatigue, fever,** pain

Nursing Discussion: **Please see discussion for zoledronic acid.**

Drug: Denosumab (Prolia, AMG 162, investigational)

Indications: Applied to FDA for treatment and prevention of bone loss in patients undergoing hormone ablation therapy for either prostate or breast cancer, and for treatment and prevention of postmenopausal osteoporosis in women

Class: RANKL inhibitor

Mechanism of Action: Denosumab, is a fully human MAb that targets RANK ligand by mimicking osteoprotegerin, which is a soluble decoy receptor for RANKL that blocks ligand binding to RANKL so it does not become activated; thus the message (signaling) is not sent to start differentiation and activation of the osteoclast.

Pharmacokinetics: Denosumab has a long half-life of 33–46 days after subcutaneous administration, which permits administration every 3–6 months. Drug is completely cleared from the body, unlike bisphosphonates, which have a potential half-life in bone of 5 years.[22]

Dosage and Administration:

- Osteoporosis: 60 mg subcutaneously every 6 month
- Metastatic cancer: 120 mg every 4 weeks subcutaneously

Available as: Per protocol

Reconstitution and Preparation: Per protocol

Drug Interactions: Unknown

Adverse Reactions:

GI: Nausea, vomiting, diarrhea

Hematologic: Infection, but rate similar to placebo

General: Feeling weak

Nursing Discussion: Denosumab offers potential advantages over bisphosphonates, including superior effect in delaying skeletal events, and while the drug's long half-life permits less frequent dosing, the drug is also cleared from the system fairly rapidly compared to the bisphosphonates, which can stay in bone for up to 5 years. ONJ has not been reported in patients receiving denosumab, and it may be because of its different mechanism of action and because it is cleared more rapidly from the body.

TARGETING APOPTOSIS

As we have seen, programmed cell death (apoptosis) is a critical safeguard to prevent the accumulation of injured or damaged cells and to prevent them from entering active cell division and sharing their defects with their progeny in daughter cells. In this way, tissue integrity, function, and efficiency of cell processes can be ensured. One of the hallmarks of cancer is avoidance of apoptosis, affording the cell immortality.

Telomerase

Telomeres are caps on the ends of chromosomes. They protect the chromosome during mitosis so that the chromosome can be copied accurately. Thus, when the two copies split, both daughter cells have intact chromosomes (Figure 4-2).

In the embryo, the embryonic stem cells express telomerase, allowing them to reattach each cut-off piece; thus the length of the chromosome remains constant and the cell can divide repeatedly. The cell keeps count of the lifetime cell divisions, and with each cell division, the ends of the chromosome are clipped off. When the chromosomes in the cell get too short, usually after about 60–70 cell divisions, the cell undergoes programmed cell death.

Figure 4-2   Telomeres protect the chromosome ends.

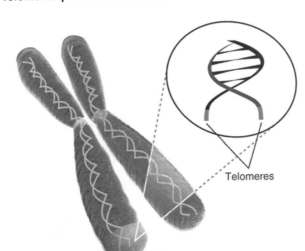

Telomeres

Data from National Cancer Institute. Scientific Progress and Future Research Directions. Appendix C: Human Embryonic Stem Cells and Human Embryonic Germ Cells. Available at http://stemcells.nih.gov /info/2001report/appendixC.asp. Accessed December 7, 2009.

Cancer again is able to subvert embryologic strategies, and many tumors make telomerase. Telomerase activity is detected in 85–90% of human tumor samples,[37] allowing these cells to escape programmed cell death or apoptosis. Alternately, some malignant cells, especially those of mesenchymal origin, are able to maintain telomere length by activating the alternative lengthening of telomeres pathway. After the maximum cell divisions, the cell goes into senescence and cannot divide. If the tumor suppressor proteins p53 and retinoblastoma protein are inactivated, then the cell can continue to divide but eventually will go into "crisis." If the cell continues to divide during crisis, then as the telomeres are shortened, the chromosome integrity is lost more and more with each cell division. The telomeres are eventually lost, exposing the chromosome ends. These unprotected ends appear to the cell as double-stranded DNA breaks, and the cell tries to fix them but may end up attaching the end of one chromosome to the end of another. Eventually, the chromosomal mistakes require the cell to undergo programmed cell death.

DePinho and Polyak identify that prior to the benign-to-malignant transition in breast cancer, the cells show marked increase in chromosomal aberrations, suggesting that telomere dysfunction drives this chromosomal instability.[38] This enables the malignant cell to have the multiple mutations and genetic abnormalities needed to become an invasive cancer. Figure 4-3 depicts the shortening telomere with successive cell divisions, the development of crisis, and the reactivation of

Figure 4-3   Crisis as cells age.

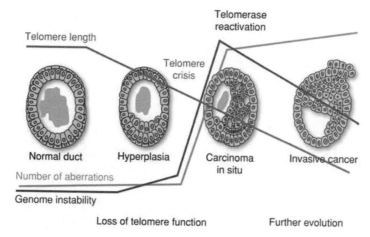

Chin K et al.[39]

telomerase resulting in breast cancer in situ tumor growth, and ultimately an invasive cancer.[39]

Apoptosis is triggered when the proteins that are proapoptotic are stronger than the antiapoptotic factors, which want to avoid apoptosis. The crucial vote is given by members of the Bcl-2 family of proteins. The process of apoptosis is mediated by two pathways, the intrinsic and the extrinsic. Both pathways come together at the end, and the intracellular enzymes called caspases will ultimately destroy the cell (Figure 4-4). This "cell suicide" does not involve inflammation from leakage of intracellular components; rather it is clean and organized, with the dismantled pieces of the cell wrapped neatly within membranes. This process is in contrast to necrosis, which involves cell swelling and leakage of the cellular contents with inflammation.

Apoptosis involves the death of a single cell, not groups or neighboring cells.[41] The cell first shrinks, and blebs appear on the intact cell membrane. The chromatin (DNA and protein) in the nucleus condenses and is broken apart in defined amounts, and the membrane of the mitochondria (cell's powerhouse) becomes permeable and releases cytochrome c.[42] This and other proapoptotic proteins cause the cell and chromatin to be wrapped in small, membrane-bound fragments called apoptotic bodies. A substance called phosphatidylserine, which normally lives in the cell's plasma membrane, becomes exposed on the surface of the membrane-wrapped packages. Its exposure is akin to wearing a sign that says "eat me" and attracts macrophages and dendritic cells, which engulf and phagocytize the packages.[43] The phagocytic cells that engulf the apoptotic bodies release cytokines (e.g., IL-10, TGFβ) that inhibit inflammation.

Figure 4-4   Intrinsic and extrinsic pathways for apoptosis.

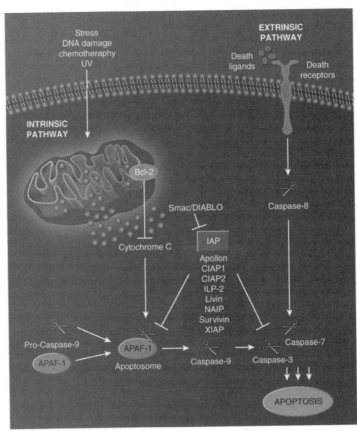

Apoptosis can occur via either the intrinsic or extrinsic pathway, which both converge at the caspase cascade. The intrinsic pathway is stimulated by p53, and involves the release of cytochrome c from the mitochondrial membrane, which then binds to APAF-1. It can be blocked by Bcl-2 and by Inhibitors of Apoptosis (IAPs). Smac/DIABLO is released from the mitochondria along with cytochrome c to block the IAPs so that apoptosis is promoted. The extrinsic pathway is independent of p53, and starts outside the cell with the attachment of pro-apoptotic ligands, such as Apo2L/TRAIL to the Death receptor on the cell surface. This recruits a protein called Fas-associated death domain (FADD) and sets up caspases to destroy the cell.

UV=ultraviolet light; Caspase=family of protective enzymes that amplify the signal for apoptosis and bring about destruction of the cell; Smac/DIABLO=Second mitochondria-derived activator of caspases/Direct IAP Binding Protein with Low PI is released from the mitochondria during apoptosis; IAP=Inhibitors of Apoptosis, a family of proteins that suppress apoptosis; CIAP1 and CIAP2=inhibit apoptosis and play a role in innate immunity; ILP-2=inhibits apoptosis induced by overexpression of Bax; Livin=apoptosis inhibitor expressed in most solid tumors; Survivin=inhibits apoptosis in the mitochondria and has a role in mitosis; XIAP=inhibits apoptosis by binding to some of the caspases; APAF-1=apoptotic peptidase activating factor 1, initiates apoptosis when cytochrome c binds to it; Apoptosome=protein structure formed when apoptosis is initiated by cytochrome c binding to APAF-1.

Table 4-2   Pro- and Antiapoptotic Factors in the Bcl-2 Family

Proapoptotic	Antiapoptotic
Bax, Bak (gatekeepers)	Bcl-2
Bok	Bcl-X$_L$
Bad, Bid	Bcl-W
Puma	Mcl-1
Noxa	Boo
Bmf	A1

Data from Goodsell DS.[45,46]; Dorsey FC, Steeves MA, Cleveland JL. Apoptosis, autophagy, and necrosis. In: J. Mendelsohn, PM Howley, MA Israel, JW Gray, CB Thompson, eds. *The Molecular Basis of Cancer.* Philadelphia, PA: Saunders Elsevier;2008:205-220.

Intrinsic Pathway

The intrinsic pathway is triggered from within the cell and involves p53 and the mitochondria. Internal stressors, inability to complete the cell cycle, detachment of the cell from the extracellular matrix, loss of survival factors, and DNA damage are triggers that will lead to intrinsic pathway-mediated apoptosis. Normally, the antiapoptotic protein Bcl-2 sits on the outer membrane of the mitochondria. When there is internal cell damage, p53 leads the way, and BAK and BAX are proapoptotic proteins that push toward apoptosis. In fact, BAX migrates to the mitochondrial membrane, where it inhibits Bcl-2, moves to the membrane, and punches holes in the membrane so that cytochrome c and a proapoptotic protein SMAC/DIABLO are released. SMAC/DIABLO interact with the inhibitors of apoptosis proteins (IAPs) so that they will not inactivate the caspase enzymes. Cytochrome c binds to an adaptor called Apaf-1 (apoptotic protease-activating factor-1), forming an apoptosome. This process requires energy in the form of *adenosine* triphosphate (*ATP*). The apoptosome regulates caspase 9 activity, which will be recruited into the apoptosome then activated, and it will then activate the caspases 3, 6, and 7.[44] The activated caspases then degrade cellular proteins, leading to cell death. Table 4-2 shows the Bcl-2 family of pro- and antiapoptotic members.

Extrinsic Pathway

The external pathway begins outside the cell, is independent of p53, and is mediated by the death receptor. There are proapoptotic receptors on the cell surface, which are turned on by proapoptotic ligands Apo2L/TRAIL (Apo2 ligand/TNF-related apoptosis-inducing ligand, which binds to the death receptor, DR4/DR5) and CD95L/FasL (which binds to the CD95/Fas receptor). When the ligand binds to its receptor, it causes the receptors to come together and induces the formation of DISC (death-inducing signaling complex) by recruiting the adaptor protein FADD (Fas-associated death domain) and the procaspases 8 and 10. Within DISC, the procaspases turn each other on, and they are then released into the cytoplasm where they can activate caspases 3, 6, and 7. The pathway then joins the intrinsic pathway. As the DISC is forming, there are antiapoptotic forces trying to inhibit its formation. These forces are the IAPs and c-FLIP, a c-FLICE inhibitory protein that works with FADD to try to block the activation of caspases. There are also decoy receptors that can block ligand binding so that the pathway is never activated.

Caspase Cascade

The intrinsic and extrinsic pathways converge at the level of caspases 3, 6, and 7. The caspases have an expanding cascade that digests the structural proteins and degrades the DNA and nuclear proteins; thus the membrane-bound packets of the degraded cell can be phagocytized.

Cancers are expert at avoiding apoptosis. For example some B-cell leukemias and lymphomas express high levels of Bcl-2, which is antiapoptotic and prevents the mitochondria from acting on any proapoptotic signals they receive.[47] Melanoma cells inhibit the gene that produces Apaf-1, again blocking the intrinsic pathway. Some lung and colon cancer cells secrete decoy proteins that bind to the FasL, so that it is unable to bind to Fas. Normally, cytotoxic T cells kill malignant cells by producing more FasL on their surface, which will bind to Fas on the surface of the target cancer cell. This normally should lead to cell death via the extrinsic pathway of apoptosis.[48] An example of an IAP that is overexpressed in a number of cancers is survivin, which is upregulated in cancer and associated with increased tumor recurrence, chemotherapy resistance, and poor survival.[49] This makes survivin a possible molecular target. In addition, using therapeutic doses of the protein Apo2L/TRAIL is being studied, as this protein binds with two proapoptotic death receptors and three antiapoptotic decoys. It also appears to induce apoptosis selectively in malignant cells but not normal cells.[50]

Thus, there is great interest in identifying targeted therapy to kill cancer cells via effective apoptosis. One example is studying ligand-based targeted therapy using recombinant human apoptosis ligand-2/TNF-related apopotosis-inducing ligand (rhApo2L/TRAIL).[51] Studies are being conducted with a new dual, proapoptotic receptor agonist that directly activates the DR4 and DR5 receptors to which the ligand Apo2L/TRAIL binds (Apomab, a fully human MAb that is an agonist of the DR5 receptor).[52] Activated DR5 then induces the DISC to initiate the extrinsic apoptotic pathway. Since Apo2L/TRAIL kills only malignant cells compared to normal ones, selective apoptosis should minimize toxicity. The TRAIL agonist mapatumumab is being studied in phase II clinical trials (liver, non–small cell lung cancer [NSCLC], lymphoma, myeloma), while AMG-655, also a TRAIL agonist, is being studied in a phase II trial of patients with colorectal, NSCLC, pancreatic, and sarcoma.[53]

A number of agents are being investigated that target Bcl-2 or other proteins and may suppress apoptosis. Because Bcl-2 protein inhibits apoptosis and makes the cells resistant to treatment with standard chemotherapy, drugs such as antisense oligonucleotides theoretically can disable Bcl-2 and restore responsiveness to chemotherapy. Oblimersen sodium is an antisense oligonucleotide that binds to Bcl-2 messenger RNA (mRNA), leading to the degradation of Bcl-2 mRNA, which then results in decreased Bcl-2 protein translation or downregulation of Bcl-2. Apoptosis is then possible, and the cancer cells should be more responsive to chemotherapy. The Bcl-2 antagonist oblimersen (Genasense) continues to be studied in phase III studies of melanoma and myeloma, while antagonists to survivin are being studied in phase II clinical trials.[53] Other pathways control apoptosis, including the P13K, ubiquitin/proteasome, and nuclear factor kappa b pathways.[46] They offer other opportunities to enhance apoptosis.

DNA REPAIR GENE MUTATIONS: OPPORTUNITIES FROM SYNTHETIC LETHALITY

The human cell is very resilient. The cells in the body undergo a million or more mutations in each cell every day, from ultraviolet rays in sunlight to the foods we eat to many other environmental exposures that cause oxidation, alkylation, hydrolysis, and mismatch of the bases.[54] Even in *one* cell cycle replication, oxidation causes thousands of DNA errors that must be repaired.[54] DNA repair is a critical process in normal cell division to correct these mistakes, and if the DNA cannot be repaired, the cell undergoes apoptosis. Mutations and the many methods of DNA repair have been reviewed. There is a process whereby if a cell cannot be fixed by one method (one gene), then another method (a backup gene) takes over so the cell does not have to die. If that other method is also nonfunctional, the cell dies. This process is called synthetic lethality, whereby the cell can live with one mutation in a repair gene, but if the backup repair gene is also mutated, the cell dies.

Recently, it was found that synthetic lethality could be used therapeutically in patients with BRCA1 and/or BRCA2 mutations.[55] BRCA1 and BRCA2 are tumor suppressor genes; they are also DNA repair genes that fix errors in the double strands of DNA by a process called homologous recombination (a way to fix or repair DNA double-strand breaks by physically cutting the DNA strands and putting them back together, as if by using scissors and glue). There are other

DNA repair genes that make a protein product that can repair DNA mistakes by a number of processes; one in particular, base-excision repair, takes over if the BRCA1 or BRCA2 genes are mutated and nonfunctional. This process requires an enzyme to cut out the mistake or error in DNA and then replace it with a newly made correct sequence, called polyadenosine diphosphate-ribose polymerase 1 (PARP1). BRCA1 and -2 breast cancer tumors show that the cells turn up the production of PARP1 (upregulate) as well as its activity in the cell. If PARP1 is inhibited, then neither repair gene can work, the cell stalls in the cell cycle, and the single-strand breaks that are not repaired accumulate. Together with the accumulated double-strand DNA breaks, these single-strand breaks cause the cell to undergo programmed cell death. This process is called *synthetic lethality*, where the cell can survive one mutated repair gene but not a second in the backup repair gene[56] (Figure 4-5).

PARP1 inhibitors have taken center stage recently with the results of early trials of olaparib (AZD2281) and BSI-201. The good news is that while blocking PARP1 in breast cancer cells will kill them, in normal cells, they are not critical; thus there is very little damage to normal cells and little toxicity.

Fong et al. reported on their success with olaparib in patients with BRCA1 or BRCA2 mutations.[57] In these patients, the BRCA mutations make the homologous-recombination repair pathway nonfunctional, which actually causes single-strand DNA breaks to accumulate in the cell; the cell is thus dependent upon the PARP1 enzyme—the backup repair pathway of single-strand breaks— to work so the cell will not have to undergo apoptosis. When PARP1 is blocked by olaparib, the cell dies. Fong et al. reported the results of a phase I trial of 60 patients with BRCA1 or -2 mutations who were refractory to prior therapy.[57] The oral drug was given daily for 2 weeks, followed by 1 week off, then escalated to a higher dose given 3 out of 4 weeks. Adverse effects were nausea, fatigue, vomiting, taste alterations, anorexia, anemia, and thrombocytopenia. Of evaluable patients, 63% had a response (defined by radiologic or tumor marker responses) or stable disease for at least 4 months. Patients without BRCA1 or -2 mutations did not respond.

Because chemotherapy works by damaging DNA, the cancer cells need PARP1 to repair the damage after chemotherapy, and this may explain how some cancers ultimately become resistant or unresponsive to specific chemotherapy agents. Thus, PARP1 inhibitors can enhance the potential of chemotherapy and radiation therapy to cause cancer cell death.[58]

In the second study, O'Shaughnessy et al. explored the efficacy of BSI-201 together with gemcitabine and carboplatin in the treatment of women with triple-negative (ER–, PR–, HER2–) breast cancer, an aggressive breast cancer subtype similar to BRCA1-mutated breast cancers.[59] Patients were randomized to receive either gemcitabine/carboplatin chemotherapy alone on days 1 and 8, or

Figure 4-5   Synthetic lethality.

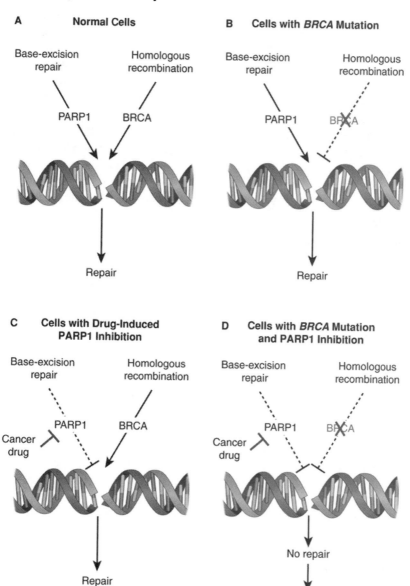

chemotherapy plus BSI-201 at a dose of 5.6 mg/kg IV every other week on days 1, 4, 8, and 11, repeated every 21 days (N = 86 of 120 planned patients). The clinical benefit rate (CBR) was determined by the number of patients with a complete response plus those who had a partial response plus those who had stable disease for 6 months or longer. The experimental group receiving BSI-201 had significantly higher CBR (52% vs. 12%), median progression-free survival (211 days vs. 87 days), and median overall survival (> 254 days vs. 169 days) compared to the control group receiving chemotherapy alone. There was no additional significant toxicity conferred by BSI-201. This appears to be a very promising strategy for attacking the Achilles' heel of BRCA1 and -2–mutated tumors. PARP inhibitors also appear to enhance the alkylating agent temozolomide's efficacy in treating brain cancers, for which it is FDA approved. This success is because base excision repair genes quickly repair the DNA damage the alkylating agent causes.[60] Thus, combining a PARP inhibitor with temozolomide may enhance the cytotoxicity so that more cells are killed.[53]

MITOTIC KINASE INHIBITORS

One of the cardinal hallmarks of cancer is unlimited cell proliferation and growth. The cell cycle is the site of cell proliferation, so it offers a very attractive therapeutic target. However, the cell cycle is complex and is driven by cyclin-dependent kinases (CDKs), which become the target. Disappointingly, though, this strategy has not been very successful, as cells develop cell-cycle–mediated resistance, and the drug cannot injure normal cells.[61] The cell gets a message to divide, often via the RAS/RAF/MAPK signaling pathway, and this raises the level of cyclin D to start turning the cell cycle on. The cell has precise machinery to ensure that the cell is copied exactly and that there are no mistakes; this is accomplished by a highly regulated cell cycle, with checkpoints and tight genetic control of the CDKs, in collaboration with cyclins that turn the cycle around. The cell is tightly regulated as it moves through all the phases of the cell cycle. The actual progression of the cell through the cell cycle occurs when cyclins rise in the cell and push the cell forward. CDK inhibitors stop the cell from moving to the next phase. For example, INK4 inhibits CDK2, -4, and -6, which are often elevated in cancer. KIP (kinase inhibitor protein) inhibits cyclin E/CDK2 and cyclin A/CDK2.[61] Certain genes are active at the checkpoint. Cyclin E and CDK2 are active in G_1/S phases. Progression through the S (synthesis) phase is directed by cyclin A/CDK2, and cyclin A with CDK1 controls G_2. CDK1/cyclin B control mitosis. The cell moves from phase to phase because as the cell moves forward, the cyclins that brought it to the phase they are leaving are tagged by ubiquitin to be degraded by the proteasome. This causes the level to fall, favoring the new cyclins that will move this next phase.

The checkpoints occur in G_1 (restriction point) when the cell decides if it is large enough and has enough food to support the cell. This phase also controls the entry into the S (synthesis) phase; the cell commits to division, it cannot turn back. The G_1/S checkpoint is controlled by the retinoblastoma tumor suppressor gene product Rb, and other checkpoints inspect the DNA for any mutations or errors. DNA repair genes are called upon to fix the mistakes if needed, as well as a mitotic checkpoint that checks that the chromosomes are aligned on the centromere correctly. If the DNA repair cannot fix the mistake, the cell is sent to apoptosis via p53 protein, which begins the intrinsic apoptotic pathway.

Therapeutic targeting of the mitotic machinery includes targeting cell cycle kinases,[62] inhibitors of checkpoint kinases,[63] and inhibitors of Aurora kinases, which control the centrosome, mitotic spindle, and other critical processes in mitosis.[64] Understanding the actual deregulation of the cell cycle in cancer has been difficult. Lapenna and Giordano discuss some of the known alterations that give direction to possible targets.[62] For example, familial melanoma cells cannot bind an INK4 inhibitor, so there is deregulation of CDK4. In melanomas, gliobastomas, and other cancers, CDK4 is overexpressed due to gene amplification; thus, RB1 (retinoblastoma protein that guards the genome) loses control over cell division. Several cancers, including breast, colorectal, and bladder, overexpress Aurora A, leading to chromosomal instability and tumorigenesis. Drugs that target these known flaws have been identified and are now undergoing phase I clinical trials. Some of the drugs, such as XL88 (EXEL-9844), are multitargeted and target CHK1, CHK2, VEGFR-2, and PDGFR. Some drugs being tested that target the Aurora kinases include[53,62]:

- AZD1152: Aurora B, highly potent and selective, induces chromosome misalignment, halts cell division, and induces apoptosis
- CYC-116: Cyclacel, a pan-Aurora inhibitor and VEGFR-2 inhibitor
- MK-0457: Targets the ATP binding site on all Aurora kinases and has synergy with docetaxel

Aurora kinases are a family of three serine/threonine kinases that are necessary for cells to divide. They help the chromasomes line up on the centromere, which must be done exactly right or the cell will be unable to divide. Aurora A moves to the centrosome where it regulates the centrosome and formation of the mitotic spindle. The detailed description of its function is shown in Table 4-3. Aurora B belongs to a bigger protein called a chromosomal passenger protein complex, and it makes sure that the chromosomes are accurately segregated. They also help during cytokinesis (division of the cytoplasm so that each daughter cell gets half of the cell's cytoplasm). Aurora A is often overexpressed. Aurora C is found only in the testes and plays a role in spermatogenesis.[53] The

Table 4-3   The Aurora Kinases

Type	Function
Aurora A	Regulates cell cycle events starting in late S phase through the M phase. Most importantly, it regulates centrosome function and mitotic spindle formation. Specifically, it is responsible for centrosome maturation, mitotic entry, centrosome separation, bipolar-spindle assembly, chromosome alignment on the metaphase plate, cytokinesis, and mitotic exit, as evidenced by increased protein levels and kinase activity starting from late G_2 through M phase, peaking in prometaphase. When Aurora A has completed its work, it is tagged by ubiquitin and degraded so that it stops functioning. During G_2, Aurora A becomes activated so it can mediate other events through interaction with p53, MBD3 (potential activator of histone deacetylase 1), and BRCA1, which can be important mediators of malignant transformation. In cancer, Aurora A does not go to the right place (localization to the centrosomes and mitotic spindle), and it is expressed at the wrong time (normally expressed during G_2 to M transition); instead, it is found throughout the cell and is active starting in G_1 and S phases of the cell cycle.
Aurora B	Aurora B's main job is to make sure the chromosomes on the mitotic spindle are placed accurately and that the cytoplasm is divided evenly between the two daughter cells (cytokinesis). It also ensures correct attachment of the microtubules. During the beginning of metaphase (prometaphase), it makes sure the centromeric proteins are stabilized and in the right places, including survivin, a protein that helps to activate it. It mediates the action of histone H3, a protein involved in chromosome condensation and mitotic entry. It also repairs incorrect microtubule attachments, as detected by tension sensors. If it cannot fix it, it senses the lack of tension in the centromere and activates the mitotic checkpoint. There is a signaling cascade that stops the cell from going from metaphase to anaphase, even when a single chromosome is not attached correctly to the mitotic spindle. Aurora B recruits specific checkpoint proteins, including Mad2. If Aurora B is mutated, or once it has done its job, it is tagged by ubiquitin, and degrades by the ubiquitin/proteasome pathway. If Aurora B does not do its job, the mitotic checkpoint does not work, resulting in more and more aneuploid cells, genetic instability, and tumor formation.
Aurora C	Aurora C is involved in spermatogenesis and is found in the testes. Its role in cancer is unknown.

Data from VanderPorten EC, Taverna P, Hogan J et al.[65]

Figure 4-6   The Aurora family.

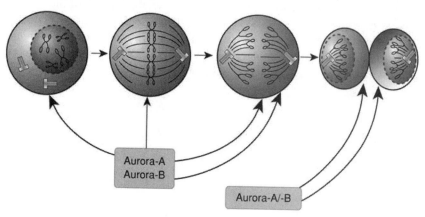

Aurora A is active in building the mitotic spindle, upon which the chromosomes line up during mitosis. Aurora B ensures that the chromosomes are aligned properly at the spindle checkpoint, as well as during cytokinesis.

Data from Jackson JR, Patrick DR, Dar MM, Huang PS. Targeted antimiotic therapies: Can we improve on tubulin agents? *Nat Rev Cancer* 2007;7(2):107-117; Fu J, Bian M, Jiang Q, Zhang C. Roles of aurora kinases in mitosis and tumorigenesis. *Mol Cancer Res* 2007;5(1):1-10.

Aurora kinases are so named because in mutated forms, the mitotic spindles that are formed resemble the Aurora Borealis.

The Aurora kinase inhibitor SNS-314 shows broad therapeutic potential with chemotherapeutics and synergy with microtubule-targeted agents in a colon carcinoma model. It is thought that Aurora kinase inhibitors will work best with chemotherapy as shown in Figure 4-6. For example, with the investigational agent SNS-314 in animal models, it worked best when followed by either docetaxel or vincristine, both spindle poisons.[65]

Although an attractive target, progress developing an effective agent has been slow. It appears that in order to block Aurora A, Aurora B must be present and active, so that dual inhibition of both A and B inhibitors will block only Aurora A and not B.[53]

Another strategy to target the mitotic machinery is with kinesin spindle protein (KSP) inhibitors. KSP helps move cellular organelles, vesicles, and microtubules to where they are needed in the cell, using ATP (the cell's energy currency). If the KSPs are disabled and cannot do their job, the cell undergoes mitotic arrest and apoptosis.[53] KSP inhibitors being studied include monastrol and ispinesib (SB-715992).

SUMMARY

Great strides have been made in understanding the importance of the microenvironment in bone metastases, and evidence suggests that halting the destructive process in fact slows cancer progression. Studies continue to find molecular flaws in apoptosis and other molecular flaws in cancer cells. However, despite the many strides and new targets, much work remains.

REFERENCES

1. Roodman GD. Mechanisms of bone metastasis. *N Engl J Med.* 2004;350(16):1655-1664.

2. Coleman RE, Rubens RD. The clinical course of bone metastases from breast cancer. *Br J Cancer.* 1987;55:61-66.

3. Lacroix M. Significance, detection, and markers of disseminated breast cancer cells. *Endocr Relat Cancer.* 2006;13:1033-1067.

4. Chiang AC, Massague JM. Molecular basis of metastasis. *N Engl J Med.* 2008;359(26): 2814-2823.

5. Jones DH, Nakashima T, Sanchez OH, et al. Regulation of cancer cell migration and bone metastasis by RANKL. *Nature.* 2006;440(30):692-696.

6. Yeung RS. The osteoprotegerin/osteoprotegerin ligand family: Role in inflammation and bone loss. *J Rheumatol* 2004;31(5):844-846.

7. Eli Lilly and Co. http://www.lilly.com/news/pdf/bone_remodeling_process_1003.pdf

8. Mundy GR. Metastasis to bone: causes, consequences and therapeutic opportunities. *Nat Rev Cancer.* 2002;2:584-593.

9. Powell GJ, Southby J, Danks JA, et al. Localization of parathyroid hormone-related protein in breast cancer metastases: increased incidence in bone compared with other sites. *Cancer Res.* 1991;51:3059-3061.

10. Chirgwin JM, Guise TA. Molecular mechanisms of tumor-bone interactions in osteolytic metastases. *Crit Rev Eukaryot Gene Expr.* 2000;10:159-178.

11. Chattopadhyay N. Effects of calcium-sensing receptor on the secretion of parathyroid hormone-related peptide and its impact on humoral hypercalcemia of malignancy. *Am J Physiol Endocrinol Metab.* 2006;290:E761-E770.

12. Bu G, Lu W, Liu CC, et al. Breast cancer derived Dickkopf1 inhibits osteoblast differentiation and osteoprotegerin expression: implications for breast cancer osteolytic bone metastases. *Int J Cancer.* 2008;123(5):1034-1042.

13. Guise TA, Mohammad KS, Clines G, et al. Basic mechanisms responsible for osteolytic and osteoblastic bone metastases. *Clin Cancer Res.* 2006;12(20 suppl):6213s-6216s.

14. Oades GM, Coxon J, Colston KW. The potential role of bisphosphonates in prostate cancer. *Prostate Cancer Prostatic Dis.* 2002;5:264-272.

15. Choi SJ, Cruz JC, Craig F, et al. Macrophage inflammatory protein 1-alpha is a potential osteoclast stimulatory factor in multiple myeloma. *Blood.* 2000;96:671-675.

16. Giuliani N, Colla S, Morandi F, et al. Myeloma cells block RUNX2/CBFA1 activity in human bone marrow osteoblast progenitors and inhibit osteoblast formation and differentiation. *Blood.* 2005;106(7):2472-2483.

17. Carducci MA, Jimeno A. Targeting bone metastasis in prostate cancer with endothelin receptor antagonists. *Clin Cancer Res.* 2006;12(2):6296s-6300s.

18. Hortobagyi GN, Theriault RL, Lipton A, et al. Long-term prevention of skeletal complications of metastatic breast cancer with pamidronate. Protocol 19 Aredia Breast Cancer Study Group. *J Clin Oncol.* 1998;16(6):2038-2044.

19. Gnant M, Mlineritsch B, Schippinger W, et al. Endocrine therapy plus zoledronic acid in premenopausal breast cancer. *N Engl J Med.* 2009;360(7):679-691.

20. Pavlakis N, Schmidt R, Stockler M. Bisphosphonates for breast cancer. *Cochrane Database Syst Rev.* 2005;3:CD003474.

21. Prolia. Drugs.com Web site. http://www.drugs.com/nda/denosumab_090218.html?printable=1. Accessed October 2, 2009.

22. Schwartz EM, Ritchlin CT. Clinical development of anti-RANKL therapy. *Arthritis Res Ther.* 2007;9(suppl 1):S1-S6.

23. Coleman RE. Targeting the tumor microenvironment: denosumab, a new RANKL inhibitor. *Breast Cancer Res.* 2009;11(suppl 1):S16. Presented at VIII Madrid Breast Cancer Conference: Latest Advances in Breast Cancer. Madrid, Spain; June 24-26, 2009.

24. Fizazi K, Bosserman L, Guozhi G, Skacel T, Markus R. Denosumab treatment of prostate cancer with bone metastases and increased urine N-telopeptide levels after therapy with intravenous bisphosphonates: results of a randomized phase II trial. *J Urology.* 2009;182(2):509-616.

25. Fizazi K, Lipton A, Mariette X, et al. Randomized phase II trial of denosumab in patients with bone metastases from prostate cancer, breast cancer, or other neoplasms after intravenous bisphosphonates. *J Clin Oncol.* 2009;27(10):1564-1571.

26. Lonning PE. Endocrine therapy and bone loss in breast cancer: time to closing in the RANK(L)? *J Clin Oncol.* 2008;26(20):4859-4861.

27. Ellis GK, Bone HG, Chllebowski R, et al. Randomized trial of denosumab in patients receiving adjuvant aromatase inhibitors for nonmetastatic breast cancer. *J Clin Oncol.* 2008;26(30):4875-4882.

28. Saad F, Smith MR, Smith B, et al. Denosumab for prevention of fractures in men receiving androgen deprivation therapy (ADT) for prostate cancer. *J Clin Oncol.* 2009;27:15s. Abstract 5056.

29. Smith MR, Ellis G, Saad T, et al. Effect of denosumab on bone mineral density (BMD) in women with breast cancer (BC) and men with prostate cancer (PC) undergoing hormone ablation therapy. *J Clin Oncol.* 2009;27:15s. Abstract 9520.

30. Shahinian VB, Kuo Y-F, Freeman JL, Goodwin JS. Risk of fracture after androgen deprivation for prostate cancer. *N Engl J Med.* 2005;352(2):154-164.

31. Kyle RA, Yee GC, Somerfield MR, et al. American Society of Clinical Oncology 2007 clinical practice guidelines update on the role of bisphosphonates in multiple myeloma. *J Clin Oncol.* 2007;17(10):2464-2472.

32. Durie BGM, Katz M, Crowley J. Osteonecrosis of the jaw and bisphosphonates. *N Engl J Med.* 2005;353:99-110.

33. Ruggiero S, Gralow J, Marx RE, Engroff SL. Practical guidelines for the prevention, diagnosis, and treatment of osteonecrosis of the jaw in patients with cancer. *J Oncol Pract.* 2006;2(1):7-14.

34. Christodoulou C, Pervena A, Klouvas G, et al. Combination of bisphosphonates and antiangiogenic factors induces osteonecrosis of the jaw more frequently than bisphosphonates alone. *Oncology.* 1009;76:209-211.

35. Dental health during cancer treatment. Zometa Web site. http://www.us.zometa.com/info/cancer _bones/dental_health.jsp. Accessed October 2, 2009.

36. American Society of Clinical Oncology (ASCO). ASCO Clinical practice guideline: The role of bisphosphonates in multiple myeloma. http://jco.ascopubs.org/cgi/content/full/20/17/3719. Accessed October 21, 2009.

37. Weinberg RA. Mechanisms of malignant progression. *Carcinogenesis.* 2008;29(6):1092-1095.

38. DePinho RA, Polyak K. Cancer chromosome in crisis. *Nat Genet.* 2004;36(9):932-934.

39. Chin K, de Solorzano CO, Knowles D, et al. *In situ* analyses of genome instability in breast cancer. *Nat Genet.* 2004;36(9):984-988.

40. Are we "Livin" or just "Survivin"? Imgenex Web site. http://www.imgenex.com/emarketing /081606_LivinorSurvivin/LivinorSurvivin_forweb.htm. Accessed October 2, 2009.

41. Susin SA, Daugas E, Ravaagnan L, et al. Two distinct pathways leading to nuclear apoptosis. *J Exp Med.* 2000;192(4):571-580.

42. Nagata S. Apoptotic DNA fragmentation. *Exp Cell Res.* 2000;256(1):12-18.

43. Li MO, Sarkasian MR, Mehal WZ, Rakic P, Flavell RA. Phosphatidylserine receptor is required for clearance of apoptotic cells. *Science.* 2003;302(5650):1560-1563.

44. Riedl SJ, Salvesen GS. The apoptosome: signaling platform of cell death. *Nat Rev Mol Cell Biol.* 2007;8:405-413.

45. Goodsell DS. The molecular perspective: Bcl-2 and apoptosis. *Oncologist.* 2002;7(3):259-260.

46. Ghobrial IM, Witzig TE, Adjei AA. Targeting apoptosis pathways in cancer therapy. *CA Cancer J Clin.* 2005;55:178-194.

47. Spurgers KB, Chari NS, Bohnenstiehl NL, McDonnell TJ. Molecular mediators of cell death in multistep carcinogenesis: a path to targeted therapy. *Cell Death Differentiation.* 2006;13:1360-1370.

48. Ashkenazi A. Targeting death and decoy receptors of the tumor necrosis factor superfamily. *Nat Rev Cancer.* 2002;2:420-430.

49. Fukuda S, Pelus LM. Survivin, a cancer target with an emerging role in normal adult tissues. *Mol Cancer Ther.* 2006;5(5):1087-1098.

50. Almasan A, Ashkenazi A. Apo2L/TRAIL: apoptosis signaling, biology, and potential for cancer therapy. *Cytokine Growth Factor Rev.* 2003;14(3-4):337-348.

51. Ashkenazi A, Holland P, Eckhardt SG. Ligand-based targeting of apoptosis in cancer: the potential of recombinant human apoptosis ligand 2/tumor necrosis factor-related apoptosis-inducing ligand (rhApo2L/TRAIL). *J Clin Oncol.* 2008;26:3621-3630.

52. Jin H, Yang R, Ross J, et al. Cooperation of the agonistic DR5 antibody Apomab with chemotherapy to inhibit orthotopic lung tumor growth and improve survival. *Clin Cancer Res.* 2008; 14:7733-7744.

53. Ma WW, Adjei AA. Novel agents on the horizon for cancer therapy. *CA Cancer J Clin.* 2009;59:111-137.

54. Lodish H, Berk A, Matsudaira P, et al. *Molecular Biology of the Cell.* 5th ed. New York, NY: WH Freeman;.2004:963.

55. DeSoto JA, Deng C-X. PARP-1 inhibitors: are they the long-sought genetic drugs for BRCA1/2-associated breast cancers? *Int J Med Sci.* 2006;3(4):117-123.

56. Iglehart JD, Silver DP. Synthetic lethality—a new direction in cancer-drug development. *N Engl J Med.* 2009;361(2):189-191.

57. Fong PC, Boss DS, Yap TA, et al. Inhibition of poly(ADP-ribose) polymerase in tumors from BRCA mutation carriers. *N Engl J Med.* 2009;361(2):123-134.

58. Virag L, Szabo C. The therapeutic potential of poly(ADP-Ribose)polymerase inhibitors. *Pharm Rev.* 2002;54:375-429.

59. O'Shaughnessy J, Osborne O, Pippen J, et al. Efficacy of BSI-201, a poly (ADP-ribose) polymerase-1 (PARP1) inhibitor, in combination with gemcitabine/carboplatin (G/C) in patients with metastatic triple-negative breast cancer (TNBC): results of a randomized phase II trial. *J Clin Oncol.* 2009;27(suppl; abstr 3):18s.

60. Trivedi RN, Almeida KH, Fornsaglio JL, et al. The role of base excision repair in the sensitivity and resistance to temozolomide-mediated cell death. *Cancer Res.* 2005;65:6394-6400.

61. Shah MA, Schwartz GK. Cell cycle modulation: an emerging target for cancer therapy. In: *Horizons in Cancer Therapeutics: From Bench to Bedside.* West Conchohocken, PA: Meniscus; 2003.

62. Lapenna S, Giordano A. Cell cycle kinases as therapeutic targets for cancer. *Nat Rev New Drug Discovery.* 2009;8:547-566.

63. Ashwell S, Zabludoff S. DNA damage detection and repair pathwasy—recent advances with inhibitors of checkpoint kinases in cancer therapy. *Clin Cancer Res.* 2006;14(13):4032-4037.

64. Carvajal RD, Tse A, Schwartz GK. Aurora kinases: new targets for cancer therapy. *Clin Cancer Res.* 2006;12(23):6869-6875.

65. VanderPorten EC, Taverna P, Hogan J, et al. The aurora kinase inhibitor SNS-314 shows broad therapeutic potential with chemotherapeutics and synergy with microtubule-targeted agents in a colon carcinoma model. *Mol Cancer Ther.* 2009; 8(4):930-939.

CHAPTER 5

Challenges in Caring for Patients Receiving Targeted Therapy

DRUG INTERACTIONS: FOCUS ON THE P450 MICROENZYME SYSTEM

P450 Microenzyme System

Many of the new oral-targeted agents are metabolized by the P450 microenzyme system. This metabolic system is an important protective system for humans and has evolved over the past 3 billion years. It is a superfamily of isoenzymes found in the endoplasmic reticulum and mitochondrial membranes of cells and functions to detoxify poisons that enter the body from ingestion or from inhalation. Thus, these isoenzymes are located in cells lining the nose, kidneys, lungs, small intestines, and liver, and in the saliva.

By definition, these isoenzymes contain heme, which binds to oxygen, thus starting the process of hydroxylation, which leads to the oxidative metabolism (breakdown) of toxins or drugs for excretion from the body. This process led to the name cytochrome, or colored cells. The P450 microenzyme system is responsible for 75% of all drugs metabolized. There are two phases of drug metabolism.[1] Phase I involves oxidation or reduction reactions that are mediated by the P450 oxidative or reductase isoenzymes. Phase II involves conjugation of a water-soluble substance to the drug, such as glucuronate, so that it will be more easily excreted in the bile or urine. In addition, this superfamily is responsible for the synthesis and breakdown of estrogen (aromatase is a P450 isoenzyme) and testosterone, cholesterol synthesis, and vitamin D metabolism.[2]

Letters and numbers are used to indicate which of the multiple pathways are involved in metabolizing a drug. The superfamily is the cytochrome family, and it is designated by CYP. This is followed by a number (which refers to the family), a letter (which refers to the subfamily), and finally by another number (which refers to the gene in that subfamily).

The isoenzyme CYP3A4 is responsible for most drug metabolism, followed by CYP2D6. In addition to the isoenzyme, however, there are differences in how people metabolize drugs, and these differences influence the drug effect. Interpersonal variation relates to the fact that people can have different copies (alleles) of the genes that code for the isoenzyme. These different copies are called polymorphisms. Sometimes, they represent ethnic variation; sometimes they are simply differences in the inherited gene copies.

In general, people metabolize drugs in one of three ways:

- Ultrarapid: The drug is broken down quickly and serum levels of the drug are low. This may mean the person needs a higher dose of the drug to get the same effect as someone who breaks it down more slowly.
- Extensive (normal)
- Poor: The drug is broken down very slowly, and high serum levels of the drug persist until the drug is finally broken down. This person will have side effects from the drug at a dose that most people tolerate; the dose will need to be decreased so the person can get the benefit without the side effects.

To understand these differences in metabolism better, consider a patient with a gene polymorphism for the UGT1A1*28* genotype who receives irinotecan. This person is not able to break down the active metabolite SN-38 easily; thus, SN-38 serum levels are high, resulting in a higher risk for bone marrow depression, neutropenia, and sepsis, and requiring a dose reduction. Another person with a normal copy of the gene would likely tolerate the given dose very well with few side effects. Another example is tamoxifen, a prodrug that needs to be metabolized by the P450 isoenzyme CYP2D6 to form the active metabolite endoxifen so it can suppress estrogen stimulation of a breast cancer cell.[2] Goetz et al. found that postmenopausal women who had undergone surgery and were receiving adjuvant hormonal therapy with tamoxifen, and who had a polymorphism in the CYP2D6 gene making them poor metabolizers, had 3.8 times the risk for developing breast cancer recurrence than extensive metabolizers over the 5-year period of the study.[3] This has led to a recommendation to test women for CYPD6 gene function prior to beginning tamoxifen therapy.

Lastly, again in patients who have a CYP2D6 deficiency, these patients are unable to convert the drug codeine to its active metabolite morphine, so they will not receive any analgesic benefit from taking codeine. An individual inherits one copy of a gene from each parent, and these copies are called alleles or gene copies. In terms of CYP2D6, people can be classified as poor metabolizers if they have two nonfunctional alleles at CYP2D6, extensive metabolizers (normal) if they have one or two functioning alleles, and ultrarapid metabolizers if they have duplicated or amplified gene copies (extra copies).[4] It is estimated that 7–10% of whites are poor drug metabolizers, while 1–7% of whites and more than 25% of Ethiopians have gene amplifications and are ultrarapid metabolizers.[4]

Some of the language surrounding this superfamily of isoenzymes can be confusing. Drugs can be metabolized by one or a few of the isoenzymes. These same drugs can also be induced (increased rate of metabolism) or inhibited (decreased rate of metabolism) by other drugs when given together. In addition, that same drug may inhibit the same enzyme that metabolizes it, as with erythromycin. Finally, a drug can be metabolized by one enzyme and inhibit another enzyme.

If a drug is being metabolized, it is called a *substrate*. If a drug inhibits the enzyme's activity so that the substrate is incompletely metabolized, it is called an *inhibitor*. This means that the drug's serum level in the patient is higher because it has not been completely broken down, and the patient is at risk for more toxicity from the persistent and higher serum levels. Two such drugs should not be given together, or the dosages should be reduced.

If a drug induces the metabolism of the substrate, it increases the metabolism of the drug, and the serum levels can be greatly reduced because the drug is broken down so fast and completely. The substrate drug dose will need to be increased unless the interacting drug can be discontinued.

Today, many patients want holistic care, and they often use botanicals. Some of these botanicals interact with chemotherapy and biotherapy. For example, St. John's wort is a CYP3A4 inducer; if it is taken by a patient being treated with irinotecan, the drug will have a significantly reduced effect. St. John's wort also interferes with most tyrosine kinase inhibitors, which are metabolized by the CYP3A4 isoenzyme. Table 5-1 summarizes these effects.

Table 5-1   Important Drug Interactions Between P450 Isoenzyme Pathways and Targeted Therapies

Drug	P450 Isoenzyme Pathway	Inducer or substrate
Bexarotene (Targretin)	CYP3A4	**CYP3A4 inhibitors:** These drugs **may increase** serum levels of bexarotene: amprenavir, aprepitant, atazanavir, cimetidine, clarithromycin, diltiazem, erythromycin, fluconazole, itraconazole, ketoconazole, gemfibrozil, grapefruit, grapefruit juice, indinavir, nefazodone, nelfinavir, ritonavir, saquinavir, telithromycin, verapamil, voriconazole. Do NOT give together with gemfibrozil; avoid coadministration with other drug(s) if possible, or monitor closely for drug side effects. **CYP3A4 inducers:** May decrease serum bexarotene concentrations: carbamazepine, dexamethasone, efavirenz, griseofulvin, modafinil, nafcillin, nevirapine, phenobarbital, phenytoin, primidone, rifabutin, rifampin, St. John's wort. Avoid coadministration if possible. If coadministered, assess need for increased bexarotene dose. Do NOT give together with St. John's wort.

(continues)

Table 5-1   Important Drug Interactions Between P450 Isoenzyme Pathways and Targeted Therapies (continued)

Drug	P450 Isoenzyme Pathway	Inducer or substrate
Bexarotene (Targretin) (continued)		**Other:** Bexarotene decreases tamoxifen plasma concentration by 35%; may also decrease serum levels of systemic hormonal contraceptives. Avoid coadministration if possible, and use two types of contraception, including one type of barrier contraceptive.
Bortezomib (Velcade)	CYP3A4, 2C19, 1A2; minor 2D6 and 2C9	**CYP3A4 inhibitors:** These drugs **may increase** serum levels of bortezomib: amprenavir, aprepitant, atazanavir, cimetidine, clarithromycin, diltiazem, erythromycin, fluconazole, itraconazole, ketoconazole, gemfibrozil, grapefruit, grapefruit juice, indinavir, nefazodone, nelfinavir, ritonavir, saquinavir, telithromycin, verapamil, voriconazole. **CYP3A4 inducers** can theoretically lower bortezomib levels: Carbamazepine, dexamethasone, efavirenz, griseofulvin, modafinil, nafcillin, nevirapine, phenobarbital, phenytoin, primidone, rifabutin, rifampin, St. John's wort. Assess for efficacy of bortezomib and need for increased drug dose. Do NOT give together with St. John's wort. Melphalan-prednisone coadministration increased bortezomib serum levels, but this is not thought to be clinically relevant. **CYP2C9 inhibitor:** Omeprazole coadministration did not affect bortezomib serum levels. Other drugs that are inhibitors or inducers of P4503A4 should be closely monitored for either toxicities or decreased efficacy.
Dasatinib (Sprycel)	CYP3A4	**CYP3A4 inhibitors:** These drugs may decrease metabolism of dasatinib, resulting in increased serum concentrations of dasatinib: amprenavir, aprepitant, atazanavir, cimetidine, clarithromycin,

Table 5-1   Important Drug Interactions Between P450 Isoenzyme Pathways and Targeted Therapies (continued)

Drug	P450 Isoenzyme Pathway	Inducer or substrate
Dasatinib (Sprycel) (continued)		diltiazem, erythromycin, fluconazole, itraconazole, ketoconazole, gemfibrozil, grapefruit, grapefruit juice, indinavir, nefazodone, nelfinavir, ritonavir, saquinavir, telithromycin, verapamil, voriconazole. Avoid coadministration; if must give together, monitor closely for drug toxicity and consider reducing dasatinib dose. **CYP3A4 inducers:** May decrease dasatinib serum levels (e.g., rifampin decreased dasatinib levels by 82%). Others: carbamazepine, dexamethasone, efavirenz, griseofulvin, modafinil, nafcillin, nevirapine, phenobarbital, phenytoin, primidone, rifabutin, St. John's wort. Assess efficacy of dasatinib and need for increased drug dose. Do NOT give together with St. John's wort. Antacids may decrease dasatinib levels; avoid coadministration or administer at least 2 hours before or after the dasatinib dose. **H_2 antagonists/proton pump inhibitors:** May decrease desatinib serum levels. Use antacids instead. **CYP3A4 substrates:** Drug is a time-dependent inhibitor of CYP3A4 and may decrease metabolism of drugs primarily metabolized by CYP3A4, such as alfentanil, astemizole, cisapride, cyclosporine, ergot alkaloids, fentanyl, terfenadine, pimozide, quinidine, simvastatin, sirolimus, and tacrolimus; therefore avoid coadministration or monitor drug closely for side effects. Single dose of dasatinib with simvastatin increases simavastatin (area under curve [AUC]) serum level by 37%.

(continues)

Table 5-1   Important Drug Interactions Between P450 Isoenzyme Pathways and Targeted Therapies (continued)

Drug	P450 Isoenzyme Pathway	Inducer or substrate
Erlotinib (Tarceva)	CYP3A4, CYP1A2	**CYP3A4 inhibitors:** Decreased metabolism of erlotinib and increased its plasma concentration when coadministered with strong inhibitors: amprenavir, aprepitant, atazanavir, cimetidine, clarithromycin, diltiazem, erythromycin, fluconazole, itraconazole, ketoconazole, gemfibrozil, grapefruit, grapefruit juice, indinavir, nefazodone, nelfinavir, ritonavir, saquinavir, telithromycin, verapamil, voriconazole. Coadministration with ketoconazole ↑ erlotinib AUC by 66%; coadministation with ciprofloxacin ↑ erlotinib AUC by 39%. Avoid coadministration. **CYP3A4 inducers:** Carbamazepine, dexamethasone, efavirenz, griseofulvin, modafinil, nafcillin, nevirapine, phenobarbital, phenytoin, primidone, rifabutin, St. John's wort. Coadministration with rifampicin ↓ erlotinib AUC by 66%. Do NOT take with St. John's wort. **CYP3A4 substrates:** Warfarin: increased INR and bleeding possible; monitor INR and decrease warfarin dose as needed. **CYP1A2 inducers:** Cigarette smoking decreases erlotinib serum levels; encourage patients not to smoke, but if unable to smoke, consider cautious erlotinib dose increase and closely monitor for side effects. pH-altering drugs: Erlotinib GI absorption is dependent on a low gastric pH; omeprazole ↓ erlotinib AUC by 46%; avoid coadministration with proton-pump inhibitors or H_2 inhibitors; use antacids if needed, and administer 2 hours before or after erlotinib. Food: ↑ erlotinib absorption to 100% (compared to dosed absorption of 60%); take drug 1 hour before or 2 hours after food intake.

Table 5-1   Important Drug Interactions Between P450 Isoenzyme Pathways and Targeted Therapies (continued)

Drug	P450 Isoenzyme Pathway	Inducer or substrate
Everolimus (Afinitor)	CYP3A4	**CYP3A4 inhibitors:** Decreased metabolism of everolimus and increased plasma concentration when coadministered with: amprenavir, aprepitant, atazanavir, clarithromycin, delaviridine, diltiazem, erythromycin, fosamprenavir, fluconazole, indinavir, itraconazole, ketoconazole, nefazadone, ritonavir, saquinavir, telithromycin, verapamil, voriconazole, grapefruit, grapefruit juice. Avoid coadministration or decrease everolimus dose. **CYP3A4 inducers:** Increase metabolism and decrease everolimus serum levels: Carbamazepine, dexamethasone, efavirenz, griseofulvin, modafinil, nafcillin, nevirapine, phenobarbital, phenytoin, primidone, rifampin, rifabutin, St. John's wort. Avoid coadministration or may need to increase everolimus dose. Do not administer with St. John's wort. Everolimus is a substrate of CYP3A4 as well as a substrate and moderate inhibitor of the multidrug efflux pump p-glycoprotein (PgP).
Gefitinib (Iressa)	CYP3A4	**CYP3A4 Inhibitors:** Decreased metabolism of erlotinib and increased its plasma concentration when coadministered with strong inhibitors: atazanavir, clarithromycin, indinavir, itraconazole, ketoconazole, nefazodone, nelfinavir, ritonavir, saquinavir, telithromycin, voriconazole, grapefruit, grapefruit juice. Coadministration with itraconazole ↑ gefitinib AUC by 88%. Avoid coadministration if possible; if not, monitor closely for gefitinib side effects. **CYP3A4 inducers:** Carbamazepine, dexamethasone, efavirenz, griseofulvin, modafinil, nafcillin, nevirapine, phenobarbital, phenytoin, primidone, rifabutin, St. John's wort. Coadministration with

(continues)

Table 5-1   Important Drug Interactions Between P450 Isoenzyme Pathways and Targeted Therapies (continued)

Drug	P450 Isoenzyme Pathway	Inducer or substrate
Gefitinib (Iressa) (continued)		rifampicin ↓ gefitinib AUC by 85%. Do NOT take with St. John's wort. If must coadminister with phenytoin or rifampicin, consider gefitinib dose increase to 500 mg PO daily if no adverse side effects, and monitor closely. **CYP3A4 substrates:** Warfarin: increased INR and bleeding possible; monitor INR and decrease warfarin dose as needed. pH-altering drugs: Erlotinib GI absorption is dependent on a low gastric pH. Ranitidine and bicarbonate ↓ gefitinib AUC by 44%. Avoid coadministration with proton-pump inhibitors, or H_2 inhibitors. Use antacids if needed, and administer 2 hours before or after gefitinib.
Imatinib mesylate (Gleevec)	CYP3A4, CYP2C9 (warfarin)	**CYP3A4 inhibitors:** May increase serum levels of imatinib mesylate: amprenavir, aprepitant, atazanavir, cimetidine, clarithromycin, diltiazem, erythromycin, fluconazole, itraconazole, ketoconazole, gemfibrozil, grapefruit, grapefruit juice, indinavir, nefazodone, nelfinavir, ritonavir, saquinavir, telithromycin, verapamil, voriconazole. AVOID coadministration or use cautiously and assess patient closely for increased imatinib toxicity. **CYP3A4 inducers** can lower imatinib serum levels. If coadministered with carbamazepine, dexamethasone, phenobarbital, phenytoin, rifampin, or rifabutin, increase imatinib dose by 50%. Do NOT give together with St. John's wort. **CYP3A4 substrates:** Imatinib interferes with CYP3A4 metabolism of the following drugs: • ↑ Simvastatin levels: monitor LDL and reduce simvastatin dose if needed. • ↑ Cyclosporine, pimozide plasma concentrations; avoid concurrent administration.

Table 5-1   Important Drug Interactions Between P450 Isoenzyme Pathways and Targeted Therapies (continued)

Drug	P450 Isoenzyme Pathway	Inducer or substrate
Imatinib mesylate (Gleevec) (continued)		• Triazolo-benzodiazepines, dihydropyridine calcium channel blockers, HMG-CoA reductase inhibit; may have ↑ serum levels; use cautiously and monitor patient closely. • Eletriptan (Repax): do not administer within 72 hours of imatinib; monitor vital signs closely. Interference with drugs metabolized by CYP2D6: if drugs metabolized by CYP2D6 are coadministered with imatinib, serum drug levels of these drugs will be elevated; coadminister cautiously and monitor patient closely. Warfarin: Do not coadminister; use low-molecular weight heparin (LMWH). Acetaminophen: ↑ serum acetaminophen serum levels.
Lapatinib (Tykerb)	CYP3A4, CYP2C8	**CYP3A4 inhibitors:** These drugs may decrease metabolism of lapatinib resulting in increased serum concentrations of lapatinib: amprenavir, aprepitant, atazanavir, cimetidine, clarithromycin, diltiazem, erythromycin, fluconazole, itraconazole, ketoconazole, gemfibrozil, grapefruit, grapefruit juice, indinavir, nefazodone, nelfinavir, ritonavir, saquinavir, telithromycin, verapamil, voriconazole. **CYP3A4 inducers:** May decrease lapatinib serum levels: carbamazepine, dexamethasone, efavirenz, griseofulvin, modafinil, nafcillin, nevirapine, phenobarbital, phenytoin, primidone, rifabutin, rifampin, St. John's wort. If must coadminister, assess efficacy of lapatinib and need for increased drug dose. Do NOT give together with St. John's wort.

(continues)

Table 5-1   Important Drug Interactions Between P450 Isoenzyme Pathways and Targeted Therapies (continued)

Drug	P450 Isoenzyme Pathway	Inducer or substrate
Lapatinib (Tykerb) (continued)		**CYP3A4 and CYP2C8 substrates:** Lapatinib inhibits both pathways so assess for toxicity in coadministered drugs that are metabolized by either pathway. PgP metabolism (transport system): if lapatinib coadministered with PgP substrates (e.g., dexamethasone, loperamide), assess for toxicity from increased substrate concentration. Conversely, lapatinib is also a substrate of PgP so that if given with an inhibitor of PgP (e.g., quinidine), lapatinib drug levels are likely to be elevated; assess for lapatinib toxicity.
Nilotinib (Tasigna)	CYP3A4	**CYP3A4 inhibitors:** These drugs may increase serum levels of nilotinib (strong): atazanavir, grapefruit, grapefruit juice, indinavir, itraconazole, ketoconazole nefazodone, nelfinavir, ritonavir, saquinavir, telithromycin, voriconazole. AVOID coadministration with strong inhibitors; if must coadminister, consider dose reduction of nilotinib and monitor patient closely for toxicity, including QT intervals on ECG. Coadminister cautiously if at all drugs that are moderate inhibitors (amprenavir, aprepitant, diltiazem, erythromycin, fluconazole, verapamil) or weak (cimitidine) inhibitors of CYP3A4; monitor closely for drug side effects. **Inducers of CYP3A4:** May decrease serum nilotinib concentrations: rifampin, phenytoin, phenobarbital, carbamazepine, dexamethasone, rifabutin, rifapentin, St. John's wort. Avoid coadministration if possible. If coadministered, assess need for increased nilotinib dose by 50%. Do NOT give together with St. John's wort. **Substrates:** Warfarin-nilotinib is a competitive substrate, so INR needs to be monitored closely

Table 5-1 Important Drug Interactions Between P450 Isoenzyme Pathways and Targeted Therapies (continued)

Drug	P450 Isoenzyme Pathway	Inducer or substrate
Nilotinib (Tasigna) (continued)		and dose adjusted frequently. Warfarin is metabolized by CYP2C9 and CYP3A4, so warfarin should be avoided if possible. Nilotinib is an inhibitor of CYP3A4, CYP2C8, CYP2C9, and CYP2D6. Nilotinib may induce CYP2B6, CYP2C8, and CYP2C9. Nilotinib is a substrate of the efflux transporter PgP; if administered with PgP inhibitors (e.g., quinidine), serum concentration of nilotinib will be increased; avoid coadministration.
Sorafenib (Nexavar)	CYP3A4, UGT1A9, CYP2C9 (warfarin)	**CYP3A4 inhibitors:** No interaction **CYP3A4 inducers:** May increase the metabolism of sorafenib and decrease its serum level: carbamazepine, dexamethasone, phenytoin, phenobarbital, rifampin, rifabutin, rifapentin, St. John's wort. Avoid coadministration if possible. If coadministered, assess need for increased sorafinib dose. Do NOT give together with St. John's wort. **Substrates:** CYP2B6 (e.g., bupropion, propofol, ifosfamide) and CYP2C8 (e.g., rapaglinide, amiodarone, ibuprofen, loperamide): substrate drug serum levels increased; monitor patient closely for drug toxicity. UGT1A1 (e.g., irinotecan) and UGT1A9 (e.g., propofol): sorafinib inhibits glucuronidation by these pathways, so substrate serum levels may be increased.

(continues)

Table 5-1   Important Drug Interactions Between P450 Isoenzyme Pathways and Targeted Therapies (continued)

Drug	P450 Isoenzyme Pathway	Inducer or substrate
Sorafenib (Nexavar) (continued)		**CYP2C9 substrate:** warfarin: potential increased INR; monitor and correct warfarin dose frequently. Chemotherapy (other) interactions: Docetaxel: ↑ 36–80% AUC; ↑ C_{max} 16–32%; coadminister with caution, if at all. Doxorubicin: ↑ 21% AUC; use together cautiously. Fluorouracil: ↑ 21–47% as well as ↓ 10% in fluorouracil AUC; use caution when coadministering with 5-FU/leucovorin.
Sunitinib (Sutent)	CYP3A4	**CYP3A4 inhibitors:** These drugs may increase serum levels of sunitinib (strong): atazanavir, clarithromycin, ketoconazole, itraconazole, grapefruit, grapefruit juice, indinavir, nefazodone, nelfinavir, ritonavir, saquinavir, telithromycin, voriconazole. AVOID coadministration with strong inhibitors; if must coadminister, consider dose reduction of sunitinib to 37.5 mg PO daily and monitor patient closely for toxicity and effect. Coadminister cautiously if at all drugs that are moderate (amprenavir, aprepitant, diltiazem, erythromycin, fluconazole, verapamil) or weak (cimitidine) inhibitors of CYP3A4; monitor closely for drug side effects. **Inducers of CYP3A4:** May decrease serum sunitinib concentrations: rifampin, phenytoin, phenobarbital, carbamazepine, dexamethasone, rifabutin, rifapentin, St. John's wort. Avoid coadministration if possible. If coadministered, assess need for increased sunitinib dose to a maximum of 87.5 mg PO daily. Do NOT give together with St. John's wort.

Table 5-1   Important Drug Interactions Between P450 Isoenzyme Pathways and Targeted Therapies (continued)

Drug	P450 Isoenzyme Pathway	Inducer or substrate
Temsirolimus (Torisel)	CYP3A4	**Strong CYP3A4 inhibitors:** May increase serum temsirolimus levels (strong): clarithromycin, itraconazole, ketoconazole, atazanavir, indinavir, nefazodone, nelfinavir, ritonavir, saquinavir, telithromycin, grapefruit, grapefruit juice, and voriconazole. Avoid coadministration; if must be given together, consider temsirolimus dose decrease to 12.5 mg weekly; when interacting drug discontinued, allow 1-week wash-out period, then resume dose taking prior to adding interactive drug. **Strong inducers:** May decrease serum temsirolimus level: dexamethasone, phenytoin, carbamazepine, rifampin, rifabutin, rifampacin, pentobarbital. If must give together, consider temsirolimus dose increase to 50 mg weekly; when interacting drug is discontinued, resume dose given prior to adding interacting drug. Teach patient NOT to take St. John's wort.
Tretinoin (ATRA, Vesanoid, All-TransRetinoic Acid)	CYP3A4, 2C8, 2E	**Strong CYP3A4 inhibitors:** May increase serum tretinoin level: atazanavir, cimetidine, clarithromycin, cyclosporine, diltiazem, erythromycin, grapefruit, grapefruit juice, indinavir, itraconazole, ketoconazole atazanavir, nefazodone, nelfinavir, ritonavir, saquinavir, telithromycin, verapamil, voriconazole. No data exist to show increased or decreased effect. However, ketoconazole was shown to ↑ tretinoin plasma AUC by 72%. Use together cautiously if at all. **Strong CYP3A4 inducers:** May decrease serum tretinoin level: dexamethasone, phenytoin, carbamazepine, rifampin, rifabutin, rifampacin, pentobarbital. No data exist to show increased or decreased effect. Use together cautiously. **Substrates:** Antifibrinolytic agents (e.g, tranexamic acid, aminocaproic acid, aprotinin): may cause fatal thrombotic complications; use together cautiously if at all.

Modified from Wilkes GM[5] with permission from the publisher.

ENCOURAGING PATIENT ADHERENCE AND PERSISTENCE

Adherence to and Persistence with Oral Anticancer Therapy

Oncology nurses have long prided themselves on their ability to develop trusting relationships with patients and to teach them, as well as their family members, effective self-care so that patients are able to minimize toxicities and adhere to their anticancer therapies. Nurses know there is a narrow therapeutic window with anticancer drugs; thus; side effects must be tolerated in cancer therapy that usually are not tolerated with general medication therapy, such as nausea, vomiting, and diarrhea, as well as side effects that present perhaps life-threatening risks, such as infection and bleeding with bone marrow suppression. However, because many of the side effects occur days from the actual drug administration, nurses have become expert at teaching patients the requisite self-care strategies to safely minimize or recover from side effects. Oncology nurses are challenged with ensuring that their patients and families receive adequate teaching to enable self-care and to minimize toxicities by early reporting and adhering to recommended interventions.

Infusion nurses have time prior to drug administration to assess tolerance of prior treatment, the effectiveness of the symptom management plan, and self-care ability. While administering treatment, they can further reinforce teaching as well as attend to other tasks, such as triaging patient phone calls to the clinic. During the same visit, nurses can discuss revisions as needed with the physician or midlevel practitioner and revise the plan as needed. This time spent with the patient and family is very important in developing a trusting relationship that is fostered with each visit and telephone call to the clinic. Oral therapies offer a slightly different challenge in that often the treatment nurses do not have an opportunity to meet, let alone develop a trust relationship with patients.

Oral therapies approved for anticancer therapy are increasing in number, and as we have seen, there are many signaling pathways that require blockade; thus, the future may hold "targeted therapy cocktails" that most likely will be oral. As more and more anticancer drugs become oral, the oncology nurse is often left in the infusion room. Because patients receiving only oral antineoplastic therapy are seen by the prescribing physician, nurses may find themselves interfacing with the patient only when they are called in for symptom management. This leaves a large gap in nursing care, and many opportunities to improve patient adherence (following exactly the prescribed instructions) and persistence (ability to continue taking the medication for a long period after the drug is started) for anticancer drug therapy are lost.[6–8] Ideally, the patient would meet the oncology staff nurse, receive teaching about the oral drug, establish a beginning trust relationship, and then develop an ongoing relationship with the nurse over the course of the oral therapy. Targeted therapies will continue to be prescribed as long as the patient is deriving benefit, which may be a number of years.

It is becoming increasingly clear that adherence to oral therapies is challenging, as is persistence with oral anticancer treatment, as evidenced by failure of patients to take their ordered oral medications exactly as prescribed for as long as it is prescribed.[9] Thus, nonadherence and inability to persist with treatment is a very important challenge. It results in ineffective treatment, increased costs (including more physician visits and higher hospitalization rates),[10] and is the single most important modifiable factor that compromises treatment outcomes.[11]

Barriers to Adherence and Persistence

The continued development of oral anticancer drugs, including such agents as multitargeted tyrosine kinases, is two part. On one hand, there is the cost of therapy and reimbursement requirements from Medicare, coupled with the fact that for those who are not cured by cancer therapy, the goal becomes to treat cancer as a chronic illness, which may last for a number of years. On the other hand, patient preference must be considered.[12] While it is recognized that patients with chronic, nonmalignant health problems may not take their medication as prescribed (e.g., the antihypertensive patient who feels well and therefore stops medication), it is a surprise that oncology patients may not adhere or persist in their recommended therapy. For example, one study showed that 15.1% of women who received tamoxifen as part of adjuvant breast cancer treatment chose to stop the tamoxifen before the treatment ended, compared to 26.7% of high-risk women who stopped therapy while taking tamoxifen to prevent breast cancer.[13] Lash et al. found that 31% of women taking tamoxifen for a prescribed 5-year course had already stopped the drug by the 5-year mark, and that this correlated with the patient's belief about the risk–benefit relationship.[14] This adherence is difficult to measure and ranges from patient self-report to pill counts to drug testing of urine (or principal excretion route). It is possible that when patients know their provider is going to measure their pill count, they are more likely to adhere to the prescribed regimen, called the Hawthorne effect.[9,15] Specifically included are cost, toxicity, ability to manage or prevent side effects, and personal factors such as ability to remember, belief in therapy, and cultural beliefs.

Reasons for patient preference of oral chemotherapy center around convenience, as the patient can self-administer the dose at home without having the inconvenience or expense of coming to the clinic—aside from scheduled visits. Often the patient believes that oral chemotherapy is less "severe," with less severe side effects than IV chemotherapy.[12,16] Conversely, patients may hold a cultural belief that only parenteral drugs will work, and though they may agree with the physician who prescribes the medication to avoid insulting the provider, at home they may become nonadherent.[17]

Moore uses the Health Belief Model to better understand patients' motivation to adhere and persist with recommended treatment, which underscores again the need to assess each patient individually and to modify the teaching plan to meet each individual's needs.[18] Central to this model are (1) the individual's own evaluation of his or her health, such as disease severity and perceived vulnerability to the cancer; (2) individual's risk–benefit assessment of the value and need for adherence to the prescribed therapy; and (3) an internal or external stimulus or "cue to action," which prompts the individual to take the medicine.[19]

Cancer is in general a disease of aging, and 77% of all cancers develop in patients aged 55 years and older.[20] In fact, the risk of developing invasive cancer is roughly 1 in 11 (8.44%) in men and 1 in 12 (8.97%) for Americans 40–59 years old, compared to 1 in 6 (15.7%) for men and 1 in 10 (10.23%) for men and women aged 60–69 years, and 1 in 3 (37.7%) and 1 in 4 (26.17%) for men and women, respectively, aged 70 years and older.[21] Along with age-related physiological changes in the ability to see, hear, and understand that affect a person's ability to carry out self-administration and care instructions, aging brings with it physiological variables that affect drug absorption, together with the risk of drug interactions and the risk of polypharmacy.

Targeted agents are combined with chemotherapy, and the self-administration regimen may be complex based on the different drug bioavailabilities when taken with food. For example, lapatinib is approved by the Food and Drug Administration to be taken with capecitabine. The lapatinib is given twice daily without food (e.g., 2 hours before or after a meal), and the capecitabine is given twice daily, 12 hours apart, within 30 minutes of a meal. In addition, the drugs have a different side effect profile, and while not generally life-threatening, they may pose serious challenges to the patient in terms of continuing therapy (persistence), with effects such as hair and skin changes from epidermal growth factor receptor (EGFR) inhibition and hand–foot reactions from the multitargeted agent sorafenib.

Cost, especially for the elderly with fixed incomes, may be a significant barrier, as is navigating the financial form challenges. The nurse should ensure that there is assistance, either by the nurse, pharmacist, or other member of the team knowledgeable about pharmaceutical drug programs, state and local aid, and other possible supports.

Another issue that may engender nonadherence is lack of understanding about drug cautions and fear of the drug. It is important to teach the patient in a supportive way to wash hands and wear gloves if handling the oral drug, but if possible to pop the drug out of the blister pack.[22] However, some drugs come in bottles, and for patients with limited dexterity, it may not be possible not to touch the pill. In addition, patients and families must be taught not to let a pregnant family member touch the drug and that any unused medicine must be returned to the pharmacy for disposal, not put down the toilet. Chan et al. did a cross-sectional survey of patients in Singapore in a single center of 126 patients receiving oral anticancer therapy.[23] They found that although 94% of patients stated they were adherent to therapy, 40% said they habitually washed their hands after administering the drug but only 1% used gloves.

The nurse assesses the patient for adherence and persistence at each interaction. Sometimes patients takes too much of the oral drug because they think if "a little is good, more is better." Conversely, patients may try to stretch the pills out if they are costly.[15] Predictors of nonadherence include the following[9]:

- Pill counts at the visit showing more or less than what should remain
- Complex treatment regimens
- Cognitive impairment, depression, or other emotional or psychological issues
- Treatment of asymptomatic disease
- Inadequate follow-up or discharge planning
- Poor patient–provider relationships
- Missed appointments
- Expensive drugs that have limited drug coverage

In summary, barriers to adherence and ability to persist with treatment can be categorized into individual patient behaviors, including cultural beliefs, drug regimen, and problems within the healthcare system[10,24]:

- *Individual patient behaviors*: Control issues, culture, health beliefs not supported by adherence, poor or inadequate social support system, denial, depression and other mental illnesses, conflicting responsibilities (e.g., self vs. family), language or cultural differences between provider and patient
- *Drug regimen*: Complex schedule, change in schedule/routine required
- *System factors*: Lack of medical support or lack of continuity of care, poor patient education and awareness about disease and treatment, lack of awareness and recognition of the problem of nonadherence by healthcare providers, poor communication/interpersonal relationship between patient and healthcare providers, high cost of medications

Developing Successful Strategies to Support Adherence and Persistence with Oral Anticancer Therapy

Nurses need the time and opportunity to assess patients' ability to self-care and their need for additional support, and to teach patients and their families drug-specific information about side effects and self-administration schedule, to answer questions, and to provide follow-up to assess adherence, problems, and tolerance of the regimen. Nurses must know about the many different drug side effects, prevention strategies to teach the patient, and management priorities. Because it is difficult for the nurse to cover all the aspects of teaching in a short time, some educational resources have suggested checklists. Projects in Knowledge recommends the following checklist to help nurses organize their patient teaching about targeted therapy[25]:

- At the start of therapy, discuss expected benefits of therapy, drug dosing and administration, what to do if a dose is missed, and how to store the oral medication.
- Discuss drug side effects—what are common, what are uncommon and should be reported right away?
- Discuss potential barriers to adherence, such as lack of motivation, side-effect management, and drug cost; provide resources for payment assistance as needed.
- Help patients create strategies to keep track of the medication and to prompt self-administration, such as a pill sorter with or without an electronic monitor, medication planner or calendar, or a timer.
- Assess whether the patient is taking any other prescription, over-the-counter, herbal or complementary medicines, such as St. John's wort, that should be stopped. Teach the patient to report any new medications they want to take BEFORE starting them.
- Discuss the need for dietary modifications, such as avoidance of grapefruit and grapefruit juice if taking drugs that are metabolized by the CYP3A4 microenzyme system.
- Teach women of childbearing age to use effective contraception to avoid pregnancy and to not breastfeed while receiving the drug; teach male patients receiving the epigenetic drugs to use effective contraception while receiving the drug.
- At follow-up visits, assess adherence to the oral regimen and any factors that interfered with adherence; offer alternatives to overcome the barrier.
- Ask if patient experienced side effects and, if so, how they were managed. Offer suggestions to improve management if needed, and answer any questions.

As discussed, many of the targeted therapy side effects are different from those caused by chemotherapy. While nurses are expert in managing diarrhea, they must learn about and become proficient in managing hypertension, EGFR-rash, and hand–foot skin reactions. In addition, they need to teach patients about potentially serious events such as bleeding and cardiac and lung toxicities. The Oncology Nursing Society has evidence-based recommendations for many symptoms such as the management of fatigue, stomatitis, and diarrhea. It is important for nurses to write specific schedules for self-administration of the drugs; for example, erlotinib should be taken at least 1 hour before or at least 2 hours after food, as it significantly increases the drug's bioavailability when the drug is taken with food. If the patient calls with increased toxicity such as diarrhea, the nurse should first ask how the patient is taking the medication (e.g., with food?). Lapatinib is given at a dose of 5 tablets daily, at least 1 hour before or 1 hour after meals, while capecitabine, which is prescribed along with lapatinib, is given twice daily 12 hours apart, within 30 minutes of a meal. Imatinib is given daily for most indications with water and a meal. Sorafenib is given twice daily, at least 1 hour before or 2 hours following food. Sunitinib is given daily with or without food for 4 weeks; the patient is then off therapy for 2 weeks, and the cycle is repeated. Thus, it is clear that a written calendar with boxes to check after the drug is given may be helpful.

Hartigan recommends that each treatment plan be individualized to the patient based on the patient's ability to learn; perceived barriers such as impaired vision, hearing, or ability to understand the nurse's instruction; and motivation.[7] Winklejohn suggests developing standardized written prescriptions, encouraging the use of patient diaries, using medication calendars with check-off boxes, and using drug-specific patient teaching sheets.[6] Many nurses suggest pillboxes, and while these in the past have been offered by pharmaceutical companies, the growing industry-wide attempt to limit vendor influence on prescribing practices has limited the ability of nurses to use these patient educational materials or boxes.

Partridge et al. summarize practical ways to enhance adherence to oral antineoplastic regimens[10]:

- Improve patient–provider communication (e.g., implement skills training for providers, use checklists for dimensions of dialogue, emphasize disease management, not cure, tailor communication to each patient, keep message simple, explain treatment plan carefully, use existing technologies that are appropriate for the patient/family, enlist help of primary care provider, develop reinforcement strategies, consider a patient newsletter addressing adherence and patient issues).
- Increase patient educational opportunities (e.g., waiting room resources, classes on oral therapy, patient support groups).
- Enhance patient role in adherence (e.g., give expectations and medication side effects as well as helpful tips on self-care and adherence, encourage open communication, and reinforce mechanism to report side effects and difficulty getting medicines).

The 2009 American Society of Clinical Oncology/Oncology Nursing Society Chemotherapy Administration Safety Standards, a consensus guideline for outpatient administration of chemotherapy (defined to include targeted agents), recommends the following[26]:

- Practice site should maintain and use standardized regimen-level preprinted forms or computer-generated forms for chemotherapy prescription writing.

- Oral chemotherapy orders should be time-limited and may not be prewritten for more than the written chemotherapy plan allows.
- Prior to starting chemotherapy, the patient should be given **written documentation**, including at a minimum information about diagnosis, goals of therapy, planned duration of chemotherapy drugs and schedule, information on potential short- and long-term side effects, emergency contact information, and plan for monitoring and follow-up.
- Written or electronic patient educational materials about oral chemotherapy should be provided before or at the time of the prescription (preparation, administration, and disposal); educational plan includes family, caregivers, and others based on the patient's ability to assume responsibility for managing self-care.
- Educational materials for patient and caregiver should be appropriate for the patient's reading level and literacy.
- The frequency of office visits and monitoring is appropriate to the agent and is defined in the treatment plan.
- Practice site should have a procedure for documentation and follow-up of patients who miss office visits or treatments.
- Toxicity assessment documentation should be available for planning subsequent treatment cycles.

As our population increases, it is likely that more multicultural patients with cancer will be treated. Avery recommends the following to maximize adherence[17]:

- Use an objective measurement of adherence, such as a patient's refill history or pill count.
- Ask patients to bring in all their medications at each visit (even if it is not their own prescribed medicine).
- Ask open-ended questions rather than *yes* or *no* questions, and use a trained interpreter when language is a barrier.
- Be proactive to get to know patients and to build a trusting relationship with them.
- Take time to explain the diagnosis, cause, and treatment regimen clearly. State the realistic expectations of side effects, dietary changes if any, and support to help patients minimize side effects and promote self-care. Elicit the patient's understanding of the disease, drug, and potential side effects.
- Explain the rationale for each medication, and label the drug with the corresponding condition or symptoms.
- Ask questions about intake of traditional medicines, herbs, fasting periods, etc., and any other cultural factors that might influence adherence.
- Providing pictures and written information in the patient's language as well as English can be helpful. Many patients have a family member who

can read English, while others can understand only very simple elements, such as numbers.

- Avoid complicated medication regimens if possible, and simplify the regimen as much as possible so the patient can comply.
- Emphasize the importance of continuing the medication even if the patient feels well.
- Suggest reminder tools such as Medisets, medication organizers, or alarm systems.
- Balance an authoritative role over the patient by being decisive, but allow for safe treatment changes based on patient's self-perceived needs.
- Have the patient tell you at the end of the appointment what you told him or her so you can assess understanding and recall.

Barefoot et al. have developed and implemented a system intended to maximize the patient's success with adherence and persistence.[27] The system proceeds as follows:

1. The physician tells the nurse that an oral anticancer agent is being prescribed.
2. The physician gets the patient's informed consent using the chemotherapy/biotherapy informed consent.
3. Orders are written on an oral anticancer order sheet, which is sent to pharmacy.
4. The pharmacy screens for interactions with the patient's current medications.
5. The patient is given an appointment for education teaching about the medication as well as safe handling, by an advanced practice nurse.
6. Pre-authorization is obtained as needed or the patient is referred for an assistance program, and pre-authorization for monitoring of laboratory values as needed is also obtained.
7. Patient is given the prescription as well as information about the drug, which is documented in the teaching note.
8. The patient is given a calendar to mark off the doses as they are taken, along with a pillbox and printed material during the educational appointment.
9. The patient's medications are added to the medication reconciliation sheet in the patient's chart.
10. The patient is asked to bring in all prescription bottles at each visit.
11. A note is placed in the follow-up appointment screen (for oral therapy) to remind secretaries that when they call the patients to confirm their next appointment, they should remind them to bring their prescription bottles.

In summary, nurses have much power to help patients and their families value and participate in adherence and persistence of treatment. Nurses assess barriers, and individually provide their patients with strategies that minimize risk of nonadherence and treatment discontinuance (nonpersistence). In addition, the nurse acts as a catalyst to change many of the institutional or health system barriers to provide effective communication and patient teaching, to reinforce learning, and to establish a trust relationship with their patients and families.

REFERENCES

1. Brunton LL, Lazo JS, Parker KL, eds. *Goodman and Gilman's The Pharmacological Basis of Therapeutics.* 11th ed. New York, NY: The McGraw Hill Companies, Inc; 2006:71-93.

2. Brauch H, Jordan VC. Targeting of tamoxifen to enhance antitumor action for the treatment and prevention of breast cancer: the 'personalized' approach. *Eur J Cancer.* 2009;45:2274-2283.

3. Goetz MP, Knox SK, Suman VJ, et al. The impact of cytochrome p450 2d6 metabolism in women receiving adjuvant tamoxifen. *Breast Cancer Res Treat.* 2007;101:113-121. doi: 10.1007/s10549-006-9428-9430.

4. Gasche Y, Daali Y, Fathi M, et al. Codeine intoxication associated with ultrarapid CYP2D6 metabolism. *N Engl J Med.* 2004;351(27):2827-2831.

5. Wilkes GM. Drug essentials: The cytochrome P450 microenzyme system and targeted therapies. *Nurse Edition.* 2009;23(2):22-28.

6. Winklejohn DL. Oral chemotherapy medications: the need for a nurse's touch. *Clin J Oncol Nurs.* 2007;11(6):793-796.

7. Hartigan K. Patient education: the cornerstone of successful oral chemotherapy treatment. *Clin J Oncol Nurs.* 2003;7(6)(suppl 6):S21-24.

8. Hollywood E, Semple D. Nursing strategies for patients on oral chemotherapy. *Oncology.* 2001;15(1)(suppl 2):37-39.

9. Ruddy K, Mayer E, Partridge A. Patient adherence and persistence with oral anticancer treatment. *CA Cancer J Clin.* 2009;59:56-66.

10. Partridge A, Kato PM, DeMichele A. Adherence to oral cancer therapies: challenges and opportunities. In: *American Society of Clinical Oncology Educational Book, 2009.* McLean, VA: American Society of Clinical Oncology; 2009.

11. De Geest S, Schafer-Keller P, Denhaerynck K, et al. Supporting medication adherence in renal transplantation (SMART): A pilot RCT to improve adherence to immunosuppressive regimens. *Clin Transplant.* 2006;20(3):359-368.

12. Weingart SN, Brown E, Bach PB, et al. NCCN task force report: oral chemotherapy. *J Natl Compr Cancer Network.* 2008;6(suppl 3):S1-S14.

13. Veronesi A, Pizzichetta MA, Ferlante MA, et al. Tamoxifen as adjuvant after surgery for breast cancer and tamoxifen or placebo as chemoprevention in healthy women: different compliance with treatment. *Tumori.* 1998;84:372-375.

14. Lash TL, Fox MP, Westrup JL, Fink AK, Silliman RA. Adherence to tamoxifen over the 5-year course. *Breast Cancer Res Treat.* 2006;99:215-220.

15. Partridge AH, Avorn J, Wang PS, Winer EP. Adherence to therapy with oral antineoplastic agents. *J Natl Cancer Inst.* 2002;94(9):652-661.

16. Aisner J. Overview of the changing paradigm in cancer treatment. Oral chemotherarpy. *Am J Health Syst Pharm.* 2007;64(9)(suppl 5):S4-S7.

17. Avery K. Medication non-adherence issues with refugee and immigrant patients. Ethnomed Web site. http://www.ethnomed.org/clin_topics/pharmacy/non_adherence.htm. Published August 2007. Accessed October 3, 2009.

18. Moore S. Facilitating oral chemotherapy treatment and compliance through patient/family focused education. *Cancer Nurs.* 2007;30(2):112-122.

19. Becker MH, Maiman LA, Kirscht JP, Haefner DP, Drachman RH. The Health Belief Model and prediction of dietary compliance: a field experiment. *J Health Soc Behav.* 1977;18:2348-366.

20. American Cancer Society. *Cancer Facts and Figures 2007.* Atlanta, GA: American Cancer Society; 2007:35.

21. American Cancer Society. *Cancer Facts and Figures 2009.* Atlanta, GA: American Cancer Society; 2009:12.

22. Bartel S. Safe practices and financial considerations in using oral chemotherapeutic agents. *Am J Health Syst Pharm.* 2007;64(9)(suppl 51):S8-S14.

23. Chan A, Leow CY, Hian SM. Patients' perspectives and safe handling of oral anticancer drugs at an Asian cancer center. *J Oncol Pharm Pract.* 2009;15(3):161-165. Abstract.

24. Partridge AH. Helping breast cancer patients adhere to oral adjuvant hormonal therapy regimens. *Comm Oncol.* 2007;4:725-731.

25. Projects in Knowledge. *Caring for Oncology Patients: Tips and Tools for Managing Targeted Therapy.* Little Falls, NJ: Projects in Knowledge Inc; 2009. In press.

26. Jacobsen JO, Polovich M, McNiff KK et al. American Society of Clinical Oncology. ASCO/ONS chemotherapy administration safety standards. *J Clin Oncol.* 2009; published ahead of print on October 14, 2009, as 10.1200/JCO.2009.25.1264, available at http://jco.ascopubs.org/cgi/doi/10.1200/JCO.2009.25.1264. Accessed October 22, 2009.

27. Barefoot BE et al. Intramuscular immunization with a vesicular stomatitis virus recombinant expressing the influenza hemagglutinin provides post-exposure protection against lethal influenza challenge. *Vaccine.* 2009.

Glossary

AKT (protein kinase B, PKB): A family of serine/threonine protein kinases produced by three genes that have important roles in a variety of cell signaling functions. The genes are *AKT1*, *AKT2*, and *AKT3*. *AKT1* produces a serine/threonine protein kinase, Akt1, which promotes cell survival by blocking apoptosis and plays a role in protein synthesis, metabolism, and angiogenesis, as well as in moving cells through the cell cycle. Akt1 is a downstream effector of the P13K pathway. In cancer, *AKT1* is considered an oncogene, and when activated, Akt1 continuously sends messages to the cell nucleus to divide and to avoid apoptosis. Akt2 is a signaling molecule in the insulin signaling pathway.

Angiogenesis: The process of making new blood vessels. It is regulated by the balance between proangiogenic and antiangiogenic factors.

Angiogenesis inhibitor: Drug that blocks the process of new blood vessel growth.

Angiopoietin-1, and -2: Proteins important in angiogenesis. They bind to Tie2 receptor tyrosine kinases—and likely also to $\alpha_v\beta_5$ integrins—and influence tumor angiogenesis, inflammation, and vascular extravasation. ANG-1 and ANG-2 have conflicting functions and, depending upon which receptor they bind to, may have antitumor vascular effects.

Anorexia: Severe loss of appetite for food.

Anthracycline: Antibiotic chemotherapy derived from *Streptomyces* bacteria species. Examples include the red-colored doxorubicin (Adriamycin) and daunorubicin (Daunomycin). They work by damaging the DNA in the cancer cells.

Antibody: A protein made by B lymphocytes in response to an invading antigen. It is made of two parts: the Fab portion that binds tightly to the antigen and the Fc portion that calls in the immune system. The antibody can directly kill the antigen, and it can call in the immune system to help in killing the antigen (e.g., complement, antibody-dependent cellular cytotoxicity).

Apoptosis: Programmed cell death or cell suicide. It does not involve inflammation as does necrosis.

Aurora kinases: Kinases that regulate the cell cycle movement from G_2 through division of the cell into two daughter cells. There are three Aurora kinases: Aurora A, B, and C. They are so called because, when mutated, the mitotic spindle is scattered like the Aurora Borealis (Northern Lights).

B-catenin: Protein located in the cytoplasm of the cell that is important in embryogenesis; in the adult, it regulates cell-to-cell adhesion. It is mutated in a number of cancers.

313

Bone morphogenetic protein (BMP): Growth factors and cytokines that can induce the formation of bone and cartilage. They interact with bone morphogenetic protein receptors (BMPRs) on the cell surface.

Bone remodeling: Process whereby old bone is removed (bone resorption) and new bone added (bone formation).

BRCA1 (breast cancer 1, early onset): A tumor suppressor gene; its gene product helps repair DNA double-strand breaks. It also helps in ubiquitination, regulation of gene transcription, and embryo development. Mutation in the BRCA1 gene increases the risk of breast cancer by up to 85% by age 70 years, and of ovarian cancer by 55%. It is thought this happens because the gene product (protein) is too small to fix DNA mutations in other genes. These errors accumulate and increase with each cell division, eventually leading to uncontrolled cell division (cancer).

BRCA2: A tumor suppressor gene. Mutation in the BRCA2 gene increases the risk of breast cancer by up to 85% by age 70 years, and of ovarian cancer by 25%.

Capecitabine: Oral chemotherapy drug that is a 5-fluouracil prodrug. It is given with bevacizumab as a first-line treatment of advanced colorectal cancer, or with lapatinib in the treatment of advanced breast cancer. One of its side effects is hand–foot syndrome.

Capillary leak syndrome: Serious side effect where fluid and proteins leak out of the tiny pulmonary capillaries into the surrounding lung tissue. This causes hypotension and can lead to multiple organ failure and shock.

CDH1 (cadherin 1, E-cadherin): Tumor suppressor gene that is the recipe for the epithelial cadherin or E-cadherin protein that helps epithelial cells stick together (cell adhesion). In addition, E-cadherin helps send messages within the cell, controls cell movement, and regulates certain gene expression. This gene is mutated in lobular breast cancer and hereditary diffuse gastric cancer.

Cell cycle: The cycle of cell division resulting in two daughter cells. There are two phases, interphase and mitosis (M phase, when the cell actually divides into two). Interphase is divided into the G_1 (gap 1), S (synthesis), and G_2 (gap 2) phases. The movement of the cell through the cell cycle is regulated by activation and inactivation of cyclin-dependent protein kinases. Only a few subsets of cells normally go through the cell cycle continuously: hematopoietic stem cells, basal cells of the skin, and cells in the basal layer of the crypts of microvilli in the colon. Some cells, including neurons, striated muscle cells, and the heart muscle cells, become permanently differentiated after leaving the cell cycle and can never divide.

Cell cycle checkpoints: Checkpoints in the cell cycle to identify cells that should not enter or complete the cell cycle due to mutations or other factors. These checkpoints are found at G_1/S, G_2/M, and the spindle assembly checkpoint.

Centrosome: Main microtubular organizing center in the cell, which also regulates cell cycle progression.

Chemokine: Protein that acts as a lure for white blood cells in inflammation and cancer. They likely play a role in luring metastatic cells to their metastatic niche where they can prosper. There are two classes: CXC, which attract neutrophils, and CC, which attract monocytes, lymphocytes, basophils, and eosinophils.

Child-Hugh score: Scale that assesses the prognosis and treatment of patients with chronic liver disease. It uses five clinical measures of liver function to determine the score, and each measure is evaluated on a 1–3 scale: bilirubin, serum albumin, INR, ascites, and hepatic encephalopathy. Class A is 5–6 points, Class B is 7–9 points, and Class C is 10–15 points. It is sometimes used in drug dosing to determine whether drug dose should be reduced or not for a particular patient with liver function abnormality.

Complete response (CR): Complete remission or disappearance of all signs of cancer for at least 1 month. It does not mean that the cancer will not return.

Congestive heart failure: A condition in which the heart muscle gets weak and cannot pump effectively so the blood backs up. It occurs first on the right side of the heart, as the right ventricle has a thin wall with low pressure, resulting in peripheral edema, tachycardia, and other signs and symptoms. After the right side of the heart fails, the left side can fail, causing blood to back up into the lungs and pulmonary edema.

Consolidation therapy: Treatment given after induction treatment to further kill cancer cells.

Cyclins: Proteins that are key regulators of the cell cycle movement. They bind to, and activate, cyclin-dependent kinases (Cdk) to push the cell through the cell cycle by raising or lowering the level of specific cyclin members D, E, A, and B. Cyclin D is G_1 phase specific and regulates the entry of cells from G_0 to G_1; it couples with Cdk4 and Cdk6, and once the cell makes it past the G_1 restriction point, it forces the cell to continue in the cell cycle by causing hypophosphorylation of the retinoblastoma protein (pRb). Cyclin E then takes over along with cyclin A, which bind Cdk2 and move the cell from G_1 into the S phase. Cyclin A starts DNA replication, then Cyclins B1 and B2, with partner Cdk1, move the cell through mitosis.

Cytokine release syndrome: Infusion reaction related to a biologic agent's killing of cells that release cytokines. Characterized by fever, rigors, hypotension, and wheezing, and may rarely be severe and fatal.

Diffusion distance of oxygen: Oxygen can diffuse on its own into tissues located 1–2 mm away (the size of the head of a pencil). For any farther distances, it must be transported by red blood cells via a capillary.

Dimerization: Once a ligand binds to a receptor tyrosine kinase, it begins to activate the receptor. To begin sending the message of instructions to the cell, the receptor must find a partner, called a dimer. The receptor can dimerize with the same receptor as it is, such as EGFR1 and EGFR1, called homodimerization, or it can partner with a neighboring family receptor such as EGFR2, called heterodimerization. Once dimerization occurs, the message is sent through the cell membrane to the inside of the cell, where it is picked up by the tyrosine kinase and sent as if by a bucket brigade to secondary messengers (other tyrosine kinases) that pass it on to the cell nucleus.

Disease-free survival, DFS: Length of time after treatment that signs of cancer are still absent.

DNA repair: The process by which the cell recognizes damage to the DNA and corrects it. How quickly the damaged DNA is repaired depends upon the kind of cell it is, how old it is, and what is going on in its external environment. If the cell is old and has accumulated a lot of damage, it cannot be fixed, so it can (1) go into permanent dormancy (senescence), (2) undergo apoptosis, or (3) undergo unregulated cell division (cancer).

Downstream: Imagine the signaling cascade is a stream taking the cell's message from outside the cell to the cell nucleus. From any point along this stream, those messengers above it are called "upstream" of it, while any messengers below it or between it and the cell nucleus are called "downstream" of it.

Echocardiogram: Diagnostic study of the heart structure and wall motion using high-frequency ultrasound. Determines left ventricular ejection fraction (LVEF). Sometimes referred to as ECHO.

Ectoderm: In the embryo, forms the outside layers of the body, such as skin, hair, sweat glands, epithelium. In addition, the brain and nervous system develop from the ectoderm.

EGFR1, erbB1, HER1: Epidermal growth factor 1 (also human epidermal growth factor receptor, HER1) or EGF receptor, a very important receptor that is overexpressed in colon cancer, rectal cancer, head and neck cancers, and NSCLC. This leads to uncontrolled cell proliferation, avoidance of apoptosis, invasion, angiogenesis, and metastasis. EGFR activation results in activation of the Ras/ERK pathway (cell proliferation), the P13K/AKT pathway (survival), and JAK/STAT pathway (survival). EGFR signaling can be blocked by EGFR inhibitors cetuximab, panitumumab, gefitinib, erlotinib, and lapatinib. Because EGFR is very active in the epidermis or skin, most toxicity is seen in this organ.

EGFR2, HER2/neu, erbB2: *See HER2/neu.*

Embolism: Enlodgement of a blood clot or other substances, such as fat globules or cancer cells, that blocks blood flow in an artery or vein.

Encephalopathy: Change in mental and cerebral functioning caused by severe hypertension, drugs, or disease.

Endoderm: In the embryo, forms all the tissues and organs involved in digestion and breathing, including the lungs, trachea, liver, pancreas, gallbladder, and thyroid and parathyroid glands.

Epigenetic code: Code based on the histone configuration and degree of methylation of DNA. It controls gene expression and whether or not the genes will be hidden (not expressed) or open (expressed). Only the open or expressed genes are transcribed to make the proteins required for normal cellular functions.

Epigenetics: Change in phenotype (appearance) related to gene expression that is not caused by inherited changes in DNA. Rather, it is caused by the regulation of gene expression by the histones about which the DNA coils, and the degree of methylation of the DNA. There is no change in the actual DNA itself. Chromatin is made up of the histone proteins and DNA. Gene expression is regulated by chromatin remodeling and the amount of methylation in the proteins. In normal embryonic cells, the pluripotent stem cell can differentiate into specialized cells and remain in a terminally differentiated state through the life of the person, a quality that occurs through epigenetics. In cancer, some tumors take advantage of epigenetics. If the DNA coils too tightly around the DNA, the gene will be closed or silenced, such as a tumor suppressor gene. In cancer, many tumor cells are hypomethylated, while in other cancers, there may be hypermethylation at specific areas called CpG islands. Cancer can be caused by epigenetic factors, such as that with diethylstilbestrol (DES).

Epithelial–mesenchymal transition (EMT): Embryologic transition from an epithelial cell with cell-to-cell adhesion and anchorage dependence to a mesenchymal type of cell that has lost cell-to-cell adhesion and can leave its home turf (anchorage independence) and migrate to another area. In cancer, it is believed cells undergo EMT to invade neighboring tissue and metastasize.

Excision repair genes: Genes that repair double-stranded DNA using at least three excision methods: mismatch repair, base excision repair, and nucleotide excision repair. If there is a mistake in only one strand of DNA, the mistake is cut out (excised), the correct section is copied from the other strand, and it is replaced in the strand.

Fas ligand (FasL): Transmembrane protein that binds to its receptor, FasR or death receptor, to cause apoptosis. It can also bind to DeR3 (decoy receptor 3), thus preventing FasL from binding to the FasR and preventing apoptosis. It is a member of the tumor necrosis factor (TNF) family.

Febrile neutropenia: A life-threatening condition caused by very low neutrophils (neutropenia) with a fever, usually indicating infection. Having too few neutrophils, the body's first line of internal defense, increases the risk of infection.

Filopodia: Spikes of cytoplasm sticking out of a cell's leading edge as it moves forward; it contains actin filaments and adheres to the tissue (substratum) in the migratory path, thus pulling the cell forward along the migratory path.

First-line therapy: Initial treatment, or standard treatment, for a given cancer, representing the best treatment at the time using available clinical trial evidence. If this does not work, or the disease recurs, it is followed by the next-best treatment, second-line, and then third-line, and so forth.

Fistula: Abnormal opening or connection between two organs, or between an organ and the surface of the body.

Gastrulation: In the embryo, a process that allows cells to migrate to positions where they will form the ectoderm (outer layer), endoderm (inner layer), and mesoderm (middle layer in between the ectoderm and endoderm). After gastrulation, the cells that will form the nervous system fold into the neural tube that will form the spinal cord. The vertebrae form from notochord made by cells in the mesoderm, which also forms the segmented body parts such as the muscles of the body wall.

Gene expression: Process by which a gene—the recipe for a protein—is "turned on" so it can be transcribed. Transcription factors locate the gene sequence in the DNA strand and turn it on so it can be copied or transcribed by messenger RNA and then taken outside the cell nucleus to make the protein.

Glioblastoma, GBM, glioblastoma multiforme, grade IV astrocytoma: Fast-growing primary brain tumor usually seen in adults, and unless completely surgically removed, likely to recur. It is highly vascular, so the antiangiogenic drug bevacizumab is FDA indicated to treat it. It is also mediated by the EGFR signaling pathway; thus, EGFR inhibitors are being studied to treat it.

Hand–foot syndrome: Syndrome involving the palms of the hands and soles of the feet, as well as any skin areas that receive repeated friction. With chemotherapy (e.g., infusional 5-FU, capecitabine) it is characterized by erythema, edema, dysesthesia, blistering, and pain compared to that caused by sorafenib or sunitinib, which is callous-like but also painful and debilitating.

Hedgehog signaling pathway: Important in the embryo, the pathway that tells the cells where they should position themselves (e.g., on the right or left, top or bottom of the embryo) so that they can develop into the right body parts, such as the fingers on a hand. In the adult, this pathway helps regulate stem cells that maintain and regenerate adult tissues. Sonic hedgehog (SHH) is the best known ligand of the Hedgehog signaling pathway, and it binds to the Patched-1 (PTCH1) and PTCH2 receptor. If the ligand is not present, PTCH1 inhibits Smoothened (SMO), which is a protein in the downstream pathway. It is thought that if the Hedgehog is abnormally activated, it may transform adult stem cells into cancer stem cells, which then orchestrate malignant transformation. Activation of the Hedgehog pathway results in increased release of proangiogenic factors (angiopoietin-1, -2) to turn on angiogenesis, cyclin D1 and B1 to turn the cell cycle on, expression of antiapoptotic genes, and decreased expression of apoptotic genes such as Fas to avoid cell death. Hedgehog signaling thus appears to also regulate angiogenesis and metastasis. It is dysregulated in basal cell cancer and is implicated in cancers of the brain, lung, breast, and prostate.

Hemoptysis: Coughing up blood from the respiratory system.

Hemorrhage: Loss of blood from injured blood vessels, often a high volume in a short time.

Hepatocyte growth factor (HGF, scatter factor [SF]): Factor secreted by mesenchymal cells that acts on epithelial and endothelial cells to regulate their growth, proliferation, motility, shape, and ability to regenerate tissue. HGF is the ligand for the proto-oncogene c-Met receptor, and this binding starts a tyrosine kinase signaling cascade to accomplish these actions. C-Met is often mutated in cancer, giving HGF a key role in malignant transformation, angiogenesis, invasion, and metastasis.

HER2 antibody drug conjugate: Monoclonal antibody directed against HER2 and linked with a cytotoxic agent.

HER2/neu, EGFR2, erbB2: Protein involved in normal cell growth. It is a receptor tyrosine kinase. The receptor is overexpressed (many extra receptors on the outside of the cell surface) or the gene is amplified (more than normal copies) in 18–20% of breast cancers, as well as some ovarian, gastric, and lung cancers.

Histone: Protein found in the chromosome that helps pack DNA into tight coils, serving as the spools around which the DNA coils. Histones together with DNA make up the nucleosome. There are six classes of histones (H1–5), and they can be either core or linker histones. They help express genes that need to be transcribed, but in order to do this, the DNA must be open so the gene can be expressed to be copied. In cancer, HDACs take an acetyl group and make the chromatin condensed (closed) so that the gene cannot be transcribed, such as a tumor suppressor gene.

Histone deacetylase inhibitor: Inhibitors that block histone deacetylases (HDAC) from taking an acetyl group; thus, the chromatin relaxes and is open so that the gene can be transcribed, such as a tumor suppressor gene. HDAC inhibitors have been shown to allow p53 tumor suppressor to be active. They cause growth arrest, differentiation, and/or apoptosis of cancer cells by altering gene expression and transcription. Vorinostat is an example of an FDA-HDAC inhibitor.

Insulin-like growth factor (IGF-1): A growth factor with anabolic effects, that is the ligand for IGF-1 receptor (IGFR, a receptor tyrosine kinase) and the insulin receptor. Studies show that increased levels of IGF increase risk for developing cancer.

Integrin: Cell receptor that binds to the extracellular matrix or other cells, and to the inner cell cytoskeleton so that the cell can communicate with its environment (transducer outside-to-inside signaling), and also tell the outside environment about the cell (inside-to-outside signaling). In addition, integrins are important in cell-to-cell adhesion, cell cycle movement, and defining the cell's shape and mobility. They work with other cellular proteins such as cadherins and cell adhesion molecules. There are a variety of integrins, and they have alpha (α) and beta (β) subunits.

Interferon (alpha, beta, gamma): A biologic response modifier that increases the body's immune response to foreign antigens. Interferons are produced by the body, or in the laboratory, and can stop cancer cell division and slow tumor growth.

Ligand: Growth factor or hormone that binds to the cell receptor on the outside of the cell, such as a receptor tyrosine kinase, to initiate a message with instructions for the cell nucleus (e.g., EGF is the ligand for EGFR).

Loss of heterozygosity, LOH: Loss of normal function of one gene copy (allele) in which the other copy was already inactivated. For example, loss of one copy of the gene may happen genetically, such as with the APC in hereditary adenomatous polyposis coloni. Then when the second copy of the gene (allele) develops a (somatic) mutation during the course of life, it results in LOH of this tumor suppressor gene.

LVEF: Left ventricular ejection fraction; normally 55–70%.

Macrophage inflammatory protein (MIP): Chemotactic cytokine (chemokine) produced by macrophages that are stimulated by bacterial endotoxins. It activates granulocytes, leading to neutrophilic inflammation. It then induces the synthesis and release of proinflammatory cytokines IL-1, IL-6, and TNFα from fibroblasts and macrophages. The two major molecules are CCL3 (MIP-1α) and CCL4 (MIP-1β).

Maintenance therapy: Treatment given after initial therapy to keep killing any new cancer cells and to keep the person in remission.

MAPK/ERK pathway: Signal transduction pathway that takes messages from the cell nucleus receptor, such as the EGFR, to the cell nucleus, telling it to divide. It uses docking proteins to activate a molecule called SOS, which then tells Ras to become active. Ras starts the bucket brigade, sending the message to the serine/threonine protein kinases that are next in line—Raf kinase, which phosphorylates and passes the message to (activates) MEK, which sends the message to (activates) mitogen-activated protein kinase (MAPK). MAPK regulates important transcription factors that turn on the cell cycle telling the cell to divide (proliferate). Transcription factors identify which genes need to be turned on, such as C-myc. In cancer, genes that should not be turned on, or that should be turned on then off, are turned on indefinitely via this MAPK so that cancer cells can continue to divide or proliferate. Sorafenib (Nexavar) is the first and only drug available to block part of this pathway, as it is a Raf kinase inhibitor.

Matrix metalloproteinases (MMPs): Family of enzymes that are very powerful destroyers of the extracellular matrix. They usually exist as proenzymes and, in a very carefully controlled way, are turned on when needed and quickly inactivated once they have done their job. In cancer, they are subverted to play an important role in carcinogenesis, angiogenesis, invasion, and metastasis.

MCP1 (monocyte chemotactic protein-1): Protein that helps to recruit monocytes to sites of infection, injury, or inflammation.

Median: Statistically, the middle value of a set of measurements.

Mesenchymal–epithelial transition (MET): Hypothesized transition of cancer cells that have used EMT to metastasize to now return to their normal appearance and behavior as an abnormal epithelial cell.

Mesoderm: In the embryo, forms the muscles, cartilage, bone, blood, and all connective tissue used in movement and support. Also forms the reproductive organs and kidneys.

Monoclonal antibody (MAb): Hybrid antibody (protein immunoglobulin) to a specific antigen, such as an antigen on a cancer cell. It is made using hybridization technology to prepare enough antibodies to treat disease. The protein can be murine (100% mouse), chimeric (both mouse, 70%, and human, 30%), humanized (mostly human, e.g., greater than 90%), and human (100% human). Risk of hypersensitivity is related to how much mouse protein is in the MAb. Infusion reactions may also occur (cytokine release syndrome). MAb-targeted therapy agents are large molecules that do not pass into the cell; they must be administered intravenously.

mTOR signaling pathway: mTOR (mammalian target of rapamycin) is a serine/threonine protein kinase, the "Grand Central Station" of the cell, responsible for regulation of cell growth, proliferation, angiogenesis (hypoxia-inducible factor), cell motility, protein synthesis, transcription, and cell survival. mTOR integrates signals from many upstream pathways (insulin growth factors IGF-1 and IGF-2, input from the external environment, cell nutrient and energy levels, and others). mTOR has two molecular complexes, each with separate function. mTOR complex 1 (mTORC1) is made up of mTOR, Raptor (regulatory associated protein of mTOR), and other proteins; its function is to sense and respond to nutrient, energy, and redox issues through protein synthesis. mTORC1 is stimulated by insulin, growth factors, oxidative stress, and amino acids (building blocks of proteins), while it is shut off by low nutrient levels, absence of growth factor stimulation, reductive stress, caffeine, and curcumin. mTORC2 is made up of mTOR, Rictor (rapamycin-insensitive companion of mTOR), and other proteins. It regulates the cytoskeleton (motility). It too is regulated by insulin, growth factors, and nutrient levels. In cancer, mTOR has been implicated in many malignant processes. Inhibition of mTOR results in cell cycle arrest so that cells cannot progress from G_1 to S phase. Examples of mTOR inhibitors are everolimus (Afinitor) and temsirolimus (Torisel).

MUGA scan: Multiple gated acquisition scan, a technique to evaluate heart function and determine the left ventricle ejection fraction (LVEF).

Myc, cMyc: the *MYC* proto-oncogene codes (is a recipe) for the myc proteins or transcription factors that bind to the DNA of other genes to show which genes need to be copied. It is very important in regulating the expression of 15% of human genes. When the *MYC* gene is mutated, it becomes an oncogene that is overexpressed and leads to the uncontrolled expression or turning on of genes involved in cell proliferation (e.g., turns up the cyclins) so malignant transformation occurs, such as Burkitt lymphoma. In addition, Myc controls genes that regulate apoptosis (downregulates Bcl-2), differentiation, and stem cell renewal. Myc communicates with important signaling pathways such as EGF, sonic hedgehog, and Wnt.

Neuropilin 1 (NRP1): Gene that makes a protein that is a membrane-bound coreceptor for VEGF and semaphoring. It plays a role in angiogenesis, cell survival, migration, and invasion.

Neuropilin 2 (NRP2): Gene that makes a protein receptor that interacts with VEGF. It plays a role in angiogenesis, cell adhesion, nervous system and heart development, and tumorigenesis.

NF-kB (nuclear factor kappa-light-chain-enhancer of activated B cells): A protein complex that acts as a transcription factor. It plays an active role in helping the cell deal with stimuli such as stress, free radicals, ultraviolet radiation, and bacterial or viral infection. It is a "first responder" to threatening stimuli to the cell and rapidly turns on genes to help the cell fight back. It regulates the immune response to infection. In cancer, abnormal regulation is linked to inflammation, cell proliferation, and survival. Because they are so powerful, they remain in an inactive state in the cell's cytoplasm, guarded by inhibitors of kB (IkBs). When needed, a signal is sent to degrade the IkBs via the ubiquitination/proteasome system, thus freeing the NF-kB to move into the cell nucleus where it turns on the expression of specific genes that help the cell to fight back, such as inflammation, immune activation, cell proliferation, or cell survival response. In cancer, because NF-kB plays such an important role in cell proliferation and survival, tumors have figured out how to make NF-kB turned on or constitutively activated all the time so that the genes for proliferation and survival are always turned on. This is accomplished by mutations in genes encoding the NF-kB transcription factors, or the IkB genes, by secreting factors that activate NF-kB.

Notch signaling pathway: Key pathway in the embryo that is critical for cell differentiation (specialization), but it is also activated in adult cells. There are four receptors, NOTCH 1–4, which have an external and internal domain. The pathway is usually turned on by cell-to-cell contact with its neighboring cells. When the ligand binds to the extracellular portion, it cleaves or separates from the internal part, which then goes into the cell nucleus and turns genes on or off. Notch signaling is important in neuron function and development, angiogenesis, heart development, pancreatic function, bone expansion during bone development, and the actin cytoskeleton. Notch signaling is abnormal in many cancers, including T-cell acute lymphoblastic leukemia.

Nucleosome: Unit made up of histones together with DNA.

Oncogene: A proto-oncogene is a normal gene that is involved in cell growth and division. When mutated, it forms an oncogene. Oncogenes turn on uncontrolled cell division (similar to a foot on the gas pedal), driving cell proliferation.

Oncogene addiction: Condition in which inactivation of a single oncogene may result in cell death.

Overall survival, OS: Percentage of patients (subjects) in a study who are still alive at a given time, such as 1 year.

Overexpression: Too much of a protein or other substance. Genes are recipes for proteins that tell the cell what to do. In cancer, many genes are mutated and make too many of some proteins, causing malignant transformation, invasion, and metastasis.

P13K, phosphatidylinositol 3-OH kinase (P13K) signaling pathway: A major signaling pathway that is key to malignant growth and proliferation. This signaling pathway includes the protein kinase Akt and interacts with the mTOR signaling pathway. They are involved in many diverse cellular functions, such as cell growth, proliferation, differentiation, motility, survival, and regulation of glucose uptake. PTEN antagonizes P13K signaling, but it is often mutated in cancer so that P13K signaling is uninterrupted.

p53: The protein made by the *TP53* gene, a transcription factor that regulates the cell cycle and acts like a tumor suppressor, called the "guardian of the genome," or "master watchman of the genome." It checks the DNA, and if mistakes are found, it halts the cell cycle progression and ensures that it is repaired by DNA repair genes; if repair is not possible, the cell is sent to apoptosis. In cancer, over 50% of solid tumors have mutated *PR53*, so that p53 is deactivated and it is unable to transcribe the genes that would either fix DNA errors or send the cell to apoptosis.

Partial response: Partial remission; at least 25% decrease in the size of a tumor that lasts for at least 1 month.

Performance status: Measure of patients' ability to perform activities of daily living, in relation to their disease. One common scale is the Karnofsky performance scale.

Phosphorylation: A process by which tyrosine kinases are given the energy needed to transmit a message to the next messenger. They use phosphorylation to turn the messenger protein on, which means it adds a phosphate group (PO_4) to the molecule, or phosphorylates it. To shut the messenger off after it has sent the message to the next messenger, a phosphatase protein dephosphorylates the messenger, or removes the phosphate group. For example, when p53 identifies DNA that cannot be fixed, it becomes phosphorylated and is able to send the cell into programmed cell death. Only under very strict conditions can this be reversed, and when it is, p53 becomes dephosphorylated, so it stops working. In cell signaling, phosphorylation and dephosphorylation are reversible, like switching the light switch on and off. Phosphorylation for other types of proteins allows them to be tagged and broken down by the ubiquitin/proteasome pathway.

Platelet-derived growth factor (PDGF): Growth factor family that plays a significant role in angiogenesis. Its receptor (PDGFR) is a receptor tyrosine kinase and can be either α or β. It plays an important role in embryogenesis, cell proliferation, migration, as well as angiogenesis. The c-Sis oncogene arises from PDGF.

Primary endpoint: The primary goal or result of a clinical study that is measured to see if one treatment is more effective than another, such as the difference in overall survival or progression-free survival between groups receiving different treatments.

Protein kinases: Enzymes that transmit messages from the membrane of the cell to the nucleus of the cell, as if by a bucket brigade.

PTEN (phosphatase and tensin homolog) gene: Gene that gives the recipe for a tumor suppressor protein found in all body tissues. This protein is a protein tyrosine phosphatase, an enzyme that removes phosphate groups from other proteins and fats. It helps regulate the cell cycle so that there is no uncontrolled cell division, and controls cell movement/migration, adhesion of cells to the surrounding matrix, and angiogenesis. It functions in a signaling pathway to bring cells into apoptosis. Mutations in the PTEN gene are commonly found in cancer, such as prostate and endometrial cancers, as well as glioblastoma, astrocytoma, and melanoma.

QTc interval: As measured by ECG (electrocardiogram, a method of graphing the heart's electrical cycle), a measure of the time between the start of the Q wave and the end of the T wave. If the heart rate is slow, the QT interval will be longer compared to a fast heartbeat when the QT interval is short. The QTc interval is corrected for heart rate. The normal QT interval is 0.30–0.44 second (0.45 second in women). Prolongation of the QT interval increases the risk for an unusual ventricular tachycardia called torsades de pointes. Other risk factors are hypomagnesemia, hypokalemia, and hypocalcemia. These electrolytes should be corrected in any patient at risk for prolonged QTc.

Radioimmunotherapy: Treatment using a radioactive source (nucleotide) attached to an antibody, usually a murine or mouse antibody.

Radioisotope: Unstable element that releases radiation energy as it breaks down.

Randomized clinical trial: Gold standard in testing treatments to see which is the best. Patients are randomized (selected by chance) to one group or the other, so the groups are balanced and similar (e.g., same number of men and women), and blinded so that the patients do not know what treatment they are receiving. This method eliminates bias in the physicians caring for the patients in the trial, as well as the physicians who read the CT or MRI scans to measure whether the patients responded to the therapy.

RANKL (receptor activator for nuclear factor kB ligand): Important ligand in bone metabolism, as it activates osteoclasts (bone resorption). It is also expressed by helper T lymphocytes and helps in maturation of dendritic cells (dendritic cell survival factor).

RAS **family of genes:** Proto-oncogenes that make proteins involved in signal transduction. Ras communicates signals from outside the cell to inside the cell and sends the message as if by a bucket brigade to the cell nucleus so that the message can be acted upon; the message usually involves the making of a specific protein for cell growth, differentiation, proliferation, and survival. Ras is called a G-protein (guanosine-nucleotide-binding protein), which makes it a binary switch that can be turned on or off. Ras works closely with the P13K signaling pathway. If the EGFR signaling pathway is abnormally turned on, it will send activation signals to Ras and down its signaling pathway. Mutations in *RAS* genes, such as K-Ras, H-Ras, and N-Ras, permanently turn on or activate this signaling pathway, so the message to divide and to avoid apoptosis is sent constantly. This mutation occurs in many cancers, such as pancreatic and some colorectal and lung cancers. Thus, if both EGFR and Ras are mutated, and an EGFR inhibitor turns off the EGFR abnormal signaling, it will not stop Ras signaling, as it is mutated and sending its own signals to the cell nucleus.

Retinoblastoma protein (pRb): Tumor suppressor protein that has a pocket to which proteins bind. It is the most important determinant of whether cells get through the G_1 checkpoint of the cell cycle, and once committed, the cell has to continue going through the cell cycle. The gene (*RB1*) that makes this protein is mutated (inactivated) by mutation of both its alleles (copies). Oncogenic proteins are produced by cells infected by the papillomaviruses, which can bind and inactivate pRb, leading to cervical cancer.

Second messengers: Signaling molecules in a signaling cascade that transfer the message to the cell nucleus from one messenger to the next messenger as if by a bucket brigade. Many protein kinases, enzymes that attach a phosphate group to either serine/threonine, or tyrosine proteins in the cell, act as second messengers.

Serine/threonine protein kinase: Protein kinases that phosphorylate serine or threonine residues on the proteins to which they are passing the message.

Signal transduction: The process of taking a message from outside the cell to the cell nucleus, involving the signaling cascade. Once the message is taken from one messenger to the next, the messenger is shut off so it cannot keep sending the same message. In cancer, the messengers may be turned on so the message is sent without normal stimulation.

Signaling cascade: A process by which a series of messengers carry the message from outside the cell through its receptor to inside the cell, and then to the cell nucleus, telling the cell what to do (e.g., divide).

Small molecule tyrosine kinase inhibitors: Small, oral agents that pass through the cell membrane and interfere with the tyrosine kinase's ability to send the cell message to the cell nucleus.

Src genes: Family of proto-oncogene tyrosine kinases that are very important in embryogenesis and cell growth, movement, and proliferation. The gene product is a tyrosine kinase protein. When the src proto-oncogene is mutated, it forms an oncogene. The src oncogene causes sarcoma and actually changed the thinking about malignant transformation.

Standard therapy: Currently accepted standard regimen for treatment of a specific cancer, based on evidence of clinical trials.

Statistically significant: Mathematical measure of whether a difference is due to chance or the treatment that is being compared. Minimal measure is $P \le .05$, which means that the likelihood that the finding of a study is due to chance alone and not the treatment is less than or equal to 5 in 100.

Stomatitis: Inflammation or irritation of the lining of the mouth

Stroma: *See tumor microenvironment.*

Synthetic lethality: Death of a cell when both the primary and backup processes are inactivated. An example is in BRCA1-mutated cancer cells; they are unable to repair DNA breaks, so depend upon PARP to fix them. When a PARP inhibitor is used, both repair processes are blocked and the cell dies.

Targeted therapy, molecular-targeted therapy: Drugs that target molecular flaws in cancer cells. The target may be on the surface of the cancer cell, such as the CD20 antigen on B lymphocytes, or the EGF receptor, which may also be on normal cells. The target may be inside the cell, such as tyrosine kinases inside the cell membrane or secondary messages taking the cell's message to the nucleus to drive proliferation, angiogenesis, and invasion. The target may also be the apoptosis machinery, and the apoptosis-inducing drug, such as bortezomib.

Taxane: Type of chemotherapy drug that works by interfering with mitosis or the phase of the cell cycle when the cell actually divides into two daughter cells. These drugs disrupt the microtubules (structures that help to move the chromosomes during mitosis), and examples are paclitaxel (Taxol) and docetaxel (Taxotere).

Telomerase: Enzyme that adds on the portion of the chromosome removed with each cell division. In early life, the embryo uses telomerase to divide repeatedly and to ensure the chromosomes do not shorten; however, in general this is turned off when the fetus is formed. Cancer cells figure out a way to turn telomerase back on so they can create an immortal cell.

Telomere: The ends of the chromosome, much like the caps of shoelaces, which protect the chromosome ends from splitting and being damaged. With each cell division, a portion of the DNA is cut off, and after 60–70 divisions, the cell can no longer divide. For cells in culture, this is called the Hayflick limit. At this point, the DNA is unstable and may harm the person if allowed to try to divide again, so the DNA repair mechanisms start to put the cell into apoptosis, called telomere crisis.

Transforming growth factor beta (TGFβ): Growth factor that controls cell proliferation and cell differentiation (specialization), and has different roles in early versus late cancer. In normal epithelial cells and early cancer, TGFβ is antiproliferative and opposes uncontrolled cell growth and division. It helps cells undergo apoptosis and also regulates the cell cycle proteins p15 and p21, which block the cyclin/CDK complex that would normally phosphorylate the retinoblastoma protein, thus moving the cell through the G_1 restriction point in the cell cycle. It also suppresses c-myc gene expression that would otherwise push the cell through the G_1 restriction point of the cell cycle. Thus it blocks the cell from advancing through the cell cycle. However, later in cancer, the TGFβ signaling pathway is mutated and can no longer control cell division. Thus, the cancer cells and surrounding stromal fibroblasts proliferate, and because they have TGFβ receptors on their cell surfaces, they increase secretion of TGFβ, which in turn continues to stimulate them, as well as suppressing immune cells and starting angiogenesis.

Tumor microenvironment, or stroma: A necessary component of tumorigenesis, invasion, and metastasis. The stroma consists of normal cells, including fibroblasts and bone marrow-derived, epithelial, immune, vascular, and smooth muscle cells, as well as tumor cells, together with the extracellular matrix. The stroma has tumor-associated macrophages, inflammatory infiltrating cells, and new blood vessels. It provides messages or cues to cancer stem cells and helps cells metastasize and set up a home in a distant site.

Tumor suppressor gene: Gene that turns cell growth and division down or off, like the brake pedal on a car. Tumor suppressor genes are often mutated in cancer, so cell proliferation is unopposed.

Tyrosine kinase: An enzyme that transfers a phosphate from adenine triphosphate (ATP, the energy source in the cell) to a tyrosine residue in a protein. In the human body, there are at least 90 protein tyrosine kinases. They are part of a larger group called protein kinases, and are divided into two classes, cytoplasmic protein kinases and transmembrane receptor-linked kinases. Kinases transfer messages received from outside the cell to the cell nucleus by phosphorylation of proteins by kinases at each step, as if by a bucket brigade. When the ligand binds to the receptor tyrosine kinase (RTK), it causes the PTK to change shape and activates the enzyme, such as making the ATP-binding site accessible. This then triggers the signal cascade or transduction of the message from outside the cell to the cell nucleus. RTKs are very important in cancer either through mutation of the gene or through chromosomal translocation resulting in an activated kinase that continues to send the message to the cell nucleus to proliferate without being activated by a ligand.

Ubiquitin/proteasome pathway: Pathway responsible for quickly tagging and degrading the proteins once they do their job so that they stop working. Proteins run the cell, and specific proteins are highly regulated so that processes like running the cell cycle and putting cells to programmed cell death are tightly controlled. The protein is tagged by ubiquitin, and then ubiquitin brings the protein to the proteasome so that it can be degraded and the component parts recycled for making new proteins.

Upstream: Imagine the signaling cascade is a stream taking the cell's message from outside the cell to the cell nucleus. From any point along this stream, those messengers above it are called "upstream" of it, while any messengers below it or between it and the cell nucleus are called "downstream" of it.

VEGF, vascular endothelial growth factor: Factor that binds to VEGFR to initiate a signaling cascade telling the endothelial cell to proliferate and migrate to form a new blood vessel to the tumor. VEGF belongs to the larger platelet-derived growth factor (PDGF) family. They are important in the embryo in making the embryonic circulatory system; in adults, they are needed for angiogenesis, making blood vessels from preexisting blood vessels. VEGF-A is the most important member. VEGF-B is active in embryogenesis. VEGF-C and -D are active in lymphangiogenesis and the lymphatic vasculature, and placenta growth factor (PIGF) is important during inflammation and cancer.

Wnt signaling pathway: Extensive signaling pathway that is very important in embryogenesis (telling the body axis how to orient, assisting gastrulation, and differentiating stem cells into specialized cells) and in some adult functions. It is mutated in many cancers. Wnt proteins bind to cell surface receptors (Frizzled family), which activates the Dishevelled family proteins, ultimately changing how much β-catenin reaches the cell nucleus. Wnt signaling pathway appears to be involved in the development of cancer stem cells.

Index

Italicized page locators indicate a figure; tables are noted with a *t*.